GENETICS OF
HUMAN TUMORS IN JAPAN

Gann Monograph on Cancer Research

The "Gann Monograph on Cancer Research" series is promoted by the Japanese Cancer Association. This semiannual series of monographs was initiated in 1966 by the late Dr. Tomizo Yoshida (1903–1973) and is now published jointly by Japan Scientific Societies Press, Tokyo and Taylor & Francis Ltd., London and Philadelphia. Each volume consists of collected contributions on current topics in cancer problems and allied research fields. The planning for each volume is done by the Monograph Committee of the Japanese Cancer Association, with the final approval of the Board of Directors. It is hoped that the series will serve as an important source of information in the field of cancer research.

The publication of these monographs owes much to the financial support given by the late Professor Kazushige Higuchi, the Jikei University School of Medicine.

Japanese Cancer Association

JAPANESE CANCER ASSOCIATION

Gann Monograph on Cancer Research No. 35

GENETICS OF
HUMAN TUMORS IN JAPAN

Edited by HIRAKU TAKEBE
JOJI UTSUNOMIYA

JAPAN SCIENTIFIC SOCIETIES PRESS, Tokyo
TAYLOR & FRANCIS LTD., London and Philadelphia

December 1988

Published jointly by
JAPAN SCIENTIFIC SOCIETIES PRESS
2-10 Hongo, 6-chome, Bunkyo-ku, Tokyo 113, Japan
ISBN 4-7622-2578-9
      and
TAYLOR & FRANCIS LTD.
4 John Street, London WC1N 2ET, UK
242 Cherry Street, Philadelphia, Pennsylvania 19106-1906, U.S.A.
ISBN 0-85066-797-6

Distributed in all areas outside Japan and Asia between Pakistan and Korea by TAYLOR & FRANCIS LTD., London and Philadelphia.

Printed in Japan

PREFACE

Genetics and cancer is an old problem in cancer medicine. The family of Napoleon Bonaparte who reportedly died of stomach cancer in 1821 and whose autopsy record confirms it is one of the oldest examples of familial cancer. Until recently, methods of studying human genetics have been limited to family analysis and little evidence has been presented for the involvement of genetic factors in human carcinogenesis. During the last decade, however, developments in cell biology and somatic cell genetics as well as molecular biology have provided powerful tools with which to study the mechanisms of carcinogenesis from genetic aspects. Epidemiological studies on populations in Japan have been carried out on some cancers possibly associated with genetic factors. Genetic epidemiology of cancer has emerged as a new field and this volume of the Gann Monograph on Cancer Research is the first attempt to review survey and research on cancer and genetics in Japan.

The volume consists of three major sections. The first 7 articles describe hereditary neoplasia. In addition to the confirmed hereditary cancers such as retinoblastoma and Wilms' tumor, tumors with possible association with a hereditary background such as neuroblastoma and neurofibromatosis are also described. Cancer-prone hereditary diseases and familial cancer are discussed in the second section. Theoretical and experimental approaches are emphasized along with epidemiological studies. The third section is entitled "Chromosomes and Gene Mutations", and two of the four articles cover atmoic bomb survivors and their children. Chromosome aberrations in leukemia and lymphoma, and oncogene mapping on chromosomes are also described.

Some of the articles in this book represent the areas or topics being most actively studied in Japan. Genetic studies on familial polyposis coli and xeroderma pigmentosum in particular were based on far more patients and families than those reported in other countries. The relatively homogeneous population in Japan may make the epidemiological data quite different from those in other more mixed populations. Comparative studies between Japan and other countries are mentioned in most of the articles in this volume.

The editors thank the contributors for their efforts in writing on a new concept of genetic epidemiology of cancer.

November 1988

H. TAKEBE
J. UTSUNOMIYA

CONTENTS

viii

OVERVIEW

GENETIC FACTORS IN HUMAN CARCINOGENESIS

Hiraku TAKEBE

*Department of Molecular Oncology and Experimental Radiology,
Faculty of Medicine, Kyoto University**

Presence of hereditary cancers and cancer-prone hereditary diseases indicates the involvement of genetic factors in human carcinogenesis. Autosomal recessively inherited cancer-prone diseases appear to have common genetic defects in processing DNA damage caused by environmental agents, and the mechanisms underlying the cancer-proneness in these diseases may play important roles in carcinogenesis in general. Recent findings on loss of heterozygosity in the genes of retinoblastoma and Wilms' tumor as well as in certain types of cancer suggest the presence of suppressors of oncogenes or antioncogenes which work recessively. Family and twin studies also support the presence of genetic predisposition to cancer in certain cancer. Genetic epidemiology of cancer as a new approach to study genetics and cancer is proposed.

There is ample evidence implicating genetic factors in human carcinogenesis. There are several hereditary diseases which have close association with high incidence of cancer. Among them, retinoblastoma, Wilms' tumor and familial polyposis coli with autosomal dominant inheritance, and xeroderma pigmentosum with autosomal recessive inheritance, have been most extensively studied genetically along with the characteristics of cancers in the patients. Table I summarizes the involvement of genetic factors in human cancer.

Cancer in general is only partially a hereditary disease. Cancers of late onset may have little association with hereditary predisposition, since they have been shown to be caused mainly be environmental factors through diet, drinking or inhaling. Studies on migrant people support this. For example, Japanese immigrants in Hawaii or California have much lower incidence of stomach cancer, but a much greater incidence of colon cancer than Japanese in Japan. The high incidence of stomach cancer in Japanese in Japan, therefore, should not be attributed to hereditary susceptibility, but to environmental factors.

Cancer-prone hereditary diseases such as familial polyposis coli or xeroderma pigmentosum are very rare, and the genetic factors underlying the etiology of these diseases may be regarded specific to these diseases. Recent studies, however, strongly suggest that such factors are related to the cause of cancer in general. Table II gives a list of possible cancer-prone populations with hereditary predisposition. Some have not been studied extensively, but the list is intended to indicate the general current impression of the relationship between cancer and hereditary factors. This chapter seeks to explain some of the characteristics of these predisposed populations with examples from studies car-

* Yoshida-konoecho, Sakyo-ku, Kyoto 606, Japan (武部　啓).

TABLE I.   Evidence and Examples of Involvement of Genetic Factors in Carcinogenesis

1. Presence of hereditary cancers (retinoblastoma, Wilms' tumor)
2. Presence of cancer-prone hereditary diseases (xeroderma pigmentosum)
3. Cancer-related specific chromosome rearrangements (Ph[1] chromosome)
4. Similarity in mechanisms between cancer and mutation
5. Oncogenes and their specific alterations in tumor cells (point mutations, rearrangements, amplification, *etc.*)

TABLE II.   Genetically High-risk Population for Cancer (Examples in Parentheses)

1. Patients with autosomal recessive cancer-prone hereditary diseases (xeroderma pigmentosum, ataxia telangiectasia, Bloom's syndrome, Fanconi's anemia)
2. Heterozygotes of the genes of the autosomal recessive cancer-prone diseases (above) (confirmed in xeroderma pigmentosum and ataxia telangiectasia, not in Fanconi's anemia)
3. Hereditary cancer of autosomal dominant inheritance (retinoblastoma, Wilms' tumor, multiple endocrine neoplasia type II)
4. Carriers of the genes of autosomally dominant cancer (above), who did not develop cancer or who were cured of cancer
5. Patients with autosomal dominantly inherited cancer-prone diseases (familial polyposis coli)
6. Patients with certain chromosome aberration syndromes (Down's syndrome)
7. Populations with elevated activity or inducibility of enzymes for metabolic activation of carcinogens, such as arylhydrocarbon hydroxylase (shown for lung cancer)
8. Populations with reduced activity of enzymes which degrade carcinogens, such as superoxide dismutase (not yet confirmed)
9. Patients with immunodeficiency diseases
10. Populations with genetically high susceptibility to cancer-related virus infection or expression (not yet confirmed)

ried out in Japan and on the Japanese population. Detailed descriptions of some of these populations are presented by various authors in this book.

Autosomal Recessive Cancer-prone Diseases

1.   Xeroderma pigmentosum

Among 4 major cancer-prone diseases of autosomal recessive inheritance (Table II), xeroderma pigmentosum (XP) has been most well characterized by clinical, cellular and molecular studies.   In addition to the chapters by Y. Fujiwara on basic research and by Satoh and Nishigori on clinical studies in this volume, a note on the mechanisms of carcinogenesis in patients with XP is provided here. Most XP patients show a deficiency in excision repair, which is believed to be an error-free type of repair. Therefore, cancer in XP may develop through the functioning of a remaining mode of repair which may be error-prone. This would be a direct analogy to the high mutability of *uvr⁻* (deficient in excision repair) bacteria by UV through SOS response or error-prone type of repair of UV damage. Although excision repair-deficient XP cells are clearly more mutable than normal cells by UV, so far there is no consistent evidence of an SOS-like response in XP cells, or in human cells in general. XP cells belonging to complementation group A are far more hypermutable than XP cells of complementation group C which are still more hypermutable than normal cells (*13*). Such differences are not reflected in skin cancer characteristics of these two groups, but are possibly related to neurological characteristics, which are normal in group C, but abnormal in most group A patients. Of all of the cancer-prone hereditary diseases, XP is the only disease with a confirmed cause of cancer, since skin cancers in patients with XP are definitely caused by ultraviolet light in sunlight.

2. Ataxia telangiectasia

Patients with ataxia telangiectasia (AT) are greatly predisposed to leukemia and malignant lymphoma. This close association with lymphoreticular malignancies is likely attributable to the immunodeficiency observed in the patients. Cells originating from AT patients are sensitive to ionizing radiation, but mutation induction by ionizing radiation is the same as that observed in normal cells given the same dose (12). The cells show considerable chromosomal instability, and chromosome aberrations are enhanced markedly by ionizing irradiation. In particular, involvement of chromosome 14 in radiation induced aberrations is noted. Possible rearrangement encompassing an immunoglobulin gene on chromosome 14 could be responsible for the high incidence of malignancy in AT patients.

3. Bloom's syndrome

Bloom's syndrome (BS) is characterized by short stature, telangiectasia, café-au-lait spots, mild immunodeficiency and high incidence of cancer. Cancer in these patients develops in a spectrum of organs, in contrast to other cancer-prone hereditary diseases with limited locations of malignancy. There are 11 confirmed Bloom's syndrome patients in Japan and two have had cancers. Cells originating from Bloom's syndrome patients have high frequencies of both spontaneous mutation and spontaneous sister chromatid exchanges, each approximately 10 fold over normal. These could be related to the cancer-proneness in Bloom's syndrome patients. Details of a recent survey on all Bloom's syndrome patients identified to date in Japan will be published elsewhere (3).

4. Fanconi's anemia

Extreme chromosome instability characterizes the cells originating from Fanconi's anemia (FA). Leukemia is the most frequent malignancy associated with the disease. The cells are very sensitive, both in cell killing and in inducing chromosome aberrations, to such DNA cross-linking agents as mitomycin C, busulfan and psoralen plus near-UV light.

No agents have been identified that cause malignancy in Fanconi's anemia despite such cellular sensitivity response and chromosomal instability. Recently we found that one DNA cross-linking agent, diepoxybutane, induced mutation in FA cells far above normal frequencies (10). This is the first indication of possible correlation between mutation and cancer in human since the UV-XP relationship which was demonstrated over ten years ago.

In summarizing the relationship between cancer and mutation as shown in Table III, it should be noted that mutation observed in the cells may not represent the mutation directly involved in carcinogenesis. The mechanism of producing mutations in the HPRT gene, which we detect as resistance to 6-thioguanine, may not be similar to that in oncogenes. Rearrangements of chromosomes may be more related to the high incidence of cancer in AT, BS, and FA patients than gene mutation.

TABLE III. Cancer in Cancer-prone Hereditary Diseases and Mutation in Cultured Cells

Disease	Deficiency	Cancer (Agent)	Mutation (Agent)
Xeroderma pigmentosum	Excision repair	High(UV)	High (UV, Chemicals)
Ataxia telangiectasia	DNA synthesis(?)[a]	High(?)	Normal or less (Gamma-rays, UV)
Bloom's syndrome	Ligase(?)	High(?)	High (Spontaneous)
Fanconi's anemia	Repair of cross-linking(?)	High(?)	High (Diepoxibutane)

[a] Reduced in suppression after X-ray irradiation.

Loss of Heterozygosity as a Possible Mechanism of Carcinogenesis

At the time of planning of this volume, the observation of the loss of heterozygosity in retinoblastoma and Wilms' tumor had just been made (1, 4). Recently, considerable work has been done on the loss of heterozygosity in cancer cells, and some of the Japanese effort should have been included in this volume. Unfortunately, the editorial process did not permit such inclusion and brief introductory comments on this phenomenon are given here.

Both hereditary retinoblastoma (Rb) and Wilms' tumor are well known for their pattern of autosomal dominant inheritance. But in analyzing the responsible genes or closely linked neighboring genes, it became clear that tumorigenesis in Rb is accompanied by loss of heterozygosity of the Rb gene. The suggestion is that the absence of a properly functioning Rb gene leads to rapid development of retinoblastoma. The genes responsible for retinoblastoma or Wilms' tumor at the loci of human chromosomes 13q14 and 11p13, respectively, could be either recessive oncogenes themselves or suppressor genes of other oncogenes. Since oncogenes identified by DNA transfection are dominant acting, the recessiveness of these genes provided a new concept for explaining the mechanism of carcinogenesis. Also, it gave a novel explanation for the apparent dominance of the gene. The pattern of dominant inheritance of both retinoblastoma and Wilms' tumor is produced by the loss of function accompanying loss of heterozygosity of recessively acting genes.

The loss of heterozygosity has been shown in cancer cells in which there is little involvement of genetic factors such as lung cancer (15). Loss of heterozygosity in colon cancer, including in patients with familial polyposis coli (7), and in osteosarcoma (14) appears to a certain extent to be related to hereditary factors.

Genetic Factors in Human Cancer in General

1. Survey on familial cancer

Surveys on familial occurrence of cancer have revealed that certain types of cancer, breast cancer in particular, is concentrated in certain families. Details of such a survey are presented by Ogawa et al. in this volume. Two orthodox approaches in estimating the relative contribution of genetic factors in carcinogenesis are possible. Comparative studies on stomach cancer incidence among affected and non-affected family members were done by Takei (11), and similar studies were also carried out by Lehtola (6) in Finland (Table IV). Takei's survey compared the patients with stomach cancer and their spouses. This was a reasonable approach since they usually share similar environmental factors. In Finland, patients with stomach cancer were matched with control persons of

TABLE IV.   Familial Studies on Stomach Cancer

Japan (Takei)		
	Relative incidence	
	Patients	Spouse
Father	1.7	1
Mother	2.5	1
Brothers	1.2	1
Sisters	1.8	1
Average	1.7	1
Total number	114/3533	66/3984
Finland (Lehtola)		
	Frequencies	
	Patients	Control
Blood relatives	3.4%	2.6%
	77/2243	59/2301

the same sex born at a similar time and place. In both surveys, incidence in the family members of the patients was slightly higher than in controls. Incidentally, the relative incidence in Finland was 1.7 when cases with diffused type stomach cancer were compared. Differences of less than two fold could not exclude the involvement of environmental factors and may be too small to conclude that the difference was due to genetic factors. Also, the relatively late onset of stomach cancer should be considered when estimating the relative contribution of environmental factors as the cause.

Another standard method of human genetics to be applied is twin study. In Sweden, extensive twin registry and cancer registry enabled Cerderlöf et al. (2) to assess possible genetic factors in cancer. So far little evidence for genetic involvement has been obtained when comparing monozygotic and dizygotic twins for their coincidences, except for cervix cancer of uterus.

2. Cancer in heterozygotes of the recessive cancer-prone diseases

In ataxia telangiectasia, Swift et al. demonstrated that blood relatives of patients had a higher incidence of cancer than did a control group, and attributed the increase to the heterozygotic AT gene (9). They also showed that XP heterozygotes had more skin cancer than controls (8). The latter case was not confirmed in families of XP patients in Japan, presumably because skin cancer is far less in Japanese than in Caucasians due to the difference in skin pigmentation. Such high susceptibility among cancer-prone genes may give rise to a considerable fraction of all cancer cases because the size of population of such heterozygotes may be a few percent of the general population.

3. Other possible predispositions to cancer

Among the predispositions listed in Table II, biochemical or metabolic factors other than DNA repair have not been investigated extensively. Correlation between activity of arylhydrocarbon hydroxylase (AHH) and lung cancer was suggested (5), but the difference in AHH activity among individuals was not significant as demonstrated among different strains of mouse and the correlation was far less clear in human than in mouse.

CONCLUSION

Hereditary predispositions to cancer may play important roles in carcinogenesis, in particular, in the mechanisms of mutagenesis. Xeroderma pigmentosum offers the best example of the involvement of genetic factors in carcinogenesis. Loss of heterozygosity is an attractive hypothesis for the major process of initiating events in addition to mutation, and may be involved not only in the cause of hereditary cancers but also in cancer in general. Further studies on familial cancer or genetic epidemiology of cancer will contribute to estimation of the quantitative involvement of genetic factors and may eventually point the way to protection from specific carcinogens to which a high-risk population is sensitive.

Acknowledgments

The author thanks Drs. Rufus S. Day, Kouichi Tatsumi and Takashi Yagi for discussion during the preparation of this manuscript. This work was supported by a Grant-in-Aid for Cancer Research from the Ministry of Education, Science and Culture, and by Nissan Science Foundation.

REFERENCES

1. Cavanee, W. K., Dryja, T. P., Philips, R. A., Benedict, W. F., Godbout, R., Gallie, B. L., Murphree, A. L., Strong, L. C., and White, R. L. Expression of recessive alleles by chromosome mechanisms in retinoblastoma. *Nature*, **305**, 779–784 (1983).
2. Cederlöf, R. and Floderus-Myrhed, B. Cancer mortality and morbidity among 23,000 unselected twin pairs. *In* "Genetic and Environmental Factors in Experimental and Human Cancers," ed. H. V. Gelboin *et al.*, pp. 151–160 (1980). Japan Sci. Soc. Press, Tokyo.
3. German, J. and Takebe, H. Bloom's syndrome. XIV. The disorder in Japan. *Clin. Genet.*, in press.
4. Koufos, A., Hansen, M. F., Lampkin, B. C., Workman, M. L., Copeland, N. G., Jenkins, N. A., and Cavanee, W. K. Loss of alleles at loci on human chromosome 11 during genesis of Wilms' tumour. *Nature*, **309**, 170–172 (1984).
5. Kouri, R. E., McKinney, C. E., Slomiany, D. J., Snodgrass, D. R., Wray, N. P., and McLemore, T. L. Positive correlation between high aryl hydrocarbon hydroxylase activity and primary lung cancer as analyzed in cryopreserved lymphocytes. *Cancer Res.*, **42**, 5030–5037 (1982).
6. Lehtola, J. Family behavior of gastric carcinoma. *Ann. Clin. Res.*, **13**, 144–148 (1981).
7. Okamoto, M., Sasaki, M., Sugio, K., Sato, C., Iwama, T., Ikeuchi, T., Tonomura, A., Sasazuki, T., and Miyaki, M. Loss of constitutional heterozygosity in colon carcinoma from patients with familial polyposis coli. *Nature*, **331**, 273–277 (1988).
8. Swift, M. and Chase, C. Cancer in families with xeroderma pigmentosum. *J. Natl. Cancer Inst.*, **62**, 1415–1421 (1979).
9. Swift, M., Sholomon, L., Perry, M., and Chase, C. Malignant neoplasm in the families of patients with ataxia-telangiectasia. *Cancer Res.*, **36**, 209–215 (1976).
10. Takebe, H., Tatsumi, K., Tachibana, A., and Nishigori, C. High sensitivity to radiation and chemicals in relation to cancer and mutation. *In* "Radiation Research," ed. E. M. Fielden *et al.*, pp. 443–448 (1987). Taylor and Francis, London.
11. Takei, K. Statistical investigations on genetic aspects of gastric carcinoma. *Jpn. J. Hum. Genet.*, **13**, 67–80 (1968) (in Japanese with English summary).

12. Tatsumi, K. and Takebe, H. γ-Irradiation induces mutation in ataxia telangiectasia lymphoblastoid cells. *Jpn. J. Cancer Res. (Gann)*, **75**, 1040–1043 (1984).
13. Tatsumi, K., Toyoda, M., Hashimoto, T., Furuyama, J., Kurihara, T., Inoue, M., and Takebe, H. Differential hypersensitivity of xeroderma pigmentosum lymphoblastoid cell lines to ultraviolet mutagenesis. *Carcinogenesis*, **8**, 53–57 (1987).
14. Toguchida, J., Ishizaki, K., Sasaki, M. S., Ikenaga, M., Sugimoto, M., Kotoura, Y., and Yamamuro, T. Chromosome reorganization for the espression of recessive mutation of retinoblastoma susceptibility gene in the development of osteosarcoma. *Cancer Res.*, **48**, 3939–3943 (1988).
15. Yokota, J., Wada, M., Shimosato, Y., Terada, M., and Sugimura, T. Loss of heterozygosity on chromosome 3, 13, and 17 in small-cell carcinoma and on chromosome 3 in adenocarcinoma of the lung. *Proc. Natl. Acad. Sci. U.S.A.*, **84**, 9252–9256 (1987).

HEREDITARY NEOPLASIA

GENETIC AND CYTOGENETIC ASPECTS OF RETINOBLASTOMA MUTATION AND ITS RELEVANCE TO THE DEVELOPMENT OF TUMOR

Masao S. Sasaki,[*1] Yosuke Ejima,[*1] Akihiro Kaneko,[*2] and Hiroshi Tanooka[*3]

Radiation Biology Center, Kyoto University,[*1] *National Cancer Center Hospital,*[*2] *and National Cancer Center Research Institute*[*3]

Retinoblastoma (Rb) occurs as a consequence of germinal or somatic mutation at q14 region of chromosome 13. Cytogenetic survey on 188 Rb patients, combined with 66 reported cases, revealed that approximately 8.4% of fresh germinal mutations were microscopically recognizable chromosome mutations: deletions or rearrangements involving 13q14. The mutation rate of these chromosome mutations was estimated to be about 0.9×10^{-6}/gamete/generation. However, there was a strong bias toward paternal origin. The chromosome mutations at 13q14 differed from the familially transmitted mutations in their cellular manifestation: *e.g.*, cultured fibroblasts carrying the latter mutations showed high susceptibility to transformation by murine sarcoma virus and enhanced generation of non-constitutional chromosome rearrangements while the cells with the former mutations behaved normally. Age-specific incidence and karyotype analyses of tumor tissues suggested that further genome reorganization was required as a prelude to malignancy for the embryonic retinal cells which already had one mutation, but generation of such genomic changes might not necessarily be independent from the first mutation.

Retinoblastoma (Rb) is a childhood tumor of the eye. Clinical observations have established that a specific mutation is associated with the development of Rb. Some tumors occur in hereditary form, where the patient inherits the Rb mutation through germ cell from a carrier parent or a healthy parent as a consequence of newly occurring germinal mutation (*81*). In the non-hereditary form, the tumors are thought to arise as a consequence of somatic mutation which took place in the embryonic retinal cells during fetal life. The hereditary patients tend to develop bilateral and predominantly multifocal tumors with significantly earlier onset as compared with non-hereditary patients, who develop invariably a single unifocal tumor in a single eye. In view of the mechanism of the development of tumors, the nature and function of the Rb mutation and its role in the carcinogenesis are particularly intriguing. Recently, DNA sequences corresponding to the Rb gene have been cloned (*25*). In a small minority of hereditary patients, the Rb mutation occurs in a form of microscopically detectable chromosome deletion or rearrangement involving chromosome 13. Such mutations can also provide useful information on the genesis of Rb.

[*1] Yoshida-konoecho, Sakyo-ku, Kyoto 606, Japan (佐々木　正夫, 江島洋介).
[*2],[*3] 5-1-1, Tsukiji, Chuo-ku, Tokyo 104, Japan (金子明博, 田ノ岡　宏).

Types and Rates of Rb Mutations

In order to study the types and rates of Rb mutations, Rb patients referred to the National Cancer Center Hospital, Tokyo, during 1979–1986 were studied for their consitutional chromosome conditions. The chromosomes were analyzed in cultured skin fibroblasts by G-banding methods of Seabright (*72*). To date, a total of 188 patients have been studied: 78 sporadic unilateral, 82 sporadic bilateral, 11 familial unilateral, and 17 familial bilateral patients. Of these, 10 were found to have constitutional chromosome mutations, all involving chromosome 13. They included 8 sporadic bilateral cases, one sporadic unilateral case and one familial bilateral case in which deleted chromosome 13 originated from an apparently normal healthy mother who had also a shortened chromosome 13 probably due to insertional rearrangement. Chromosome 13 abnormalities in the sporadic cases included one each of the case with deletion of a region q14–q21, q14–q22, q12–q14, two cases with deletion of q14, a case with del(13)(q14)/normal mosaicism, and one each of the case with t(13; 6)(q14; q13) and t(13; 10)(q14; q22) reciprocal translocation.

A similar study in Japanese patients has been made by Motegi *et al.* (*56*). They found 8 cases with chromosome abnormalities involving chromosome 13 in 66 patients. In their cases, del(13)(q14)/normal mosaicism was relatively common, being found in 5 cases. The others included 2 cases with *de novo* del(13)(q14) deletion and a case with t(13; 18)(q14; q12) translocation. Table I summarizes the combined data on the chromosome constitutions of a total of 254 patients studied in these two investigations.

It should be noted that these study populations are rather biased toward the bilaterally affected patients because of the management plans in these hospital and do not represent the breakdown of Rb patients in general. Based on the national registration of Rb patients during the period 1975–1979 and supplemented by a search using questionnaires and death certificates, Kaneko (*33*) estimated annual incidence to be 6.73×10^{-5} or one out of 14,859 live births. The ratio of bilateral to unilateral cases was 1: 2.61. Of those, 4.4% constituted familial cases, either bilaterally (2.5%) or unilaterally affected (1.9%). Therefore, in the sporadic cases, the ratio is 1: 2.75. When the data in Table I are calculated according to this ratio, the incidence of Rb patients with chromosome 13 anomalies in sporadic cases is estimated to be $[(15/122)+(2/92) \times 2.75]/[1+2.75]=4.87 \times 10^{-2}$ or 4.87%. This incidence in Rb patients is comparable with some previous estimates made by literature surveys (*45, 51, 83*), and also with that of relatively large scale population studies of Cowell *et al.* (*16*), where the expression of esterase D, a gene closely linked to the Rb locus (*75*), was studied in 200 British patients, 4.5% of

TABLE I. Summary of Cytogenetic Data of Consecutive Surveys of 254 Rb Patients[a]

Heredity	Tumor laterality	Chromosome constitutions		Total
		Normal	Abnormal	
Sporadic	Unilateral	90	2	92
	Bilateral	107	15	122
Familial	Unilateral	14	0	14
	Bilateral	25	1	26
Total		236	18	254

[a] The data include 66 cases reported by Motegi *et al.* (*56*).

whom were shown to have deletion involving esterase D locus. However, Dryja *et al. (20)* were unable to detect deletion cases in an analysis of 51 patients by esterase D determination. Low incidence of deletion has also been reported by Salamanca-Gómez *et al. (66)*. They found three sibs in a family exhibiting deletion at 13q14 in a cytogenetic survey of 110 Rb patients.

It is generally recognized that, in the sporadic cases, virtually all of the bilateral patients and 10–12% of the unilateral patients are due to the fresh mutations which occurred in the germ cells of their parents *(74, 81)*. Assuming that 10% of the sporadic unilateral cases are due to the germinal mutation, the incidence of Rb patients due to fresh germinal mutations is calculated to be 2.19×10^{-5}. Provided that the probability of mutation is equal for two germ cells, the mutation rate as defined by [number of sporadic cases caused by germinal mutation] divided by [$2 \times$ total number of mates in the population] is estimated to be 1.09×10^{-5}/gamete/generation. This is also comparable with the estimate of the mutation rates in populations from England, USA, Switzerland, Germany, Hungary, The Netherlands, Japan, France, and New Zealand which are in a range 5×10^{-6} to 12.3×10^{-6} *(17, 24, 47, 71, 80)*. Chromosomally abnormal cases in Table I include 6 cases with mosaicism, which is caused by somatic mutation acquired during embryonal development, and a familial case in which chromosome mutation is thought to be inherited from germ cells of a grandparent. The remaining 11 cases are due to the *de novo* chromosome mutations. They constitute about 2.98% of all Rb patients, and 8.4% of the Rb patients which are thought to be caused by germinal mutation. Therefore, the mutation rate for apparently recognizable chromosome mutations is estimated to be 0.92×10^{-6}/gamete/generation.

Origin of the Chromosome Mutations

Eleven patients with *de novo* chromosome mutations and their parents were studied for parental origin using Q-band fluorescent heteromorphisms of chromosome 13 as heritable markers. Results are shown in Table II, where patients with chromosome 13 anomalies of *de novo* origin other than those in Table I are also included. They are chro-

TABLE II. Types of Constitutional Chromosome Abnormalities and Their Parental Origin

Patient	Sex	Tumor laterality[a]	Chromosome abnormality	Parental origin[b]
RBNaYo	F	B	del (13) (q12q22)	Paternal
RBFuTo	M	B	del (13) (q14q22)	n.e.
RBKuKe	F	B	del (13) (q14q21)	Paternal
RBSuNa	F	B	del (13) (q14q21)	Paternal
RBOhMa	M	U	del (13) (q12q14)	Paternal
RBNiSa	M	B	del (13) (q14)	Paternal
RBObEm	F	B	del (13) (q14)	Maternal
RBYaMa	M	B	46, XY/46, XY, del (13) (q14)	n.e.
RBOhNa	F	B	t (13; X) (q12; p22)	Paternal
RBWaTa	M	B	t (13; 6) (q14; q13)	Paternal
RBNaMi	F	B	t (13; 10) (q14; q22)	Paternal
RBOhYu	M	B	t (13; 18) (q14; q12)	n.e.
RBTsHi	M	B	del (13) (q14) mat	—

[a] B, bilateral; U, unilateral.
[b] n.e., not examined.

mosomally biased cases being referred to the hospital for the possible involvement of constitutional chromosome abnormalities. Parental origin was successfully established in 9 cases with *de novo* chromosome mutations. In some of these, parental origin was further confirmed by the pattern of electrophoretic mobility of esterase D in erythrocytes and/or lymphocyte cytosol polypeptide 1 (LCP1), which was also closely linked to the Rb locus (*38*) in EB virus transformed lymphoblastoid cells. In 8 out of 9 informative cases, the chromosome mutations were of paternal origin, and in the remaining one case of maternal origin.

A similar strong bias toward paternal origin has also been noticed for non-Robertsonian-type chromosome rearrangements in several selected cases of inborn errors (*14*) and Prader-Willi syndrome (*11, 60*). A deletion or mutation of gene(s) within the 13q14 is thought to be an underlying mechanism in the development of at least some retinoblastomas (*8*). If submicroscopic deletions also constitute the origin of a significant proportion of the Rb patients (*22, 37, 42*), the predominance of the paternal origin may raise a problem as to the significant contribution of errors in paternal meiotic processes in Rb mutation, and sex difference in types and rates of new mutations.

The etiology of the Rb still remains to be elucidated. Our study indicates that deletion at 13q14 occurs in a significant portion of Rb patients. It should be noted that deletion at 13q14 can also be found as mosaicism in a significant portion of Rb patients (*45, 55*) and, moreover, the proportion of those abnormal cells examined in peripheral blood lymphocytes varies among patients (*56*) and tends to decrease with age (*57*). These lines of evidence, together with the presence of deletion at submicroscopic level (*22, 25, 42*), the deletion or rearrangement at 13q14 in somatic as well as germ cells may constitute a more common etiology of Rb than previously thought.

In Prader-Willi syndrome, in which approximately 50% of the patients appear to have a rearrangement involving chromosome 15, particularly deletion at 15q11 (*43*), the involvement of nomadic DNA sequences such as transposable elements has been proposed as a possible basis of such site-specific chromosomal perturbation (*63*). As suggested previously (*67, 68*), a similar condition may be possible as a testable proposition for the etiology of Rb.

Cellular Manifestations of the Rb Mutations

Recently, it has been reported that cultured skin fibroblasts from some Rb patients are sensitive to the cell killing by X-ray irradiation (*3, 61, 62, 83–86*). This finding is particularly interesting in view of the inherent tendency of the Rb patients to develop tumors after radiation therapy (*32, 34, 65*). In a series of experiments with cultured skin fibroblasts obtained from hereditary or deletion-type Rb patients as well as patients with trisomy for whole or a part of chromosome 13, Weichselbaum *et al.* (*83, 84*) and Nove *et al.* (*61, 62*) came to a hypothetical postulation of "repair locus" at band 13q14. The repair locus is close to the Rb locus, and its deletion or triplication has been suggested to alter cellular radiosensitivity. The increased radiosensitivity of the Rb cells has been a matter of considerable debate. The increased radiosensitivity has not been found in other experiments (*23, 40, 54, 89*). In the study using fibroblasts from various forms of Rb patients, we were unable to find any increase in the radiosensitivity as determined by clonogenic survival after X-ray irradiation (*23*). They covered Rb patients of hereditary and non-hereditary forms, unilateral and bilateral affection, deletion, and

TABLE III. List of Cell Strains Tested for Cellular Radiosensitivity

Strain	Sex	Tumor laterality	Remarks
Sporadic Rb (Fig. 1B)			
RB13	F	B	
RB22	M	B	
RB23	F	U	
RB24	M	B	
RB25	F	U	
RB89	F	B	Malignant fibrous histiocytoma
Ramilial Rb (Fig. 1C)			
RB14	M	B	
RB15	F	U	Mother of RB14
RB17	M	B	
RB18	F	U	Mother of RB17
RB37	M	B	
RB39	M	U	
RB60	M	B	
RB84	M	U	
RB95	M	B	Malignant fibrous histiocytoma
RB97	F	U	
RB107	M	B	
D-deletion Rb (Fig. 1D)			
RB1	F	B	46, XX, del (13) (q12q22)
RB9	F	B	46, X, t (13; X) (q12; p22)
RB16	M	B	46, XY, del (13) (q14q22)
RB26	M	B	46, XY/46, XY, del (13) (q14)
RB32	M	B	46, XY, del (13) (q14)

triplication of a region 13q14, but no evidence has been obtained for the presence of the "repair locus" on chromosome 13. The normal response of the Rb fibroblasts to ionizing radiation has also been found for the repair and replication of DNA after irradiation (15, 82, 87), induction of mutations (82), and micronuclei formation by radiation (28).

We further extended the experiment on the cellular radiosensitivity. The patients tested are listed in Table III. They included 6 patients with sporadic Rb, 11 with familial Rb, and 5 Rb patients with chromosome 13 abnormalities. The experimental procedures were the same as those of Ejima et al. (23). The results are shown in Fig. 1. It is evident that in no case did fibroblasts from Rb patients, whether they were sporadic or familial, unilateral or bilateral chromosome 13 abnormality or not, show the increased cellular radiosensitivity. On the contrary, familial Rb and some sporadic Rb having normal constitutional karyotype were rather radioresistant as compared with the normal controls and Rb patients with chromosome 13 abnormalities. A similar trend has been also observed by Harnden et al. (29). A tendency toward rather enhanced radioresistance has been also noted in cultured skin fibroblasts from other dominantly inherited diseases such as familial polyposis coli (our unpublished data) and neurofibromatosis (39).

The reason the occasional radiosensitivity is found in some experiments while rather enhanced radioresistance in others is not clear. The conditioning of the cells before and after irradiation as well as the amount of serum in the medium has been sug-

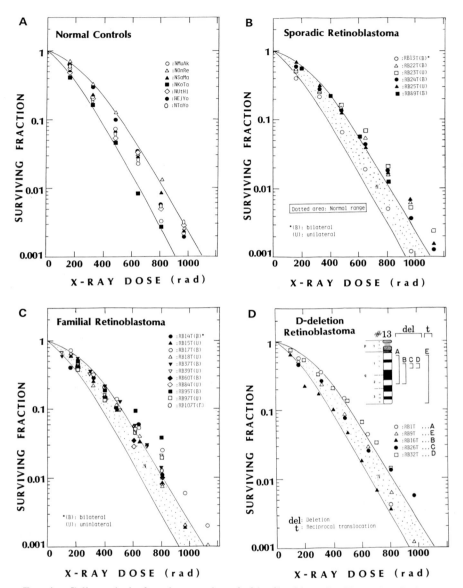

FIG. 1.   Cell survival of various strains of skin fibroblasts by X-ray irradiation
          For information on each patient, see Table III.

gested as one factor (4). The difference in the amount of cells failing to enter S phase among cell strains (59) may also have some relevance.

Recently, Miyaki *et al.* (53) found that cultured skin fibroblasts from hereditary (familial) Rb patients were highly susceptible to morphological transformation by murine sarcoma virus (MSV) while those from Rb patients with deletion in chromosome 13 showed the same susceptibility as normal controls and sporadic unilateral (non-hereditary) cases. These observations indicate that the autosomal dominant trait that predisposes to cancer can be manifested as some abnormal cellular characteristics in response to the insult of certain exogeneous agents.

Chromosomal Instability Associated with Rb Mutations

Some of the cancer predisposing diseases of recessive inheritance such as ataxia telangiectasia, Fanconi's anemia, and Bloom's syndrome are characterized by the elevated frequencies of spontaneous chromosome breakage. However, in general, such chromosomal instability has not been observed in Rb patients (*26, 35, 54*) although slight increase in aneuploidy, gaps, and breaks has been noted in sporadic unilateral cases (*17, 19*). Most of the sporadic unilateral Rb patients are non-hereditary. Therefore, increased chromosomal instability to chromosome breakage may not be related to the Rb gene. Morten (*54*) reported increased sensitivity to chromosome aberration formation by X-ray in peripheral blood lymphocytes from 10 out of 11 Rb patients. However, Nagasawa and Little (*59*) found normal chromosomal sensitivity to X-ray in cultured skin fibroblasts derived from Rb patients.

In spite of the absence of increased level of chromosomal fragility as expressed by open breaks, it has been shown by detailed banding techniques that cultured skin fibroblasts obtained from some Rb patients show abnormally increased frequency of cells with chromosome rearrangements (*67*). The chromosome rearrangements are reciprocal translocations and inversions, and non-constitutional mutant karyotypes are frequently observed. As seen in Table IV, such chromosomal rearrangements (mutant karyotypes) were observed in some of the sporadic Rb having normal constitutional karyotype and

TABLE IV.   Frequencies of Cells with Non-constitutional Chromosome Abnormalities in Cultured Skin Fibroblasts from Patients with Rb

Heredity	Patient	Tumor laterality	Constitutional karyotype	No. of cells analyzed	No. of cells with non-constitutional mutant karyotypes (%)
Sporadic	GM1142	B	46, XX, del (13) (q14q22)	50	0
	RBNaYo	B	46, XX, del (13) (q12q22)	60	0
	RBNiSa	B	46, XY, del (13) (q14)	50	0
	RBYaMa	B	46, XY/46, XY, del (13) (q14)	80	0
	RBOhNa	B	46, X, t (13; X) (q12; p22)	100	0
	Total			340	0 (0)
	RBMaMa	B	46, XX	50	19 (38.0)
	RBTaRi	B	46, XX	40	4 (10.0)
	RBYoHi	B	46, XY	50	2 (4.0)
	RBIuRi	B	46, XX	40	0
	RBTaTo	B	46, XY	40	0
	RBKoMa	B	46, XY	28	0
	RBNaNo	U	46, XY	50	35 (70.0)
	RBTaMi	U	46, XX	50	0
	RBYaMe	U	46, XX	50	0
	Total			390	60 (15.4)
Familial	RBIt-Mo	U	46, XX	60	5 (8.3)
	RBUtSi	B	46, XY	37	3 (8.1)
	RBAs-Mo	U	46, XX	50	9 (18.0)
	RBAsKe	B	46, XY	50	1 (2.0)
	Total			197	18 (9.1)

all of four familial cases. Interestingly, cells with such non-constitutional mutant karyo-types were not found in the Rb patients having constitutional chromosome 13 abnor-malities. The enhanced generation of the chromosome rearrangements in skin fibro-blasts has also been observed in other patients carrying the cancer predisposing gene of the dominant trait such as familial leukemia (70), medullary thyroid cancer syndrome (70), familial polyposis coli (18, 67, 77), Peutz-Jeghers' syndrome (67, 77), Gardner's syndrome (67), familial colon cancer (68), prokeratosis of Mibelli (46, 79), nevoid basal cell carcinoma syndrome (30), and familial melanoma (31).

It is interesting to note that none of five patients with constitutional chromosome 13 abnormalities showed any increase in such chromosomal instability. This finding is comparable with the susceptibility to transformation by MSV (53). If the chromosomal instability and susceptibility to transformation by MSV found in the cultured fibro-blasts of Rb patients are the reflection of the Rb mutation, the discrimination by type of germinal mutation suggests that the familially transmitted Rb mutations and the majority of fresh germinal mutations are essentially different from the germinal muta-tion of the deletion type. Inactivation of the gene by different mechanisms is highly likely (67).

Hereditary Rb patients have an increased propensity to develop tumors other than Rb, like osteosarcoma, fibrosarcoma, soft tissue sarcoma, etc. (32, 34, 65). These second tumors have long been attributed to radiation therapy. However, the second primary tumors also develop at sites far distant from the irradiated site and also in bilateral pa-tients who received no radiation (1, 2). Since the first report by Lele et al. (44), more than 40 Rb patients with constitutional chromosome 13 abnormalities have been re-ported. Yet, none of these patients has been described as having the development of second tumors. However, most of these papers were not primarily focused on the de-velopment of second tumors, and therefore the susceptibility of such patients to the second tumors remains to be elucidated. The development of second tumors in heredi-tary Rb patients has been thought to be a pleiotropic effect of the Rb gene (34). The underlying mechanisms of the development of second tumor are not known, but the Rb gene-mediated mutator function as expressed by the enhanced generation of varie-gated chromosome rearrangements and susceptibility to transformation by MSV could have some relevance if such gene effects are tissue specific. In this respect, the follow-up investigation of the Rb patients with constitutional chromosome 13 abnormalities is particularly intriguing.

Role of Rb Mutation in the Development of Tumor

There is debate whether one mutational event is enough to explain malignant trans-formation in Rb. A difference in the age at diagnosis between bilateral and sporadic unilateral Rb patients is well documented. A multistage stochastic model of carcino-genesis based on the age-specific incidence may provide some information on the number of independent events necessary for tumor development (5). From an analysis of 23 sporadic bilateral and 25 sporadic unilateral patients, Knudson (36) showed that the age-specific incidence as expressed by the cumulative log of fraction of cases not yet diagnosed was linear (one-hit type) for bilateral cases while it was quadratic (two-hit type) for sporadic unilateral cases. This led Knudson (36) to a hypothesis that two mutations by independent hits are required for the Rb tumor to develop. In bilateral

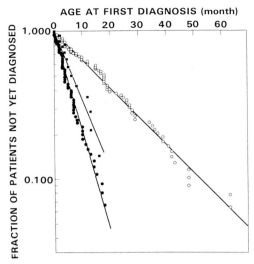

FIG. 2.   Comparison of the age-specific incidence among three groups of Rb patients as expressed by the change in the fraction of patients not yet diagnosed by
indicated age
    ○ sporadic unilateral; ● sporadic bilateral; ■ Rb patients with constitutional
chromosome 13 abnormalities.

(hereditary) cases, one mutation is already present as a germinal mutation and only one
more somatic mutation is required, whereas in sporadic unilateral (non-hereditary)
cases two successive somatic mutations are required. However, the shape of regression
curves is also influenced by other factors such as knowledge among parents on the disease, diagnostic efficiency, etc.. Bonaiti-Pellie et al. (9, 10) analyzed the age distribution
of 604 cases and found that the age-specific incidence for unilateral cases fitted a third
order regression curve rather than a second order curve. Figure 2 shows the regression
curves of cumulative log survival (fraction of cases not diagnosed) for 71 sporadic bilateral, 75 sporadic unilateral patients and 13 Rb patients with constitutional chromosome
13 abnormalities. As seen in the figure, it is evident that sporadic unilateral cases also
show the best fit to the linear regression curve. The regression coefficient (λ) and mean
latency period ($1/\lambda$) for three types of Rb patients were obtained by fitting the survival
fractions to the simple exponential function $S = e^{-\lambda t}$ with t (month) in age at diagnosis
(Table V). Our data thus do not render support for the two-hit hypothesis, but are
rather in line with the idea that only one mutational event is enough for Rb tumor to
develop (48–50, 81) or if two or more mutations are required they may not be independent from the first mutation.
    Advanced Rb tumor rarely occurs in newborn babies, and the development of Rb
tumor in adult is also rare. Therefore, the retinal cells at risk for malignant transformation must be present at a specific stage during development, probably as early as the
5th month of fetal life (52). In the development of Rb tumor, the contribution of hit
during postnatal life is not readily explained. If the second mutation is required, it must
also occur in fetal retinal cells. Instead of the two-hit hypothesis, Matsunaga (50) proposed a host resistance model as an alternative hypothesis in that one mutational event
was enough and inherited host resistance played an important role in the manifestation

TABLE V. Comparison of Coefficients and Mean Latency Periods of
Three Groups of Sporadic Rb

Heredity	No. of patients	Coefficient (λ)	Latency (month) ($1/\lambda$)
Unilateral	75	0.044	22.6
Bilateral	71	0.155	6.5
Chromosome 13 abnormality	13	0.103	9.3

Relationship between fraction of patients not yet diagnosed (S) and age at first diagnosis (t in month) was fitted to $S = \exp(-\lambda t)$.

of the Rb mutation as tumor. According to his model, the crucial event initiating tumor formation in the gene carrier is an error in differentiation and manifestation as tumor development is influenced by inherited host resistance which has multifactorial threshold character.

From an analysis of 27 Rb patients with chromosome 13 abnormalities collected from the literature, Matsunaga (51) showed that the chromosome 13 abnormalities, notably 13q−, have lower carcinogenic potential than mutant Rb gene as manifested by significant difference in the distribution of tumor laterality, whereas the degree of expressivity as manifested by latency period did not differ significantly. Although a small number of cases were involved, our data suggest that the tumors seem to appear with longer latency period in the Rb patients with chromosome 13 abnormalities than in those with mutant Rb gene. The difference between the two results may be accounted for by ascertainment of the bias coming from the recognizable patterns of phenotypes other than tumor. The small deletions or reciprocal translocations that constitute a significant fraction of our cases do not manifest as congenital abnormalities while larger deletions are usually accompanied by developmental retardation and some other congenital malformations, which may constitute factors to facilitate the recognition of ocular tumor.

The lower carcinogenic potential of the Rb mutation by chromosome structural rearrangement could be due to the growth disadvantage of the cells with deletion or the effect of recessive lethal of deletion associated with the mitotic recombination of chromosome 13. However, there is no simple relationship between the size of deletion and age at diagnosis. Recent studies using esterase D isoenzyme pattern and DNA restriction fragment length polymorphism (RFLP) revealed that loss of heterozygosity of chromosome 13 including 13q14 occurred in a significant fraction of Rb tumors (12, 13, 20, 27). All or a part of normal chromosome 13 including 13q14 is missing from the tumor while all or a part of chromosome 13 carrying the Rb mutation is duplicated resulting in a homozygosity for the mutation (58). Such loss of heterozygosity has been found in about 50% of primary Rb tumors (21). Its role in the development of Rb tumor is still not clear, but it will result in a cell lethal when the Rb mutation is given as a large deletion or translocation.

Chromosomal Mechanisms of the Development of Rb Tumor

In hereditary Rb patients, all of the embryonic retinal cells contain Rb mutation, or they are initiated, and constitute the cells at risk. However, only a few of these cells give rise to tumors. The crucial event engendering tumorigenicity is particularly intriguing. Evidence indicates that the Rb tumor originates from primitive multipotent retinal cells which are still capable of differentiating into both glial and neuronal cells (41, 78). The number of developing retinal cells at risk decreases rapidly as the retina matures.

The two-mutation model proposed by Knudson (36) assumes the second somatic mutation. The homozygosity of the Rb mutation mentioned above is presumed to be the second mutation necessary to transform the initiated cells to neoplastic. However, almost simultaneous appearance of tumors in both eyes in hereditary Rb cannot readily be explained by a simple stochastic hit model, and led Matsunaga (50) to postulate the host resistance model, in which errors in differentiation constitute a prelude to the neoplastic transformation and the manifestation of tumors is influenced by inherited host resistance.

Information on the chromosome changes in Rb tumors has been accumulated. Special concern was focused on chromosome 13, and actually the deleted chromosome 13 was found in some tumors (7). However, later studies showed that the deletion of chromosome 13 was not so common as had been thought in the early stage of study and the majority of tumors showed two normal chromosomes 13 (76). Karyotype abnormalities have been observed in virtually all of the Rb tumors studied so far. Squire et al. (76) studied 27 Rb tumors and found that duplication of 1q and 6p was very common, being observed in 21/27 and 15/27, respectively. Duplication of 1q, i.e., +1q, is present as a translocation of an extra copy of long arm of chromosome 1 onto another chromosome, and that of 6p is observed as an isochromosome, i.e., +i(6p), usually 4 copies of 6p being present. Table VI summarizes the chromosome abnormalities in 36 primary Rb tumors studied in our laboratory (69). Again, +1q abnormality was most common and found in 81% of tumors. The +i(6p) abnormality is unique in Rb tumor and very rarely seen in other types of tumors. Seven tumors (19%) had +i(6p). Altogether, 32 out of 36 tumors (89%) had either +1q or +i(6p), and 2 had both abnormalities. In 11 tumors, these abnormalities were only non-constitutional karyotype changes, indicating a significant role in tumor development. Double minutes were found in 6 tumors (17%). There was no difference in types and frequencies of chromosome aberrations between unilateral and bilateral tumors or between familial and sporadic cases.

Triplication of 1q is not specific to Rb tumor, and has been described in a variety of other human neoplasms (6). In some instances, particularly in hematological disorders, the +1q has been observed only in the late stage of karyotypic evolution, and thus has been evaluated as an event related with a malignant progression or proliferation rather than the initial event responsible for the development of tumors (64). However,

TABLE VI. Summary of Chromosome Abnormalities in 36 Primary Rb Tumors

Chromosome abnormality	Tumor laterality		
	Sporadic unilateral	Bilateral	Total (%)
+1q	14	15	29 (80.6)
+i(6p)	6	1	7 (19.4)
13q−	3	2	5 (13.9)
DM	2	4	6 (16.7)

DM, double minutes.

in some human tumors, aberration of chromosome 1 is assumed to represent specific and possibly initiating changes (6). We have noticed that, in sporadic unilateral Rb tumors, the same +1q abnormality (same translocation) was observed in all cells from a single tumor (monoclonal in terms of the formation of +1q abnormality), whereas at least 10 out of 18 bilateral tumors showed polyclonal appearance of such +1q abnormality (69). The observation gives a cytogenetic basis for the unifocal origin of tumors in sporadic unilateral patients and multifocal origin in hereditary Rb, and implies that in the development of Rb tumor, the generation of an extra copy of 1q (or, equally, 6p) is an early event and plays an important, or even crucial, role in the tumorigenic conversion of the retinoblasts which already have one Rb mutation.

It is generally accepted that carcinogenesis is a progressive multistep process. The Rb gene is considered as a tissue-specific suppressor of regulatory gene (50, 58). One can speculate that its diminished expression at a particular stage of retinal development, probably at the differentiation stage, leads some residual primitive retinal cells to step toward the exuberant proliferation by acquiring genome rearrangement. Such genome rearrangement may not necessarily be independent from the first mutation at 13q14. The reinforcement of malignant property may be possible by the gain of an extra copy of 1q or 6p with yet unknown mechanisms or by further loss of normal allele. In some instances, homozygosity may have an evolutionary rather than an etiological role. In the mouse T-cell leukemia, loss of heterozygosity at H-2 locus takes place as an adaptive response to the immunological environment (73). Similar allele loss by homozygosity has been observed in the adaptive response of cultured human lymphoblastoid cells to a selective environment for drug resistance (88). It is thus natural that the condition of the host resistance is a strong determinant in the expressivity of the Rb gene.

Acknowledgments

This work was in part supported by a Grant-in-Aid for Scientific Research from the Ministry of Education, Science and Culture, and by a Cancer Research Grant from the Ministry of Health and Welfare of Japan.

REFERENCES

1. Abramson, D. H. Treatment of retinoblastoma. *In* "Retinoblastoma," ed. F. C. Blodi, pp. 63–93 (1985). Churchill Livingstone, New York, Edinburgh, London, Melbourne.
2. Abramson, D. H., Ellsworth, R. M., and Zimmerman, L. E. Nonocular cancer in retinoblastoma survivors. *Trans. Am. Acad. Ophthalmol. Otolaryng.*, **81**, 454–457 (1976).
3. Arlett, C. F. and Harcourt, S. A. Survey of radiosensitivity in a variety of human cell strains. *Cancer Res.*, **40**, 926–932 (1980).
4. Arlett, C. F. and Priestley, A. Defective recovery from potentially lethal damage in some human fibroblast strains. *Int. J. Radiat. Biol.*, **43**, 157–167 (1983).
5. Ashley, D.J.B. The two "hit" and multiple "hit" theories of carcinogenesis. *Br. J. Cancer*, **23**, 313–328 (1969).
6. Atkin, N. B. Chromosome 1 aberrations in cancer. *Cancer Genet. Cytogenet.*, **21**, 279–285 (1986).
7. Balaban, G., Gilbert, F., Nichols, W., Meadows, A. T., and Shields, J. Abnormalities of chromosome 13 in retinoblastoma from individuals with normal constitutional karyotypes. *Cancer Genet. Cytogenet.*, **6**, 213–221 (1982).
8. Benedict, W. F., Murphree, A. L., Banerjee, A., Spina, C. A., Sparkes, M. C., and Sparkes,

R. S. Patient with 13 chromosome deletion: evidence that the retinoblastoma gene is a recessive cancer gene. *Science*, **219**, 973–975 (1983).

9. Bonaiti-Pellie, C., Briard-Guillemot, M. L., Feingold, J., and Frezal, J. Mutation theory of carcinogenesis in retinoblastoma. *J. Natl. Cancer Inst.*, **57**, 269–276 (1976).

10. Briard-Guillemot, M. L., Bonaiti-Pellie, C., Feingold, J., and Frezal, J. Etude genetique du retinoblastome. *Humangenetik*, **24**, 271–284 (1974).

11. Butler, M. G. and Palmer, C. G. Parental origin of chromosome 15 deletion in Prader-Willi syndrome. *Lancet*, **i**, 1285–1286 (1983).

12. Cavenee, W. K., Dryja, T. P., Phillips, R. A., Benedict, W. F., Godbout, R. Gallie, B. L., Murphree, A. L., Strong, L. C., and White, P. L. Expression of recessive alleles by chromosomal mechanisms in retinoblastoma. *Nature*, **305**, 779–784 (1984).

13. Cavenee, W. K., Hansen, M. F., Nordenskjold, M., Maumenee, I., Squire, J. A., Phillips, R. A., and Gallie, B. L. Genetic origin of mutations predisposing to retinoblastoma. *Science*, **228**, 501–503 (1985).

14. Chamberlin, J. and Magenis, R. E. Parental origin of *de novo* chromosome rearrangements. *Hum. Genet.*, **53**, 343–347 (1980).

15. Cleaver, J. E., Char, D., Charles, W. C., and Rand, R. Repair and replication of DNA in hereditary (bilateral) retinoblastoma cells after X-irradiation. *Cancer Res.*, **42**, 1343–1347 (1982).

16. Cowell J. K., Rutland, P., Marcelle, J., and Hungerford, J. Deletions of the esterase D locus from a survey of 200 retinoblastoma patients. *Hum. Genet.*, **72**, 164–167 (1986).

17. Czeizel, A. and Gárdonyi, J. Retinoblastoma in Hungary. *Humangenetik*, **22**, 153–158 (1974).

18. Delhanty, J.D.A., Davis, M. B., and Wood, J. Chromosome instability in lymphocytes, fibroblasts and colon epithelial like cells from patients with familial polyposis coli. *Cancer Genet. Cytogenet.*, **8**, 27–50 (1983).

19. De Nunez, M., Penchaszadeh, V. B., and Pimentel, E. Chromosome fragility in patients with sporadic unilateral retinoblastoma. *Cancer Genet. Cytogenet.*, **11**, 139–141 (1984).

20. Dryja, T. P., Bruns, G.A.P., Gallie, B., Petersen, R., Green, W., Rapaport, J. M., Albert, D. M., and Gerald, P. S. Low incidence of deletion of the esterase D locus in retinoblastoma patients. *Hum. Genet.*, **64**, 151–155 (1983).

21. Dryja, P. D., Cavenee, W., White, R., Rapaport, J. M., Petersen, R., Albert, D. M., and Bruns, G.A.P. Homozygosity of chromosome 13 in retinoblastoma. *N. Engl. J. Med.*, **310**, 550–553 (1984).

22. Dryja, T. P., Rapaport, J. M., Joyce, J. M., and Petersen, R. A. Molecular detection of deletions involving band q14 of chromosome 13 in retinoblastomas. *Proc. Natl. Acad. Sci. U.S.A.*, **83**, 7391–7394 (1986).

23. Ejima, Y., Sasaki, M. S., Utsumi, H., Kaneko, A., and Tanooka, H. Radiosensitivity of fibroblasts from patients with retinoblastoma and chromosome 13 anomalies. *Mutat. Res.*, **103**, 177–184 (1982).

24. Fitzgerald, P. H., Stewart, J., and Suckling, R. D. Retinoblastoma mutation rate in New Zealand and support for the two-hit model. *Hum. Genet.*, **64**, 128–130 (1983).

25. Friend, S. H., Bernards, R., Rogelj, S., Weinberg, R. A., Rapaport, J. M., Albert, D. M., and Dryja, T. P. A human DNA segment with properties of the gene that predisposes to retinoblastoma and osteosarcoma. *Nature*, **323**, 643–646 (1986).

26. Gainer, H. St. C. and Kinsella, A. R. Analysis of spontaneous, carcinogen-induced and promoter-induced chromosomal instability in patients with hereditary retinoblastoma. *Int. J. Cancer*, **32**, 449–453 (1983).

27. Godbout, R., Dryja, T. P., Squire, J., Gallie, B. L., and Phillips, R. A. Somatic inactivation of genes on chromosome 13 is a common event in retinoblastoma. *Nature*, **304**, 451–453 (1983).

28. Godbout, A. D., Heddle, J. A., Gallie, B. L., and Phillips, R. A. Radiation sensitivity of fibroblasts of bilateral retinoblastoma patients as determined by micronucleus induction *in vitro*. *Mutat. Res.*, **152**, 31–38 (1985).

29. Harnden, D. G., Morten, J., and Featherstone, T. Dominant susceptibility to cancer in man. *Adv. Cancer Res.*, **41**, 165–255 (1984).

30. Hepple, R. and Hoehn, H. Cytogenetic studies on cultured fibroblast-like cells derived from basal cell carcinoma tissue. *Clin. Genet.*, **4**, 17–24 (1973).

31. Jaspers, N. G., Roza-de Jongh, E.J.M., Donselaar, I. G., Van Velzen-Tillemans, T. M., Van Hemel, J. O., Rumke, Ph., and Van der Kamp, A.W.M. Sister chromatid exchanges, hyperdiploidy and chromosomal rearrangements studied in cells from melanoma-prone individuals belonging to families with the dysplastic nevus syndrome. *Cancer Genet. Cytogenet.*, **24**, 33–43 (1987).

32. Jensen, R. D. and Miller, R. W. Retinoblastoma: epidemiological characteristics. *N. Engl. J. Med.*, **285**, 307–311 (1971).

33. Kaneko, A. Incidence of retinoblastoma in Japan from 1975 to 1979. *Atarashii Ganka*, **1**, 729–730 (1984) (in Japanese).

34. Kitchen, E. D. and Ellsworth, R. M. Pleiotropic effect of the gene for retinoblastoma. *J. Med. Genet.*, **11**, 244–246 (1974).

35. Knight, L. A., Gardner, H. A., and Gallie, B. L. Absence of chromosome breakage in patients with retinoblastoma. *Hum. Genet.*, **51**, 73–78 (1979).

36. Knudson, A. G. Mutation and cancer: statistical study of retinoblastoma. *Proc. Natl. Acad. Sci. U.S.A.*, **68**, 820–823 (1971).

37. Knudson, A. G., Meadows, A. T., Nichols, W. W., and Hill, R. Chromosome deletion and retinoblastoma. *N. Engl. J. Med.*, **295**, 1120–1123 (1976).

38. Kondo, I. and Hamaguchi, H. Evidence for the close linkage between lymphocyte cytosol polypeptide with molecular weight of 64,000 (LCP1) and esterase D. *Am. J. Hum. Genet.*, **37**, 1106–1111 (1985).

39. Kopelovich, L. and Rich, R. F. Enhanced radiotolerance to ionizing radiation is correlated with increased cancer proneness of cultured fibroblasts from precursor states in neurofibromatosis patients. *Cancer Genet. Cytogenet.*, **22**, 203–210 (1986).

40. Kossakowska, A. E., Gallie, B. L., and Phillips, R. A. Fibroblasts from retinoblastoma patients: enhanced growth in fetal calf serum and a normal response to ionizing radiation. *J. Cell Physiol.*, **111**, 15–20 (1982).

41. Kyritsis, A. P., Tsokos, M., Triche, T. J., and Chader, G. J. Retinoblastoma—origin from primitive neuroectodermal cells? *Nature*, **307**, 471–473 (1984).

42. Lalande, M., Donlon, T., Petersen, R. A., Liberfarb, R., Manter, S., and Latt, S. A. Molecular detection and differentiation of deletions in band 13q14 in human retinoblastoma. *Cancer Genet. Cytogenet.*, **23**, 151–157 (1986).

43. Ledbetter, D. H., Riccardi, V. M., Albert, S. D., Strobel, R. J., Kennan, B. S., and Crawford, J. D. Deletion of chromosome 15 as a cause of the Prader-Willi syndrome. *N. Engl. J. Med.*, **364**, 325–329 (1981).

44. Lele, K. P., Penrose, L. S., and Stallard, H. B. Chromosome deletion in a case of retinoblastoma. *Ann. Hum. Genet.*, **27**, 171–174 (1963).

45. Liberfarb, R. M., Bustos, T., Miller, W. A., and Sang, D. Incidence and significance of a deletion of chromosome band 13q14 in patients with retinoblastoma and in their families. *Ophthalmology*, **91**, 1695–1699 (1984).

46. Machino, H., Miki, Y., Teramoto, T., Shiraishi, S., and Sasaki, M. S. Cytogenetic studies in a patient with prokeratosis of Mibelli, multiple cancers and a *forme fuste* of Werner's syndrome. *Br. J. Dermatol.*, **111**, 579–586 (1984).

47. Matsunaga, E. Parental age and sporadic retinoblastoma. *Annu. Rep. Jpn. 1st. Genet.*, **16**, 121–123 (1965).

48. Matsunaga, E. Hereditary retinoblastoma: penetrance, expressivity and age of onset. *Hum. Genet.*, **33**, 1–15 (1976).

49. Matsunaga, E. Hereditary retinoblastoma: delayed mutation or host resistance? *Am. J. Hum. Genet.*, **30**, 406–424 (1978).

50. Matsunaga, E. Hereditary retinoblastoma: host resistance and age of onset. *J. Natl. Cancer Inst.*, **63**, 933–939 (1979).

51. Matsunaga, E. Retinoblastoma: host resistance and 13q- chromosomal deletion. *Hum. Genet.*, **56**, 53–58 (1980).

52. Matsunaga, E. Inherited tissue resistance to the gene for retinoblastoma. *In* "Genetic and Environmental Factors in Experimental and Human Cancer," ed. H. V. Gelboin *et al.*, pp. 161–173 (1980). Japan Sci. Soc. Press, Tokyo.

53. Miyaki, M., Akamatsu, N., Ono, T., and Sasaki, M. S. Susceptibility of skin fibroblasts from patients with retinoblastoma to transformation by murine sarcoma virus. *Cancer Lett.*, **18**, 137–142 (1983).

54. Morten, J.E.N. Cellular studies on retinoblastoma. *Int. J. Radiat. Biol.*, **49**, 485–494 (1986).

55. Motegi, T. High rate of detection of 13q14 deletion mosaicism among retinoblastoma patients (using more extensive methods). *Hum. Genet.*, **61**, 95–97 (1982).

56. Motegi, T., Kaga, M., Yanagawa, Y., Kadowaki, H., Watanabe, K., Inoue, A., Komatsu, M., and Minoda, K. A recognizable pattern of the midface of retinoblastoma patients with interstitial deletion of 13q. *Hum. Genet.*, **64**, 160–162 (1983).

57. Motegi, T. and Minoda, K. A decreasing tendency for cytogenetic abnormality in peripheral lymphocytes of retinoblastoma patients with 13q14 deletion mosaicism. *Hum. Genet.*, **66**, 186–189 (1984).

58 Murphree, A. L. and Benedict, W. F. Retinoblastoma: clue to human oncogenesis. *Science*, **223**, 1028–1033 (1984).

59. Nagasawa, H. and Little, J. B. Comparison of kinetics of X-ray induced cell killing in normal, ataxia telangiectasia and hereditary retinoblastoma fibroblasts. *Mutat. Res.*, **109**, 297–308 (1983).

60. Niikawa, N. and Ishikiriyama, S. Clinical and cytogenetic studies of the Prader-Willi syndrome: Evidence of phenotype-karyotype correlation. *Hum. Genet.*, **69**, 222–227 (1985).

61. Nove, J., Little, J. B., Weichselbaum, R. R., Nichols, W. W., and Hoffman, E. Retinoblastoma, chromosome 13, and *in vitro* cellular radiosensitivity. *Cytogenet. Cell Genet.*, **24**, 176–184 (1979).

62. Nove, J., Nichols, W. W., Weichselbaum, R. R., and Little, J. B. Abnormalities of human chromosome 13 and *in vitro* radiosensitivity. *Mutat. Res.*, **84**, 157–167 (1981).

63. Riccardi, V. M. The Prader-Willi syndrome (PWS) as a "transposable elements" disorder. *Am. J. Hum. Genet.*, **33**, 117A (1981).

64. Rowley, J. D. Mapping of human chromosomal regions related to neoplasia: Evidence from chromosomes 1 and 17. *Proc. Natl. Acad. Sci. U.S.A.*, **74**, 5729–5733 (1977).

65. Sagerman, R. H., Cassady, J. R., Tretter, P., and Ellsworth, R. M. Radiation induced neoplasia following external beam therapy for children with retinoblastoma. *Am. J. Roentgenol.*, **105**, 529–535 (1969).

66. Salamanca-Gómez, F., Luengas, F., and Antillon, F. Genetic and cytogenetic studies in children with retinoblastoma. *Cancer Genet. Cytogenet.*, **13**, 129–138 (1984).

67. Sasaki, M. S. Dominantly expressed procancer mutations and induction of chromosome rearrangements. *Prog. Mutat. Res.*, **4**, 75–84 (1982).

68. Sasaki, M. S. and Ejima, Y. Procancer class of genes and generation of chromosome mutation. *Gann Monogr. Cancer Res.*, **27**, 85–94 (1981).

69. Sasaki, M. S., Ejima, Y., Kaneko, A., and Tanooka, H. Tumorigenic chromosomal changes during the development of retinoblastoma. Proc. Jpn. Cancer Assoc., The 45th Annual Meeting, p. 267 (1986).

70. Sasaki, M. S., Tsunematsu, Y., Utsunomiya, J., and Utsumi, J. Site-directed chromosome rearrangements in skin fibroblasts from persons carrying genes for hereditary neoplasms. *Cancer Res.*, **40**, 4796–4803 (1980).
71. Schappert-Kimmijser, J., Hemmes, G. D., and Nijland, R. The heredity of retinoblastoma. *Ophthalmology*, **151**, 197–213 (1966).
72. Seabright, M. A rapid banding technique for human chromosomes. *Lancet*, **ii**, 971–972 (1971).
73. Shen, F. W., Chaganti, R.S.K., Doucette, L. A., Litman, G. W., Steinmetz, M., Hood, L., and Boyse, E. A. Genomic constitution of an H-2: T1a variant leukemia. *Proc. Natl. Acad. Sci. U.S.A.*, **82**, 6447–6450 (1984).
74. Sorsby, A. Bilateral retinoblastoma: A dominantly inherited affliction. *Br. Med. J.*, **2**, 580–583 (1972).
75. Sparkes, R. S., Sparkes, M. C., Wilson, M. G., Towner, J. W., Benedict, W. F., Murphree, A. L., and Yunis, J. J. Regional assignment of genes for human esterase D and retinoblastoma to chromosome band 13q14. *Science*, **208**, 1042–1044 (1980).
76. Squire, J., Gallie, B. L., and Phillips, R. A. A detailed analysis of chromosomal changes in heritable and non-heritable retinoblastoma. *Hum. Genet.*, **70**, 291–301 (1985).
77. Takai, S., Iwama, T., and Tonomura, A. Chromosome instability in cultured skin fibroblasts from patients with familial polyposis coli and Peutz-Jeghers' syndrome. *Jpn. J. Cancer Res.*, **77**, 759–766 (1986).
78. Taylor, H. R., Carroll, N., Jack, I., and Crock, G. W. A scanning electron microscopic examination of retinoblastoma in tissue culture. *Br. J. Ophthalmol.*, **63**, 551–559 (1979).
79. Taylor, A.M.R., Harnden, D. G., and Fairburn, E. A. Chromosomal instability associated with susceptibility to malignant disease in patient with prokeratosis of Mibelli. *J. Natl. Cancer Inst.*, **51**, 371–378 (1973).
80. Vogel, F. Neue Untersuchungen zur Genetik des Retinoblastoms. V. *Mensch. Vererb. Konstit.-Lehre*, **34**, 205 (1957).
81. Vogel, F. Genetics of retinoblastoma. *Hum. Genet.*, **52**, 1–54 (1979).
82. Wang, Y., Parkes, W. C., Wigle, J. C., Maher, V. M., and McCormick, J. J. Fibroblasts from patients with inherited predisposition to retinoblastoma exhibit normal sensitivity to the mutagenic effects of ionizing radiation. *Mutat. Res.*, **175**, 107–114 (1986).
83. Weichselbaum, R. R., Nove, J., and Little, J. B. Skin fibroblasts from a D-deletion type retinoblastoma patient are abnormally X-ray sensitive. *Nature*, **266**, 726–727 (1977).
84. Weichselbaum, R. R., Nove, J., and Little, J. B. X-ray sensitivity of diploid fibroblasts from patients with hereditary or sporadic retinoblastoma. *Proc. Natl. Acad. Sci. U.S.A.*, **75**, 3962–3964 (1978).
85. Weichselbaum, R. R., Nove, J., and Little, J. B. X-ray sensitivity of fifty three human diploid fibroblast cell strains from patients with characterized genetic disorders. *Cancer Res.*, **40**, 920–925 (1980).
86. Weichselbaum, R. R., Tomkinson, K., and Little, J. B. Repair of potentially lethal X-ray damage in fibroblasts derived from patients with hereditary and D-deletion retinoblastoma. *Int. J. Rad. Biol.*, **47**, 445–456 (1985).
87. Wood, W. G., Lopez, M., and Kalvonjian, S. L. Normal repair of gamma radiation induced single- and double-strand DNA breaks in retinoblastoma fibroblasts. *Biochim. Biophys. Acta*, **698**, 40–48 (1982).
88. Yandell, D. W., Dryja, T. P., and Little, J. B. Somatic mutations at a heterozygous autosomal locus in human cells occur more frequently by allele loss than by intragenic structural alterations. *Somatic Cell Mol. Genet.*, **12**, 255–265 (1986).
89. Zampetti-Bosseler, F. and Scott, D. Cell death, chromosome damage and mitotic delay in normal human, ataxia telangiectasia and retinoblastoma fibroblasts after X-irradiation. *Int. J. Radiat. Biol.*, **39**, 547–558 (1981).

Gann Monograph on Cancer Research 35, 1988

CLINICAL ASPECTS OF RETINOBLASTOMA IN JAPAN

Akihiro Kaneko

Department of Ophthalmology, National Cancer Center Hospital*

Six clinical aspects of retinoblastoma in Japan were reviewed: incidence, reasons for the first medical visit, age at the first diagnosis, treatment and results of conservative therapy, survival rate and incidence, and problems of retinoblastoma students learning in schools for the blind.

Japanese incidence of retinoblastoma was about one case per 15,000 live births in the period from 1975 to 1979. Most patients visited ophthalmological clinics because of leukocoria. The success rate of conservative therapy of Reese Group V cases in the National Cancer Center Hospital, Tokyo, was 33%. This was comparable to the rates of therapy centers in developed countries.

Incidence of Retinoblastoma (4)

The incidence of retinoblastoma in Japan from 1975 to 1979 was investigated using the National Registration of Children with Retinoblasotma, questionnaires sent to all eye hospitals which had not joined the National Registration and death certificates filed with the Ministry of Health and Welfare of Japan. The number of determined cases was 596, of which 508 were from the National Registration, 84 from the questionnaires, and 4 from the death certificates. There were 429 unilateral cases (213 boys and 216 girls), and 167 bilateral cases (98 boys and 69 girls); this was one bilateral case to 2.6 unilateral cases. The incidence of bilateral cases in boys was 1.4 times that in girls. This difference was not statistically significant.

No histopathological diagnosis was available in 20 unilateral and 10 bilateral cases because of conservative therapy, refusal of enucleation of the eye by parents or other reasons.

Familial cases numbered 26, 4.4% of the total; they consisted of 15 bilateral cases (10 boys and 5 girls) and 11 unilateral cases (2 boys and 9 girls).

The average annual incidence was 119 cases of which 86 were unilateral and 33 were bilateral. The average annual number of live births in this period was 1,768,200. Accordingly, the incidence of retinoblastoma from 1975 to 1979 was one case per 14,859 live births.

Reasons for the First Medical Visit of Retinoblastoma Patients (7)

The reasons for the first visit of retinoblastoma patients to eye clinics, according to the statistics on 463 patients with this condition who were registered by the National Registration of Children with Retinoblastoma in 1975, are shown in Table I. Leukocoria (white pupil) is a phenomenon in which a white light reflex is observed within the pupil.

---

* 5-1-1, Tsukiji, Chuo-ku, Tokyo 104, Japan (金子明博).

TABLE I. Reasons for the First Medical Visit of Retinoblastoma Patients (Japan, 1975)

1.	Leukocoria (cat's eye)	75%
2.	Strabismus	12
3.	Disorder of conjunctiva and/or cornea	6
4.	Poor vision	3
5.	Fundus examination	1
6.	Others	3

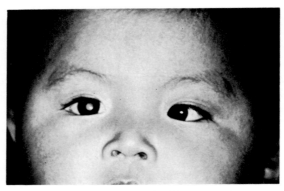

FIG. 1. Leukocoria and strabismus of a retinoblastoma patient
This 5-month-old baby showed not only white light reflex (leukocoria) in her right eye but also strabismus due to the loss of visual function. Fundus examination revealed bilateral retinoblastoma.

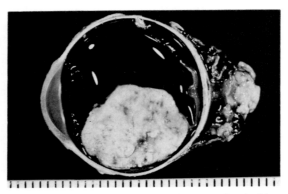

FIG. 2. Cross section of the eyeball enucleated because of retinoblastoma
Retinoblastoma (14 mm × 12 mm) which developed from the retina occupied about half of the vitreous space.

Retinoblastomas are usually white tumors. When they grow in the vitreous cavity to a size where they near the lens, their white surfaces can be seen from the outside, especially in the darkness. Strabismus is an abnormal position of the eye due to the disruption of the macula by the tumor. Disorders of the conjunctiva or the cornea are hypermia of the conjunctiva or cloudiness of the cornea caused by secondary glaucoma or uveitis due to the tumor. Poor vision is recognized in bilateral cases by abnormal behavior of infants with low visual acuity, when visual functions of both eyes are destroyed by the tumor. The fundus examination is usually coincidental. Premature babies or babies with a family history of retinoblastoma are offered the opportunity to be checked by fundus examination. No exopthalmos has been found in Japan as the initial sign of retinoblastoma.

Age at the First Diagnosis of Retinoblastoma

Average age at the time of the first diagnosis of retinoblastoma was determined from the 596 cases recorded from 1975 to 1979. Without a family history of retinoblastoma, there were 27.1 ± 22.0 unilateral cases and 10.9 ± 10.3 bilateral cases. With a family history, there were 30.2 ± 18.5 unilateral cases and 9.9 ± 8.6 bilateral cases. Since no statistically significant difference was found in the two groups, parents with retinoblastoma should be more thoroughly made aware of the hereditary characteristics of the condition and the need for fundus examinations as early as possible for newborn infants.

Treatment of Retinoblastoma

Modalities of treatment of retinoblastoma depend on the stage of the tumor. Enucleation of the eyeball is indicated for suspected extraocular extension or loss of visual function. The first case of conservative therapy of retinoblastoma in Japan was reported in 1916 by Professor Jujiro Koomoto in Tokyo, who used X-ray irradiation. However, the first systematic trial of conservative therapy was started by the National Cancer Center Hospital in Tokyo in 1964. Our recent treatment modalities for conservative therapy of retinoblastoma are external beam irradiation with a 6-MeV linear accelerator, photocoagulation with a Xenon arch coagulator, cryotherapy with a cryoprobe cooled to about $-80°C$, episcleral plaque irradiation using Stallard's cobalt 60 applicator and chemotherapy. The rate of cure using conservative therapy in the National Cancer Center Hospital is shown in Table II. Visual results of these treatments are shown in Fig. 3.

Reese Group V includes massive tumors involving over half the retina and tumors with vitreous seeding. The success rate of conservative therapy on Reese Group V retinoblastoma is as low in our hospital as in any other in the world (1, 3). One of the main factors for low visual acuity after conservative therapy is an irradiation cataract if the tumor does not involve the macular region.

TABLE II.   Cure Rates of Conservative Treatment of Retinoblastoma

Reese group	Ellsworth (1965–1972) % (cases)	Kaneko (1973–1982) % (eyes)
I	91 (43)	94 (18)
II	83 (35)	89 (19)
III	82 (56)	82 (11)
IV	62 (21)	92 (13)
V	29 (75)	33 (15)
Total	75 (230)	79 (76)

Cure was determined more than 5 years after the first treatment.

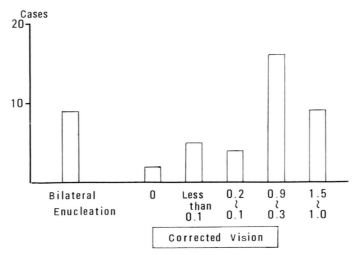

FIG. 3. Results of conservative treatment of retinoblastoma 1973–1979 (National Cancer Center Hospital)
These visual results were determined more than 5 years after the first treatment. Deceased patients were excluded from these statistics.

Survival Rate for Retinoblastoma (2)

Survival rates for retinoblastoma differ according to the degree of advancement of the tumor, as is true in other malignancies. Using 255 cases which were registered in the National Registration of Retinoblastoma and followed up for more than 5 years, survival rates were determined. Figures 4 and 5 show the results. When tumors were limited to within the eyeball and no evidence of optic disc invasion was found, the 5-year-survival was 98%. When tumors were limited to within the eyeball but no definite denial of optic disc invasion was possible, the 5-year-survival became 87%. With ex-

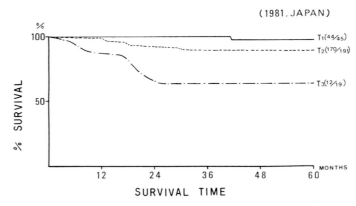

FIG. 4. Survival curves for 255 cases of retinoblastoma (1981, Japan)
T_1, tumors confined within the eyeball and no involvement of the optic disc; T_2, tumors confined within the eyeball and involvement of the optic disc or suspicion of involvement of the optic disc; T_3, tumors extending outside of the eyeball. Classification according to fundus examination and clinical findings.

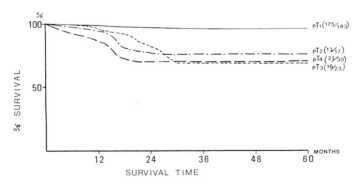

FIG. 5. Survival curves for 253 cases of retinoblastoma (1981, Japan)
pT_1, tumor(s) confined to the retina and no choroidal invasion; pT_2, tumor(s) invading the choroid but no scleral invasion; pT_3, a) tumor beyond the lamina cribrosa but not at the line of resection; b) intrascleral invasion; pT_4, a) tumor at the line of resection of the optic nerve; b) extrascleral invasion.
Classification according to histopathological findings.

traocular invasion which was clinically obvious, it dropped to 67%. For 253 cases for which histopathological information was available, 5-year-survival rates are shown in Fig. 5. Optic nerve invasion beyond the lamina cribrosa and scleral invasions were ominous signs.

Incidence and Ophthalmological Problems of Retinoblastoma Students Learning in Schools for the Blind (5)

A questionnaire concerning retinoblastoma students was sent to all 71 schools for the blind in Japan and covered the followings 9 items: name, sex, date and year of birth, visual acuity, state of the eyeballs, state of the prosthesis, grade of intelligence, abnormality of the body, and heredity. Teachers of nursing or parents were asked to complete the entries. All schools were cooperative with this investigation. We found 162 cases of bilateral retinoblastoma, 5 cases of unilateral and one case of undefined laterality. Bilateral retinoblastoma was found in 2.1% of all blind students in these schools (Table III). These cases were estimated to account for 32–38% of the annual incidence of bilateral retinoblastoma in Japan (Table IV). The eyeballs were preserved unilaterally or bilaterally in 32% of the bilateral cases (Table V). However, 52% of the eyeballs were shrunken, and 75% of these patients had visual acuity of less than 0.01. No prosthesis was used in 12% of the enucleated sockets. Only 50% of the users of

TABLE III. Incidence of Bilateral Retinoblastoma in Students in Japanese Schools for the Visually Handicapped (1981)

	Number of students	Number with bilateral retinoblastoma	Percentage
Kindergarden	186	14	7.5
Elementary school	1,818	77	4.2
Junior high school	1,272	32	2.5
Postgraduate course	4,554	39	0.9
Total	7,830	162	2.1

TABLE IV. Ratio of Students with Bilateral Retinoblastoma in Schools for the Visually
Handicapped to Total Bilateral Retinoblastoma Cases (1981)

Annual incidence of bilateral retinoblastoma	33.4
Average number of students with bilateral retinoblastoma in grade one of elementary schools for the visually handicapped	12.8 (38%)
Average number of students with bilateral retinoblastoma in grade one of junior high schools for the visually handicapped	10.7 (32%)
Average number of students with bilateral retinoblastoma in grade one of compulsory education schools for the visually handicapped	12.1 (36%)

TABLE V. Status of Eyeballs in Students with Bilateral Retinoblastoma in
Japanese Schools for the Visually Handicapped (1981)

Status	Number of cases (%)		
	Male	Female	Total
Both eyes enucleated	73 (72)	37 (62)	110 (68)
One eye enucleated	25 (25)	21 (35)	46 (28)
Both eyes preserved	4 (3)	2 (3)	6 (4)

prostheses were satisfied with their prosthesis. The improvement of conservative therapy of retinoblastoma and careful after-therapy of enucleated sockets are necessary to decrease the incidence and ophthalmological problems of retinoblastoma students in schools for the blind.

Acknowledgment

This work was supported by a Grant-in Aid for Cancer Research from the Ministry of Health and Welfare of Japan.

REFERENCES

1. Ellsworth, R. M. Various aspects of retinoblastoma. International Symposium on Intraocular Tumors, Schwerin (1981).
2. Kaneko, A. A proposal for TNM classification of retinoblastoma. *Folia Ophthalmol. Jpn.*, **33**, 350–353 (1982).
3. Kaneko, A. Recent advances in treatment and study of retinoblastoma. *Folia Ophthalmol. Jpn.*, **34**, 442–451 (1983).
4. Kaneko, A. Incidence of retinoblastoma in Japan from 1975 to 1979. *Atarashii Ganka*, **1**, 137–138 (1984) (in Japanese).
5. Kaneko, A. The incidence and ophthalmological problems of retinoblastoma students learning in schools for the blind of Japan. *Acta Soc. Ophthalmol. Jpn.*, **88**, 162–166 (1984).
6. Koomoto, J. X-ray therapy of glioma retinae. *Rinsho Ganka*, **12**, 185 (1917) (in Japanese).
7. Minoda, K. National Registration of Retinoblastoma Children in 1975. *Acta Soc. Ophthalmol. Jpn.*, **80**, 1648–1657 (1976).

MULTIPLE ENDOCRINE NEOPLASIA TYPE 2

Shin-ichiro TAKAI,[*1] Akira MIYAUCHI,[*2] Tetsuro MIKI,[*3]
Hideo TATEISHI,[*1] Isamu NISHISHO,[*1] Kazuyoshi MOTOMURA,[*1]
and Takesada MORI[*1]

The Second Department of Surgery, Osaka University Medical School,[*1]
Department of Surgery, Kagawa Medical School,[*2] *and Department of*
Medicine and Geriatrics, Osaka University Medical School[*3]

Multiple endocrine neoplasia type 2 (MEN 2) syndrome is an autosomal dominant disorder which is characterized by the association of
medullary thyroid carcinoma (MTC) and pheochromocytoma. In accord
with other component diseases, this syndrome is subdivided into types
2A and 2B. Among 271 patients with MTC in Japan at least 48 have
MEN 2A (17.7%), 6 have MEN 2B (2.2%) and there are 38 familial MTC
cases (14.0%). Twenty-two kindred at high risk for MEN 2A and 12
kindred with familial MTC alone are known. MEN 2 syndrome is consistent with Knudson's two-mutational-event theory for oncogenesis. Recently the locus for the gene predisposing to MEN2A was assigned to
chromosome 10 by linkage analysis using restriction fragment length polymorphisms (RFLPs) in European Caucasian kindreds. We confirmed it in
Japanese kindreds. The structure and function of MEN 2A will be clarified
in the near future.

Multiple endocrine neoplasia (MEN) is a syndrome which is characterized by association of tumors or hyperplasia of certain endocrine glands. The combination of
glands involved is not random but fixed according to the type of syndrome. Three types
of MEN are recognized at present and the endocrine tumors (or hyperplasia) involved
and their prevalence rates are shown in Table I (*2, 20, 22, 25*). MEN 2A is a syndrome
characterised by the association with medullary thyroid carcinoma (MTC) and peo-
chromocytoma with occasional parathyroid adenopathy. Patients with MEN 2B have
characteristic phenotypes due to mucosal neuromas (*3*).

Familial occurrence of the disease due to autosomal dominant inheritance is known
in all three types of MEN. Among these three types, MEN 2A has been studied most
intensively in an attempt to find the predisposing gene.

Clinical Aspects

1) Medullary thyroid carcinoma

There are two kinds of epithelial cells in the thyroid gland, *i.e.*, follicular cells and
C cells. Thyroid follicular cells are epithelial cells which line the thyroid follicles and
secrete thyroxine and triiodothyronine.

[*1, *3] 1-1-50, Fukushima, Fukushima-ku, Osaka 553, Japan (高井新一郎, 宮内　昭, 三木哲郎, 立石秀郎,
西庄　勇, 元村和由, 森　武貞).
[*2] Miki-cho, Kagawa 761-07, Japan (宮内　昭).

TABLE I. Three Types of Multiple Endocrine Neoplasia

Type	Endocrine gland (tumor or abnormality)	Prevalence (%)	
		Japan[a]	U.S.A.[b]
MEN 1	Pituitary (adenoma)	34–73	65
	Parathyroid (hyperplasia)	80–92	88
	Pancreas (islet cell tumor)	40–81	81
MEN 2A	Thyroid (MTC[c])	100	100
	Adrenal medulla (Pheo.)	94	48
	Parathyroid (adenoma?)	23	23–70
MEN 2B	Nerves (mucosal neuroma)	100	80–100
	Thyroid (MTC)	100	100
	Adrenal medulla (Pheo.)	67	20–36
	Marfanoid habitus		
	Ganglioneuromatosis of digestive tract		
	Megacolon		
	Pes cavus		

[a] From ref. *20*.

[b] Data for MEN 1 from ref. *2*, for MEN 2A and 2B from ref. *22* (lower value) and ref. *25* (higher value).

[c] MTC stands for medullary thyroid carcinoma.

Pheo., pheochromocytoma.

The second type of epithelial cells, C cells, are very few in number and scattered solitarily between the thyroid follicles, so they are also called parafollicular cells. C cells produce and secrete a peptide hormone called calcitonin, a serum calcium-decreasing hormone.

MTC is the cancer derived from C cells, and produces calcitonin in excess; determination of plasma calcitonin levels is useful in diagnosis of this tumor. In addition to calcitonin, MTC can secrete various peptide hormones such as adrenocorticotrophic hormone (ACTH), melanophore-stimulating hormone (MSH), somatostatin, vasoactive intestinal polypeptide and nerve growth factor (*22, 26*). In some cases with sufficiently high levels of such hormones, specific symptoms due to the excess hormone may modify the clinical course of the patient. However, serum calcium levels are never lower than normal in spite of a high plasma concentration of calcitonin, because continuously high levels of calcitonin do not affect the calcium level, although an acute rise of calcitonin decreases the amount of calcium. If parathyroid adenopathy is present (MEN 2A), hypercalcemia will be demonstrated.

Intractable diarrhea is a characteristic symptom of this tumor, but it is a symptom seen only in rather advanced cases. In Japan, intractable diarrhea is less frequent than in other countries (*15*).

MTC occurs both sporadically and familially. Sporadic MTCs are usually unilateral, but familial (hereditary) MTCs are always bilateral due to the multicentric occurrence of the tumors.

2) Pheochromocytoma

Pheochromocytoma is a tumor derived from the adrenal medulla, and produces an excess of catecholamines. The rate of catecholamine secretion is autonomous and unpredictable, causing an abrupt rise in blood pressure which is sometimes life-threatening.

In the patient with MEN 2, pheochromocytomas are also multicentric and bilateral, but the unilateral adrenal gland may be much larger than the other gland in some patients. MTC usually precedes the pheochromocytoma in MEN 2.

3) Parathyroid adenopathy

Hyperfunction of parathyroid gland(s) may be associated in the patient with MEN 2A. The nature of parathyroid adenopathy in MEN 2A is still debatable. In contrast to MEN 1 syndrome where all 4 parathyroid glands are always swollen and hyperplastic, often only a single parathyroid gland is hyperplastic in MEN 2A.

Since parathyroid hyperfunction is not found in patients with sporadic MTC and is rarely found in MEN 2B, it is believed that hyperfunction of parathyroid glands is also a direct effect of an abnormal gene rather than secondary hyperplasia due to calcitonin excess.

4) Mucosal neuromas and other skeletal abnormalities

Patients with MEN 2B have characteristic phenotypes due to mucosal neuromas which include bumpy lips, small nodules on the tongue, everted eyelids and a very slender body with long thin extremities resembling Marfan's syndrome (3, 26).

Besides these easily recognisable external abnormalities, the digestive tract is also involved, diverticulosis of colon and megacolon are examples of other abnormalities (5, 15, 20, 22, 25, 26). Constipation is a symptom from which MEN 2B patients often suffer. Difficulties in suckling may be the earliest symptom of this syndrome (13). This alimentary tract symptom probably results from ganglioneuromatosis throughout the entire digestive tract.

5) Diagnosis and treatment of MEN 2

Aspiration biopsy and cytological diagnosis (ABC) is very useful in diagnosis of thyroid tumors, and MTC also can be identified by this method (18). In high risk families, annual examination of children by plasma calcitonin assay, especially with stimulation tests using calcium or gastrin, is very important in the early diagnosis of MTC (22, 25, 26, 32). In patients with hereditary MTC, total thyroidectomy must be carried out because MTCs are always multicentric in the hereditary type of this tumor.

The treatment policy for pheochromocytomas in MEN 2 is still debatable. The Mayo group insisted that bilateral total adrenalectomy should be carried out in MEN 2 patients (26). Others recommended a more conservative approach for the treatment of pheochromocytomas in MEN 2 (30). Our policy is also somewhat conservative, because pheochromocytomas in MEN 2 are rarely malignant and glucocorticoid replacement after total adrenalectomy is rather troublesome (27).

Epidemiological Aspects

1) MTC and MEN 2 in Japan

Nationwide surveys were carried out by the Japanese Association for Thyroid Surgery in 1976 (15) and 1981 (27), and 242 cases of MTC were registered and analysed. In 1986, a follow-up study of those cases was performed. One of the authors (A. M.) analysed 271 cases composed of those 242 cases and 29 new cases found in Kuma Hospital after 1981 (20).

TABLE II.   MTCs and MEN 2 in Various Countries

	Japan[a]	Mayo Clinic A[b]	Mayo Clinic B[c]	MDAH[d]	Norway[e]
No. of cases	271	139	124	161	57
MTC in all thyroid cancers	1.5%	8.2%		8.7%	3.4%
Male: female in all MTC	1: 2.7	1: 1.3		1: 1.06	1: 1.6
MEN 2A	48 (17.7%)	15 (10.8%)	27 (21.8%)	31 (19.3%)	
MEN 2B	6 (2.2%)	14 (10.1%)	14 (11.3%)	5 (3.1%)	
Familial MTC only	38 (14.0%)		39 (31.5%)		
Male: female in familial cases[f]	1: 2.5		1: 1		

[a] Data obtained by nationwide surveys (20).
[b] Data from Mayo Clinic (6).
[c] Data from Mayo Clinic (25).
[d] Data from M. D. Anderson Hospital (22).
[e] From ref. 21.
[f] For Japanese series, all MEN 2A, 2B, and familial MTC were included.
In the Mayo series, sporadic cases of MEN 2B were excluded.

TABLE III.   Kindred at High Risk for MEN 2A or MTC in Japan[a]

Components found in the kindred[b]	Number of kindred	Number of patients	Incomplete cases among kindred MTC+Pheo.	MTC+HPT	MTC alone
All components	6	14	6	1	1
MTC+Pheo.	16	35	24	—	11
MTC alone	12	26	—	—	26
Total	34	75	30	1	38

[a] From ref. 20.
[b] Kindred is classified by the member who has the most components.
HPT, hyperparathyroidism.

There were 48 cases of MEN 2A, 6 cases of MEN 2B and 38 patients with MTC alone belonging to high risk families for this tumor (Table II) (20). Among patients with MEN 2A, 11 cases were sporadic, i.e., the patient was the only person affected in his or her family; the remaining 37 patients belonged to 22 kindred (Table III). Most patients with MEN 2B (5 out of 6) were sporadic and the remaining case was reported to have siblings with elevated calcitonin but without the characteristic phenotype, leaving some doubt about the familial nature of this patient.

The breakdown of patients belonging to high risk families is shown in Table III. There were 12 kindreds where all affected members suffered from MTC alone. Some of these 12 might in reality be MEN 2A families (19, 20) because mild pheochromocytoma or hyperparathyroidism could be overlooked, or would appear later on. But some of those families may also possibly be kindred at high risk for MTC alone, because one such family was reported in the literature (8).

Figure 1 shows some examples of Japanese kindred which we are studying. Since the autosomal dominant mode of inheritance is apparent, it is curious that a marked female preponderance is found in the Japanese series (Table II). The progression of MTC seemed much slower in some male patients in Japan, because no clinical symptoms or only subtle signs of the disease were found in some male members in Fig. 1 who were

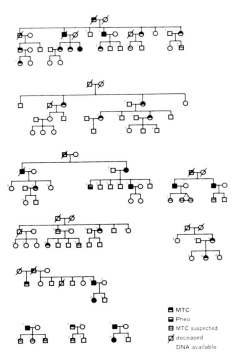

FIG. 1. Japanese kindred at high risk for MEN 2A (or MTC)
Affected members were diagnosed by histological examination of thyroid tumors or
proved to have high basal or stimulated calcitonin levels in their serum. Pheochromocytomas were also proved by operation or clinical and biochemical examinations
including urinary catecholamine excretion.
    Only a small portion of the affected members shown in this figure were included
in the analysis of Japanese MTC (20). These pedigrees were found by screening
the relatives of patients registered at the survey.

judged to be affected by calcitonin level. Obvious MTCs were usually found in daughters or female sibs of those affected males with few clinical signs of MTC. Male to female
ratio of the affected family members in the Fig. 1 was 1: 1.25. In the second and third
generations of the families illustrated in Fig. 1, there were 16 affected persons among
38 males (42%) and 20 affected persons among 37 females (54%). Therefore, the over-
looking of those male patients with very mild clinical disease may account for the female
preponderance found in the Japanese series.

2) *Comparison with MTC and MEN 2 in other countries*
    MTC in all thyroid cancers is lower in Japan than in the U.S.A. and Norway (Table
II). The incidence of thyroid cancers is also slightly lower in Japan than in other countries, for example, based on the Cancer Registry it was 0.5–0.6 and 2.0–2.1 for male and
female 100,000 populations, respectively in Japan, 1.1–1.9 and 2.9–4.9 in the U.S.A. and
1.5 and 3.7 in Norway (31). Therefore, the incidence of MTCs is clearly very low in
Japan.
    As shown in Table II, MEN 2A and 2B accounted for 17.7% and 2.2% of all MTC
in the Japanese series (20). Similar results were reported from M. D. Anderson Hospital

(*22*). From the Mayo Clinic somewhat different results were reported (*6, 25*): compared to an earlier report (*6*), the number of MEN 2A cases markedly increased and 39 patients with MTC alone were also found in high risk families in a later report (Table II) (*25*). The latter report included many patients who were found at earlier stages by screening of members of MEN 2A kindred by calcitonin assay.

3) Estimation of total number of patients with MEN 2 in Japan

According to the data from mass screening of thyroid cancer, the prevalence rate was 0.13% in the general population in Japan (*9*). Therefore, two MTC patients are found per 100,000 population, since MTC accounts for 1.5% of all thyroid cancers. As the total population of Japan is 120,000,000, the number of MTC patients must be about 2,400. About 20% of these MTC are MEN 2A or 2B (Table II), so that the total number of MEN 2 cases must be about 480. If familial cases of MTC alone are actually considered to be MEN 2, there are about 800 MEN 2 patients in Japan.

Pathogenetic and Genetic Studies

1) C Cell hyperplasia and adrenal medullary hyperplasia as precursor for tumorigenesis in MEN 2

In the thyroid specimen from patients with hereditary MTC, small clusters of C cells are usually found outside frank MTCs. These C cell hyperplasias are considered to be precursors of MTCs in MEN 2 or hereditary MTC. Similarly, hyperplasia of adrenal medullary cells precedes pheochromocytomas in MEN 2.

2) Knudson's two mutational event theory for oncogenesis and MEN 2

From the analysis of age at onset of retinoblastomas, Knudson proposed a theory for oncogenesis (*14*): i) two-mutational events are necessary for oncogenesis, and ii) in hereditary cases, one of the two mutations has been transmitted from the affected parent to kindred.

Early onset and multicentric occurrence of hereditary tumors may well be accounted for by Knudson's theory.

C cell hyperplasia and adrenomedullary hyperplasia preceding MTC and pheochromocytoma in MEN 2 patients, and age at onset curves for these two tumors are consistent with Knudson's two-mutational-event theory (*5, 12*).

Both thyroid C cells and catecholamine-producing cells of adrenal medulla derived from the neural crest, a mutation of the gene responsible for differentiation of both cells is considered to predispose a person to MEN 2.

3) Nature of the second mutation in MEN 2

Studies on retinoblastoma clarified the nature of the second mutation of this tumor to be loss of wild-type allele on the homologous chromosome. Namely, retinoblastoma results from elimination of both normal alleles at the locus for this disease by one of several chromosomal mechanisms (*4*).

It seems reasonable to assume that MEN 2 results from the same mechanism, because MEN 2 shares several characteristics with retinoblastoma as discussed earlier. If this assumption is correct, the second mutation in C cells and/or adrenomedullary cells should be loss of activity of the wild-type allele at the MEN 2A locus.

4) Genetic studies on MEN 2

Cytogenetic studies and linkage analyses are being used to determine the gene predisposing to MEN 2.

Babu *et al.* reported that an interstitial deletion at the short arm of chromosome 20 was seen constitutionally in patients with MEN 2A and 2B (*1*). But their findings have not been confirmed by other researchers (*7, 11*), and linkage studies using DNA probe excluded close linkage between the MEN 2A and loci on the short arm of chromosome 20 (*10, 23, 29*).

Only one report has been published on the chromosome analysis of MTC cells because cell culture of this tumor is difficult. Wurster-Hill *et al.* reported that hypodiploid modal number of chromosomes and loss or structural abnormalities of chromosome 22 were found in all three MTCs from two patients in common (*33*).

Linkage analyses using restriction fragment length polymorphisms (RFLPs) have been made on several MEN 2 kindreds by some groups including us (*10, 23, 29*). At the second workshop on MEN 2 in September of 1986, it was reported that about 30% of the human genome had been excluded from close linkage with the MEN 2 locus (*23*). In 1987, the close linkage between MEN 2A and interstitial retinol-binding protein 3 (RBP 3) loci was found in European Caucasian kindreds (*16, 24*). We have confirmed the close linkage of these 2 loci in Japanese MEN 2A kindreds (to be published). The gene predisposing to MEN 2A must reside on chromosome 10, since RBP 3 has been assigned to the pericentromere region of this chromosome (10 p 11-q 11).

Regarding deletion of genes in the tumor of MEN 2A, we found loss of heterozygosity in 2 pheochromocytomas and an MTC using probes on chromosome 22 (*28*). Loss of genes on chromosome 1 was also reported in MTCs and pheochromocytomas (*17*). We are now studying loss of heterozygosity in tumors of MEN 2A using RBP 3.

Considering the rapid advancement in this field, the isolation and sequencing of the MEN 2A gene should be done in the near future.

Acknowledgment

This study was supported by a Grant-in-Aid for Special Project Research, Cancer-Bioscience, from the Ministry of Education, Science and Culture of Japan.

REFERENCES

1. Babu, V. R., Van Dyke, D. L., and Jackson, C. E. Chromosome 20 deletion in human multiple endocrine neoplasia type 2A and 2B: a double-blind study. *Proc. Natl. Acad. Sci. U.S.A.*, **81**, 2525–2528 (1984).

2. Ballard, H. S., Frame, B., and Hartsock, R. J. Familial multiple endocrine adenoma— peptic ulcer complex. *Medicine*, **43**, 481–516 (1964).

3. Carney, J. A., Sizemore, G. W., and Hales, A. B. Multiple endocrine neoplasia, type 2b. *In* "Pathobiology Annual 8," ed. H. L. Ioachim, pp. 105–153 (1978). Raven Press, New York.

4. Cavenee, W. K., Dryja, T. P., Phillips, R. A., Benedict, W. F., Godbout, R., Gallie, B. L., Murphree, A. L., Strong, L. C., and White, R. L. Expression of recessive alleles by chromosomal mechanisms in retinoblastoma. *Nature*, **305**, 779–784 (1983).

5. Cerny, J. C., Jackson, C. E., Talpos, G. B., Yott, J. B., and Lee, M. W. Pheochromocytoma in multiple endocrine neoplasia type II: An example of the two-hit theory of neoplasia. *Surgery*, **92**, 849–852 (1982).

6. Chong, G. C., Beahrs, O. H., Sizemore, G. W., and Woolner, L. B. Medullary carcinoma of the thyroid gland. *Cancer*, **35**, 695–704 (1975).

7. Emmertsen, K., Lamm, L. U., Rasmussen, K. Z., Elbrønd, O., Hansen, H. H., Henningsen, K., Jorgensen, J., and Petersen, G. B. Linkage and chromosome study of multiple endocrine neoplasia IIa. *Cancer Genet. Cytogenet.*, **9**, 251–259 (1983).

8. Farndon, J. R., Leight, G. S., Dilley, W. G., Baylin, S. B., Smallridge, R. C., Harrison, T. S., and Wells, S. A. Familial medullary thyroid carcinoma without associated endocrinopathies: a distinct clinical entity. *Br. J. Surg.*, **73**, 278–281 (1986).

9. Furihata, R. and Maruchi, N. Epidemiological studies on thyroid cancer in Nagano prefecture, Japan. *In* "Thyroid Cancer," ed. C. E. Hedinger, pp. 79–81 (1969). Springer-Verlag, Berlin.

10. Goodfellow, P. J., White, B. N., Holden, J.J.A., Duncan, A.M.V., Sears, E.V.P., Wang, H. S., Berlin, L., Kidd, K. K., and Simpson, N. E. Linkage analysis of a DNA marker localized to 20p12 and multiple endocrine neoplasia type 2A. *Am. J. Hum. Genet.*, **37**, 890–897 (1985).

11. Ikeuchi, T., Takai, S., Miki, T., Tateishi, H., and Nishisho, I. High-resolution banding analysis of No. 20 chromosomes from patients with multiple endocrine neoplasia type 2. *Proc. Jpn. Cancer Assoc.*, 226 (1985).

12. Jackson, C. E., Block, M. A., Greenwald, K. A., and Tashjian, A. H., Jr. The two-mutational-event theory in medullary thyroid cancer. *Am. J. Hum. Genet.*, **31**, 704–710 (1979).

13. Jones, B. A. and Sisson, J. C. Early diagnosis and thyroidectomy in multiple endocrine neoplasia, type 2b. *J. Pediatr.*, **102**, 219–223 (1983).

14. Knudson, A. G., Jr. Mutation and cancer: statistical study of retinoblastoma. *Proc. Natl. Acad. Sci. U.S.A.*, **68**, 820–823 (1971).

15. Kosaki, G., Takai, S., Miyauchi, A., and 45 others. Medullary carcinoma of the thyroid in Japan. *Gan no Rinsho* **24**, 799–812 (1978) (in Japanese).

16. Mathew, C.G.P., Chin, K. S., Easton, D. F., Thorpe, K., Carter, C., Liou, G. I., Fong, S.-L., Bridges, C.D.B., Haak, H., Nieuwenhuijzen Kruseman, A. C., Schifter, S. Hansen, H. H., Telenius, H., Telenius-Berg, M., and Ponder, B.A.J. A linked genetic marker for multiple endocrine neoplasia type 2A on chromosome 10. *Nature*, **328**, 527–528 (1987).

17. Mathew, C.G.P., Smith, B. A., Thorpe, K., Wong, Z., Royle, N. J., Jeffreys, A. J., and Ponder, B.A.J. Deletion of genes on chromosome 1 in endocrine neoplasia. *Nature*, **328**, 524–526 (1987).

18. Miyauchi, A. Practical aspect of aspiration biopsy cytology—Medullary carcinoma and anaplastic carcinoma of the thyroid. *Naibunpitsugeka (Endocr. Surg.)* **1**, 141–147 (1984) (in Japanese).

19. Miyauchi, A., Masuo K., Ogihara, T., Takai, S., Matsuzuka, F., Kuma, K., Maeda, M., Kumahara, Y., and Kosaki, G. Urinary epinephrine and norepinephrine excretion in patients with medullary thyroid carcinoma and their relatives. *Folia Endocrinol. Jpn.*, **58**, 1505–1516 (1982).

20. Miyauchi, A. and Takai, S. Multiple endocrine neoplasia types 1 and type 2 in Japan. *Naibunpitsugeka (Endocr. Surg.)*, **3**, 433–439 (1986) (in Japanese).

21. Normann, T., Gautvik, K. M., Johannessen, J. V., and Brennhovd, I. O. Medullary carcinoma of the thyroid in Norway. Clinical course and endocrinological aspects. *Acta Endocrinol.*, **83**, 71–85 (1976).

22. Saad, M. F., Ordonez, N. G., Rashid, R. K., Guido, J. J., Hill, C. S., Jr., Hickey, R. C., and Samaan, N. A. Medullary carcinoma of the thyroid. A study of the clinical features and prognostic factors in 161 patients. *Medicine*, **63**, 319–342 (1984).

23. Simpson, N. E. and Kidd, K. K. Where is the locus for multiple endocrine neoplasia type 2A? *Henry Ford Hosp. Med. J.*, **35**, 168–171 (1987).

24. Simpson N. E., Kidd, K. K., Goodfellow, P. J., McDermid, H., Myers, S., Kidd, J. R.,

Jackson, C. E., Duncan, A.M.V., Farrer, L. A., Brasch, K., Castiglione, C., Genel, M., Gertner, J., Greenberg, C. R., Gusella, J. F., Holden, J.J.A., and White, B. N. Assignment of multiple endocrine neoplasia type 2A to chromosome 10 by linkage. *Nature*, **328**, 528–530 (1987).

25. Sizemore, G. W., Carney, J. A., and Heath, H., III. Epidemiology of medullary carcinoma of the thyroid gland: A 5-year experience (1971–1976). *Surg. Clin. N. Am.*, **57**, 633–645 (1977).

26. Sizemore, G. W., Van Heerden, J. A., and Carney, J. A. Medullary carcinoma of the thyroid gland and the multiple endocrine neoplasia type 2 syndrome. *In* "Surgery of the Thyroid and Parathyroid Glands," ed. E. L. Kaplan, pp. 75–102 (1983). Churchill Livingstone, New York.

27. Takai, S., Miyauchi, A., Matsumoto, H., Ikeuchi, T., Miki, T., Kuma, K., and Kumahara, Y. Multiple endocrine neoplasia type 2 syndromes in Japan. *Henry Ford Hosp. Med. J.*, **32**, 246–250 (1984).

28. Takai, S., Tateishi, H., Nishisho, I., Miki, T., Motomura, K., Miyauchi, A., Kato, M., Ikeuchi, T., Yamamoto, K., Okazaki, M., Yamamoto, M., Honjo, T., Kumahara, Y., and Mori, T. Loss of genes on chromosome 22 in medullary thyroid carcinoma and pheochromocytoma. *Jpn. J. Cancer Res.*, **78**, 894–898 (1987).

29. Tateishi, H., Takai, S., Nishisho, I., Miki, T., Motomura, K., Okazaki, M., Miyauchi, A., Ikeuchi, T., Yamamoto, K., Hattori, T., Kumahara, Y., Matsumoto, H., Honjo, T., and Mori, T. Studies of multiple endocrine neoplasia type 2A syndrome: Linkage analyses and comparison of constitutional and tumor genotypes. *Henry Ford Hosp. Med. J.*, **35**, 157–160 (1987).

30. Tibblin, S., Dymling, J. F., Ingemansson, S., and Telenius-Berg, M. Unilateral *versus* bilateral adrenalectomy in multiple endocrine neoplasia IIA. *World J. Surg.*, **7**, 201–208 (1983).

31. Waterhouse, J. and others. eds. "Cancer Incidence in Five Continents," Vol. III, pp. 520–523 (1976). IARC Scientific Publications No. 15, IARC, Lyon.

32. Wells, S. A., Jr., Baylin, S., and Gann, D. S. Medullary thyroid carcinoma. Relationship of method of diagnosis to pathologic staging. *Ann. Surg.*, **188**, 377–383 (1978).

33. Wurster-Hill, D. H., Noll, W. W., Bircher, L. Y., Pettengill, O. S., and Grizzle, W. A. *Cancer Genet. Cytogenet.*, **20**, 247–253 (1986).

Gann Monograph on Cancer Research 35, 1988

PATHOLOGICAL AND GENETIC ASPECTS OF ADENOMATOSIS COLI IN JAPAN

Joji UTSUNOMIYA

Second Department of Surgery, Hyogo College of Medicine*

Pathological and genetic aspects of adenomatosis coli (AC) are reviewed principally based on the data published by the author and his collaborators and the related literature, mainly of Japan. The data are presented in sufficient detail to make the original papers written in Japanese informative for foreign researchers.

Adenomatosis coli can be subdivided into common and specific rare variants. The former includes simple AC (familial polyposis coli) which may be further subdivided into the profuse and sparse types, and Gardner symptoms which may be further subdivided into the complete and incomplete types. The specific rare subtypes of AC are Turcot and Zanca syndromes. Neoplastic involvement of the upper gastrointestinal (GI) tract is the principal phenotypic manifestation of the AC gene and does not indicate genetic heterogeneity. Age specific prevalence analysis of the common type variants revealed a history of AC which may be somewhat influenced by environmental factors. Genetic backgrounds of Japanese AC were quite similar to those reported by the British and Americans.

Accumulated studies have revealed that there are several types of familial large bowel cancer roughly divided into hereditary gastrointestinal polyposes (HGIP) and non-polyposis familial large bowel cancers which include cancer family syndrome and its related conditions. Morson's pathological classification of intestinal polyposis among neoplastic class, *i.e.*, adenomatosis coli (AC), and a hamartomatous one including Peutz-Jeghers syndrome and juvenile polyposis show four important principal characteristics: familial occurrence, tendency to produce malignant lesions, involvement throughout the gastrointestinal (GI) tract, and association with other lesions (Table I). Therefore, they can be reasonably termed "hereditary gastrointestinal polyposes" (*53*).

Adenomatosis coli (also called familial adenomatous polyposis) indicates a condition in which more than 100 adenomas are distributed throughout the large bowel, regardless of familial occurrence or association with extracolonic lesions (*6, 48*). This disorder is the most important among HGIP, because of its extremely high risk of large bowel cancer, its relatively high incidence and its predominant familial occurrence, often appearing in a large number of kindred.

This article describes pathological and genetic aspects of AC based primarily on the author's studies and on other reports from Japan.

---

* 1-1, Mukogawa-cho, Nishinomiya, Hyogo 663, Japan (宇都宮譲二).

TABLE I. Classification of the Gastrointestinal Polyposes

Classification			Site of polyposes			Cancer high risk	Mode of inheritance
Genetic	Histological	Nomenclature	st.	si.	li.		
Hereditary	Neoplastic	Adenomatosis coli	+	+	+	+++	AD
		Familial polyposis coli					
		Gardner syndrome					
		Turcot syndrome					(AR)
		Zanca syndrome					
	Hamartomatous	Peutz-Jeghers syndrome	+	+	+	+	AD
		Juvenile polyposis	+	+	+	+	AD
		Cowden disease	+	+	+	+	AD
Non-hereditary	Inflammatory	Inflammatory polyposis	−	−	+	−	−
		Lymphoid polyposis	−	+	+	−	−
	Unclassified	Metaplastic polyposis	−	−	+	−	−
		Cronkhite-Canada syndrome	+	+	+	±	−

st, stomach; si, small intestine; li, large intestine; AD, autosomal dominant; AR, autosomal recessive.

Central Register of Polyposes

In 1972, the author was involved with an AC case in which some of the patient's relatives had previously been reported twice in the literature as independent families 42 years and 13 years earlier. He consequently realized the necessity of a central register for collecting information on AC families throughout the nation and for maintaining this record over the generations. The Center for Analyzing Familial Polyposis (the Polyposis Center) was established at Tokyo Medical and Dental University in 1975 for a 7 year period, the limit stipulated by national law (48, 49). Since 1982 when the author left there, the activity has been maintained under the name of the Research Center for Polyposes and Intestinal Diseases.

Information on the probands of HGIP as well as non-polypotic familial cancer has been collected through five different sources: inquiries to hospitals throughout the nation, autopsy records, published literature, voluntary visits by patients, and the Japanese Society for Large Bowel Cancer Research. For each family, an exact pedigree map, a "working pedigree," has been constructed using the koseki, the national family register which has been traditionally maintained for more than 80 years. In order to identify family members, a permanent coding system was devised (38, 48). The affected members are identified through hospital records, death certificates, and communication with their family members. The Center sends a list of these high risk people to local physicians who register the cases in order to promote the examinations of local family members. By this means, increasing members of the fusion of two or more linked pedigrees has been recognized (Table II) and this has accelerated ascertainment of the pedigrees.

In 1982, when the author moved to his present institution, Hyogo College of Medicine, the Center had registered 472 families (697 cases) of AC, 131 families (146 cases) of Peutz-Jeghers syndrome and many with other polyposes (Table III). A family survey had been completed on 327 AC families with 4,847 members, and had revealed the presence of 854 affected and 3,545 persons at high risk as possible AC gene carriers. Some

TABLE II. Frequency of Pedigree Linkage in AC Families
Registered at the Polyposis Center, 1982

	~1961	~1972	~1976	~1979	~1983	Total
Registered family	45	122	168	128	99	562
Pedigree linkage	1	12	25	14	20	72
%	2.2	9.8	14.9	10.9	20.2	12.8

TABLE III. Number of Registered Cases (Family) of Hereditary Polyposes
and Related Conditions at the Polyposis Center, 1982 (55)

Resource	Adenomatosis coli	Multiple adenomas	P-J syndrome	Juvenile polyposis	Familial cancer of the colon
Jpn. Soc. LBC[a]	169 (111)	62 (62)	23 (20)	2 (1)	16 (15)
Questionnaire	182 (148)	91 (91)	70 (67)	2 (2)	41 (35)
Literature	82 (58)	7 (7)	7 (7)	0 (0)	7 (4)
Autopsy records	23 (17)	30 (30)	8 (8)	0 (0)	0 (0)
Voluntary Registr.	241 (138)	6 (6)	38 (29)	6 (6)	15 (10)
Total	697 (472)	196 (196)	146 (131)	10 (9)	79 (64)

[a] Japanese Society for Large Bowel Cancer Research.
P-J syndrome, Peutze-Jeghers syndrome.

of the material from pathological, genetic and, epidemiological analyses used in several published reports are reviewed in the following.

Pathology

1. Lesions of the large bowel
1) Polyps
   A) Number of polyps: We observed two distinct groups of patients with adenomatous polyps in the large bowel, by dividing cases at the number of around 100 (48) as Bussey described (6). Therefore, cases with less than 100 adenomas are hereafter termed "multiple adenomas," to differentiate them from AC.
   On the resected specimen, there are two heterogenous classes of AC in number of polyps, the profuse type and the sparse type (15). The criteria for delineating these clusters were a total count of 5,000 polyps, or unit amount under macroscopic observation of 10/cm², and microscopically, two adenomatous foci detected within 1 cm² of a histological section or adenomatous foci estimated to occupy 20% of the total area of the section (adenoma percent) (15). Radiologically, double contrast barium enema revealed that the boundary range distinguishing these two types was 6–9 polyps/cm² in adults and 3–6/cm² in children (18).
   B) Polyp size: Small polyps (less than 5 mm in diameter) constituted over 80% of the polyps on the specimen (15) (Table IV). Cases with one or more polyps of more than 1 cm diameter were associated with advanced cancer somewhere in the large bowel at a frequency of 47%, whereas in cases in which the lesions were 5 mm or less, malignancy was never detected (15).

TABLE IV. Frequency of Cancer in Adenoma in AC and Non-polypotic Adenomas

Size (mm)	AC		Adenomas	
	n (%)	Cancer (%)	n	Cancer (%)
Utsunomiya et al. (19)				
0–5	3,593 (90.1)	65 (1.8)	189	3 (1.6)
6–10	289	57 (19.7)	127	19 (15.0)
11–20	71	23 (32.4)	49	22 (44.9)
21–	31	10 (32.3)	7	5 (71.4)
Total	3,984	155 (3.9)	372	49 (13.2)
Fujisawa et al. (8)				
0–5	6,763 (94.7)	7 (0.1)	171	0 (0)
6–10	326	9 (2.8)	74	10 (13.5)
11–20	44	8 (18.2)	35	15 (42.9)
21–	12	7 (58.2)	29	20 (69.0)
Total	7,145	31 (0.4)	309	45 (14.6)
Iwama (15)				
0–5	15,708 (97.7)	7 (0.04)	—	
6–10	270	1 (0.3)	—	
11–20	81	6 (7.4)	—	
21–	25	12 (48)	—	
Total	16,084	26 (0.2)	—	

TABLE V. Frequency of Large Bowel Cancer at Diagnosis (55)

Group	Male			Female			Total		
	Case	Cancer (+)		Case	Cancer (+)		Case	Cancer (+)	
	n	n	%	n	n	%	n	n	%
Proband	197	131	66.5	127	87	68.5	324	218	67.3
Call-up	87	26	29.9	43	11	25.6	130	37	28.5
Total	284	157	55.3	170	98	57.6	454	255	56.2

C) Histology: Malignant potential of the adenomas of AC did not seem to be significantly different from the usual solitary adenomas of the large bowel (8, 15, 19) (Table IV). Cytokinetic studies revealed that an abnormal cellular proliferation pattern exists in the crypts of apparently non-adenomatous mucosa (14). Sialomucin properties of the non-adenomatous mucosa of AC were different from those of the normal colon (25). There was found an abnormal histochemical distribution of the lectin (UEA-1) binding site in the flatt rectal mucosa of AC patients (19).

2) Cancer

Advanced cancer of the large bowel was found in 56.2% of the total patients at the time of diagnosis. The frequency was much less in the call-up cases (28.5%) than in the proband (67.3%) (Table V). Their subsite distribution within the bowel was similar to that of the usual colorectal cancer in both the Japanese and the British series (Table VI). Relative incidence of cancer of the sigmoid colon versus that of the rectum (S/R ratio) also increased by times in AC patients as seen in general colorectal cancer in Japan (Table VII). Multiple lesions were found in 38.0% of the AC cancers which was extremely high frequency compared with the 4.5% in general colorectal cancer (Table VIII).

TABLE VI.   Subsite Distribution of Large Bowel Cancer

Subsite	Japan				England			
	AC Polyposis Center (55) (1982)		General population Jpn. Soc. LBC (1977–1981)[a]		AC St. Marks Hosp. (6) (1974)		General population Smiddy and Goligher (34) (1957)	
	n	%	n	%	n	%	n	%
Caecum	8	2.5	—	5.7	13	4.5	101	6.1
Ascending colon	31	9.9	—	7.6	4	1.4	48	2.9
Hepatic flexure	—	—	—	—	8	2.8	29	1.8
Transverse colon	39	12.5	—	7.2	18	6.3	77	4.7
Splenic flexure	—	—	—	—	16	5.6	50	3.0
Descending colon	26	8.3	—	4.5	—	—	—	—
Sigmoid colon	82	26.2	—	24.5	63	22.0	350	24.0
Rectum	131	41.9	—	45.1	141	49.3	944	57.4
Anal canal	—	—	—	5.1	—	—	—	—
Unclassified	—	—	—	—	23	8.0	—	—
Total	313	100.0	18,915	100.0	286	100.0	1,644	100.0

[a] Report from Japanese Society of Large Bowel Cancer Research.

TABLE VII.   Time Trend of Registered AC Cases at the Polyposis Center (55)

	~1970	1971	~1977	1978	~1981
Registered cases	164		307		123
Call up cases	4.9%		27.4%		31.7%
Sex ratio	1.69		1.36		0.95
Average age at diagnosis	38.4		38.3		38.2
S/R ratio of cancer[a]	0.78		0.83		0.95

[a] Relative frequency of cancer of sigmoid colon *versus* that of rectum.

TABLE VIII.   Multiplicity of Large Bowel Cancer

	AC (229 cases)		General population[a] (24,616 cases)	
	n	%	n	%
Single	142	62.0	23,504	95.5
Multiple	87	38.0	1,112	4.5
2	40	46.0	895	80.5
3	21	24.1	148	13.3
4	4	4.6	39	3.5
over 5	22	25.3	30	2.7

[a] The 16th Meeting of Japanese Society of Large Bowel Cancer Research.

2.   Lesions of the upper GI tract
1) Gastric lesions

A) Polyps: Gastric polyps were detected in 66.7% of the cases seen personally and were assumed to be an integral phenotypic manifestation of the AC gene (44), because they were distributed in all of the families studied; similar results were reported from other institutes (12, 43). An increasing number of reports from other countries suggests

TABLE IX.   Gastric Polyps in AC

Reporter	Place (year)		Incidence of polyps				Proportion of adenomas	
			in case		in family			
			n	%	(n	%)	n	%
Japanese literature								
Utsunomiya et al. (44)	Tokyo	(1974)	10/15	66.7	(6/6	100.0)	4/6	66.7
Ushio et al. (43)	Tokyo	(1976)	10/15	66.7	(7/8	87.5)	0/6	0
Iida and Ohmae (12)	Kyushu	(1978)	18/25	72.0	(14/16	87.5)	9/18	50.0
Utsunomiya (56)	Hyogo	(1986)	16/20	80.0	(12/15	80.0)	10/16	62.5
Jpn. Soc. LBC Res.[a]	Japan	(1986)	115/309	37.1	—		43/96	44.8
Literature[b]	—	(1977–1985)	99/200	49.5	—		—	—
Western literature								
Ranzi et al. (30)	Italy	(1981)	6/9	66.7	—		4/6	66.7
Jarvinen et al. (16)	Finland	(1983)	21/34	61.7	—		4/21	19.0
Burt et al. (4)	U.S.A.	(1984)	7/11	63.6	—		1/7	14.3
Shemesh et al. (32)	Israel	(1985)	7/14	50.0	—		7/7	100.0
Tonelli et al. (42)	Italy	(1985)	6/24	25.0	—		3/6	50.0
Bülow et al. (3)	Denmark	(1985)	13/26	50.0	—		1/13	7.7
Western total			60/118	50.8	—		20/60	33.3

[a] Summed data of reports at the 26th Meeting of the Japanese Society for Large Bowel Cancer Research.
[b] Fourteen literature references reporting on gastric polyps in AC.

that the phenomenon is not specific to Japanese (Table IX). Histologically there are two types of polyps: adenomatous (44) and hamartomatous polyps of the fundic gland (59). Neither is specific to AC (11), although the fundic gland polyp of AC was suggested to have some histochemically different characteristics than those found in the general population (27). Adenomatous lesions were found in 44% of the cases with gastric polyps in the Japanese series, while in an accumulated series of western reports this figure was 33% (Table IX). Intestinal metaplasia which is seen more frequently in the Japanese stomach than in the western may be responsible for this difference (59). Although the fundic gland polyps do not appear to carry any malignant potential, we saw evidence of malignant foci associated with the adenomatous lesion (56).

B) Cancer: Fifteen or more cases of AC with gastric cancer have been reported in Japan; in some cases, these are multiple (59). Incidence of gastric cancer in AC patients either synchronous or metachronous has been reported to be from 2.1% to 5.0% (Table X).

2) *Duodenal lesions*

A) Polyps: Histologically verified small adenomas were detected in almost all of the cases examined by endoscopic biopsy or at autopsy (12, 59). Similar evidence was found in studies in western countries (Table XI). The adenomas are distributed mainly in the second portion of the duodenum and Vaters papilla was involved with a frequency of 50% in the patients biopsied (12, 59). We recently observed a case with large adenomas confined both at main and accessory papillae which suggested increased neoplastic potential around the orifices of the pancreatic duct.

B) Cancer: Duodenal carcinoma occurring in AC has been reported in 9 cases in the Japanese literature and the frequency was reported to be 0.6 to 1.9% (Table XII).

TABLE X.　Gastric Cancer in AC

Reporter	Place	(Year)	Total cases	Cases with gastric cancer		
				n	%	Age
Japanese literature						
Ushio et al. (43)	Tokyo	(1984)	44	2	4.5	47.0
Watanabe et al. (59)	Kyushu	(1976)	22	3	13.6	36.7
Jpn. Soc. LBC Res.[a]	—	(1987)	329	7	2.1	48.5
Polyposis Center	—	(1987)	1,564	33	2.1	—
Literature[b]	—	(1977–1985)	301	15	5.0	—
Western literature						
Murphy et al. (22)	Mexico	(1962)	—	1	—	15
Schurig et al. (33)	W. Germany	(1968)	—	1	—	51
Jones and Nance (17)	U.S.A.	(1977)	—	1	—	62
Pauli et al. (29)	U.S.A.	(1980)	—	1	—	68
Desigan et al. (7)	U.S.A.	(1986)	—	1	—	53

[a] Summed data of reports of the 26th Meeting of Japanese Society for Large Bowel Cancer Research.
[b] Twenty-four literature references reporting on gastric cancer in AC.

TABLE XI.　Duodenal Polyps in AC

Reporter	Place	(Year)	Incidence of polyps		Proportion of adenomas	
			n	%	n	%
Japanese literature						
Iida and Ohmae (12)	Kyushu	(1977)	12/13	92.0	12/12	100
Ushio et al. (43)	Tokyo	(1976)	9/10	90.0	5/9	55.6
Utsunomiya (56)	Hyogo	(1986)	18/24	75.0	18/18	100
Jpn. Soc. LBC Res.[a]	—	(1986)	60/253	18.8	—	—
Western literature						
Ranzi et al. (30)	Italy	(1981)	6/9	66.7	6/6	100
Jarvinen et al. (16)	Finland	(1983)	20/33	60.6	16/20	80
Burt et al. (4)	U.S.A.	(1984)	8/11	72.3	7/8	89
Shemesh et al. (32)	Israel	(1985)	14/14	100.0	14/14	100
Bülow et al. (3)	Denmark	(1985)	13/26	50.0	12/10	92.3
Tonelli et al. (42)	Italy	(1985)	14/24	58.3	14/14	100
Western total			75/117	64.1	69/75	92

[a] Summed data of reports of the 26th Meeting of the Japanese Society for Large Bowel Cancer Research.

TABLE XII.　Duodenal Cancer in AC

Reporter	Year	Total cases	Cases with duodenal cancer		
			n	%	Age
Japanese					
Jpn. Soc. LBC Res.[a]	1987	319	6	1.9	46.5
Polyposis Center	1987	1,564	10	0.6	—
Reported cases	1987	—	9	—	38.1
Other countries					
Watne et al. (58)	1975	280	2	0.7	27.0
Bussey (5)	1972	127	—	4.0	—

[a] Summed data of reports of the 26th Meeting of the Japanese Society for Large Bowel Cancer Research.

3) Jejunal and ileal lesions

Polyps or adenomas were found in the jejunum of 8 cases and in the ileum of 4 cases, out of a total of 16 cases endoscopically examined at operation (*28*).

Thus, it is clear that adenomatous involvement throughout the GI tract is a consistent phenotypic manifestation of the AC gene and not a observation specific to Japanese. The possibility of environmental modifying factors superimposing on the AC genotype should also be considered.

3.   Extra-GI associated lesions and variant syndrome

It has been recognized that the AC patient can manifest various neoplastic lesions in tissues or organs other than the GI tract, and some of these are considered to be a marker of genetically distinctive variants of AC. The three syndromes identified to date are Gardner's, Turcot's, and Zanca's.

1) Gardner syndrome (GS)

Gardner (*9*) reported a family with superficial hard tumors (osteoma) and soft tumors (desmoid, fibroma) in association with adenomatous polyposis, and this combination is thus identified by his name. Although a complete type of GS was observed in about 7% in both the series examined personally by the author and in registry records, an incomplete type of GS was found more frequently (35.7%) in the former than in the latter (18.4%) (Table XIII). The evidence indicates there is a considerable number of cases with GS which might be overlooked at examination.

Panoramic X-ray examination of the jaw disclosed radiopaque lesions (occult osteomatous lesion) in 94% of the AC patients (*46*). Autopsy of one case revealed that these lesions were endosteomas. Their pathogenesis has been speculated to be an excess of the repair process occurring in the jawbone (*10*). The nature of the lesions themselves is not specific to AC, but their multiple occurrence was characteristic (*10*). They had a positive relationship with the superficial stigmata of GS (*10*). As will be discussed later in the genetic section, GS, particularly in its complete form, may possess a specific and distinct genotype, but there are many clinically indistinguishable transitional cases between complete GS and simple AC (familial polyposis coli); therefore, those two can be grouped as common subtypes of AC while the Turcot and Zanca syndromes are rare subtypes.

2) Turcot syndrome

An association of tumors of central nervous system (CNS) and polyposis (*36*) has been reported in several families in Japan. The syndrome appears to have a more heterogenous character than GS; the mode of transmission was apparently recessive, the age of onset much younger, and the adenomas were larger and scantier than in other ACs (*13*).

TABLE XIII.   Proportion of Gardner Syndrome

GS	Registered cases				Cases seen personally (45)	
	in 1974 (45)		in 1981 (39)			
	n	%	n	%	n	%
Cases without GS	203	92.3	388	74.1	16	57.1
Cases with one GS	15	6.8	96	18.3	10	35.7
Cases with both GS	2	0.9	40	7.6	2	7.1
Total	220	100.0	524	100.0	28	100.0

GS, Gardner stigmata.

3) Zanca syndrome

Zanca described a non-familial case with two small adenomas in the colon associated with multiple cartilaginous exostosis of the long bones (MCE), and believed the condition to be a hereditary one (*60*). Since no similar case has been reported, the combination has been considered rather as coincidental. A recent paper (*20*), however, has strongly suggested that this might be a genetically distinctive variant of AC, reporting a case of a 41-year old male who had a typical course of MCE and underwent colectomy for a cancer associated with diffuse adenomatous polyposis of the colon. His father who suffered with classical MCE died of colonic cancer associated with polyposis and one of his aunts was also known to have MCE.

Natural History and Cancer Risk

1. Stages of disease

The natural history of AC can be divided into three stages for the large bowel lesion: the latent, adenoma, and cancer stages.

Age specific incidence and prevalence of affected individuals were calculated in 53 selected sets of the siblings with affected parents; all known members were examined for polyps (*53*). Polyps were estimated to achieve a clinically detectable size in 80% of the gene carriers at between 5 and 10 years of age, because this was the age at which they

TABLE XIV.   Age Specific Incidence and Prevalence of Affected Individuals in
53 Sets of Examinations of All Siblings of an Affected Parent (*53*)

Age	0~	5~	10~	15~	20~	25~	30~	Total
Examined	1	15	25	25	24	16	11	117
Manifested	0	6	8	14	12	6	4	50
Incidence (%)	0	40.0	32.0	56.0	50.0	37.5	36.4	42.7
Prevalence (%)	0	37.5	34.1	42.4	44.4	43.3	42.7	42.7

TABLE XV.   Age Distribution of Symptom Onset in Adenomatosis Patients (298 cases) (*52*)

Age	Male		Female	
	Cancer (−) cases (P)	Cancer (+) cases	Cancer (−) cases (P)	Cancer (+) cases
0–4	1 (.02)	3	1 (.02)	—
5–9	5 (.10)	4	4 (.11)	2
10–14	7 (.22)	4	7 (.27)	1
15–19	10 (.40)	2	5 (.38)	7
20–24	14 (.64)	11	13 (.67)	12
25–29	8 (.78)	21	7 (.82)	14
30–34	6 (.88)	15	3 (.89)	18
35–39	2 (.91)	17	1 (.91)	7
40–44	3 (.97)	11	2 (.96)	10
45–49	2 (1.0)	12	1 (.98)	4
50–54	—	3	—	3
55–	—	11	1 (1.0)	3
Total	58	114	45	81

Proband and call-up cases included.

TABLE XVI. Age Distribution of Adenomatosis Patients Living or Dead at
the Time of Confirmation (677 cases) (52)

Age	Male		Female	
	Living	Dead (P)	Living	Dead (P)
0–4	—	—	—	—
5–9	5	—	3	—
10–14	12	2 (.01)	2	1 (.00)
15–19	14	1 (.01)	13	1 (.01)
20–24	10	4 (.02)	13	6 (.03)
25–29	21	14 (.06)	13	7 (.06)
30–34	28	24 (.14)	17	28 (.17)
35–39	27	27 (.24)	12	21 (.28)
40–44	20	38 (.41)	11	33 (.44)
45–49	12	33 (.58)	10	24 (.58)
50–54	9	19 (.69)	7	15 (.69)
55–59	7	22 (.81)	2	20 (.82)
60–64	7	9 (.88)	4	12 (.89)
65–69	1	6 (.93)	2	8 (.95)
70–74	2	8 (.98)	—	3 (.98)
75–	1	2 (1.0)	1	3 (1.0)
Total	176	209	110	182
Unknown	1	—	27	—

Proband and secondary cases included.

TABLE XVII. Calculation of Prevalence Rate of Large Bowel Cancer (452 cases) (52)

Age (t)	Male					
	Cases diagnosed	Cancer (−) cases	Cancer (+) cases	Summed cases of cancer by age	Total cases observed	Prevalence (P)
0–4	—	—	—	—	—	—
5–9	6	6	—	—	284	—
10–14	10	10	—	—	278	—
15–19	25	21	4	4	268	.015
20–24	25	20	5	9	247	.036
25–29	38	19	19	28	227	.123
30–34	38	16	22	50	208	.240
35–39	44	9	35	85	192	.443
40–44	34	12	22	107	183	.585
45–49	24	5	19	126	171	.737
50–54	15	3	12	138	166	.831
55–59	11	1	10	148	163	.908
60–64	8	1	7	155	162	.957
65–69	3	1	2	157	161	.975
70–74	2	2	—	—	160	—
75–	1	1	—	—	158	—
Total	284	127	157	—	—	—

Continued . . .

TABLE XVII. Continued.

Age (t)	Female					
	Cases diagnosed	Cancer (−) cases	Cancer (+) cases	Summed cases of cancer by age	Total cases observed	Prevalence (P)
0–4	—	—	—	—	—	—
5–9	5	5	—	—	170	—
10–14	8	4	4	4	165	.024
15–19	14	12	2	6	161	.037
20–24	25	14	11	17	149	.114
25–29	29	17	12	29	135	.215
30–34	23	4	19	48	118	.407
35–39	19	10	9	57	114	.500
40–44	19	3	16	73	104	.702
45–49	12	—	12	85	101	.842
50–54	5	1	4	89	101	.881
55–59	5	—	5	94	100	.940
60–64	5	1	4	98	100	.980
65–69	1	1	—	—	99	—
70–74	—	—	—	—	—	—
75–	—	—	—	—	—	—
Total	170	72	98	—	—	—

TABLE XVIII. Age at Different Risk or Prevalence of Various Stages (24)

	Risk	Japan		England[a]	
		Male	Female	Male	Female
Symptom onset	10%	10.3	9.7	10.8	12.3
	50	22.5	21.3	25.5	25.0
Adenoma diagnosis	10	12.8	12.1	12.5	11.8
	50	27.7	24.7	26.7	25.1
Large bowel cancer diagnosis	1	16.0	13.1	17.5	12.4
	10	29.5	23.8	27.3	24.6
	50	42.0	39.8	41.9	40.7
	90	58.7	65.7	55.1	56.3
Death	10	32.8	32.8	29.4	29.4
	50	50.1	49.4	45.4	44.7

[a] Modified from the data by Veale (57) and Ashley (2).

were detected in 40% of possible dominant gene carriers (53) (Table XIV). The latent stage is therefore estimated to be an average of approximately 7 years. Using the well documented registered cases, age specific cumulative incidence rate or prevalence of symptom onset, diagnosis of polyposis, diagnosis of large bowel cancer and death were calculated (52) as shown in Tables XV, XVI, and XVII. From these data, ages at different risk or prevalence for various clinical stages were estimated as in Table XVIII.

2. Factors affecting natural history and cancer risk

The age specific prevalence of large bowel cancer of British patients calculated from the data of St. Marks Hospital presented in an article by Veale (57) is similar to the Japa-

TABLE XIX.   Cause of Death Other than Large Bowel Disease
in Parents of Patients with Adenomatosis (37)

	A group	B group
Gastric cancer	5 (17.9%)[a]	4 (7.7%)[a]
All cancers	16 (57.1)[b]	8 (15.4)[b]
Total deaths	28 (100.0)	52 (100.0)

A group: parent confirmed or highly suspected as gene carrier.
B group: parent among whose offspring a single member is affected.
[a] $\chi^2 = 1.88$, [b] $\chi^2 = 15.11$.

nese series (54), while Japanese males appear to have a slightly slower progression in their natural history compared with the males in the British series (24, 54) (Table XVIII).

By sex, both the adenomas and the cancers manifested themselves several years younger in females than in males in both Japan and Britain (Table XVIII). Average age of patients with cancer was 39.5 years for males, 36.8 years for female, and 38.3 overall.

Average age of cancer occurrence in the profuse polyps type was 34.0 years which was about 8 years younger than that of the sparse polyps type (41.8 years). However, the sparse type in the GS group produced cancer at an average age of 37.1 years which was younger by 6 years than the sparse type without GS (43.3 years) (41). No time trend in these values was apparent during the period of the study (Table VIII).

3.   Malignancy of other organs

While a patient should live longer after surgical treatment, malignant lesions may occur in various organs other than the large intestine. Gastric cancer was reported in 2.1–5.3% of the patients (Table X) and duodenal cancer in 6 and 1.9% (Table XII). Death rate by gastric cancer was significantly higher in a family member with AC than in control (37) (Table XIX). Their actual prevalence needs to be clarified in the future, but currently available data suggest that these cancers might develop in slightly older ages than does large bowel cancer, but apparently earlier than in the general population. The average age at death due to gastric cancer was 43.6 years old in the 12 Japanese cases (Table X) and 49.8 years old in the 5 non-Japanese; that of duodenal cancer was 41.1 years (Table XII). The apparent ability of small bowel adenomas to develop many years after colectomy is one more vexing aspect of the natural history of AC (26, 35).

Genetics

1.   Incidence

The frequency of individuals carrying AC at birth was estimated to be $0.45 \pm 0.5 \times 10^{-4}$ or 1/22,222 (23). Comparable data from Western countries was 1/23,930 in England (57), 1/7, 437 in U.S.A. (31), and 1/7,646 in Sweden (1).

2.   Sex ratio

The male/female ratio showed male cases significantly more numerous, being 1.38 or 352/256 in our total series, and similarly 1.31 in the St. Marks (57) and 1.48 in the Reed series (31). In call-up cases, however, there was no significant sex difference; the ratios were 1.18 or 73/62 in ours and 1.08 in the St. Marks series (57). The decreasing trend of the ratio in recent cases (Table VIII) indicates the increased chances of detecting female carriers.

The infant death rate among siblings of patients was found to be significantly higher than that in controls. This increase in mortality was more predominant in females than in males (47), indicating that the female gene carrier might be less resistant to various diseases in infancy and suggesting that it might be related to the earlier manifestation of the disorder in females.

3. Non-familial cases

The proportion of non-familial cases was 41.5% in the 1981 series which is similar to 45% in the St. Marks study (57). This value has been decreasing since the beginning of our study in 1968 when it was 64%, suggesting progress in the ascertainment of family members through the Center's activity (40).

4. Relative fitness

This was calculated to be 0.88 in our series as below (45), while it was 0.8 in Veale's (57) and 0.78 in Reed's (31).

$$F = \frac{\text{Average number of an affected member's offspring 18 years or older}}{\text{Average number of a non-affected member's offspring 18 years or older}}$$

$$= \frac{\dfrac{134}{54}}{\dfrac{212}{75}} = \frac{2.48}{2.87} = 0.88$$

5. Penetrance

There were 126 selected pedigrees in which family analysis determined parents of the proband to be obligate gene carriers. In 111 pedigrees, or 88.1% of these, one of the parents was found to be affected. If parents who had died of suspected gastrointestinal malignancy were included in the analysis, the penetrance of our series was 93.7%. The remaining four parents had died by accidental or unknown causes before the age of 52. If they are also included as affected, the actual value is almost 100% !(37). The comparative value was 80% in Veale's (57), and 90% in Reed's series (31).

6. Segregation ratio

Families in which all offspring of affected patients were examined were analyzed. As shown in Table XIV, the observed segregation ratio (θ) was 0.427 in our series. The data of Veale was 0.361 (57) and that of Reed was 0.400 (31). The adjusted segregation ratio (A) was calculated in our series as follows:

$$A = \frac{\theta}{P} = \frac{0.427}{0.937} = 0.456 \quad \text{P: penetrance}$$

7. Genetic heterogeneity
1) Age

Veale demonstrated that there were two peaks in the distribution of the age of diagnosis (57). He speculated that there existed two heterogenous forms based on the

TABLE XX.   Correlation among Relatives of Age at Death (50)

Sib/sib	n	r	Parent/child	n	r	Uncle/nephew etc.	n	r
Brother/brother	27	0.63**	Father/son	15	0.34	Uncle/nephew	12	0.47
Brother/sister	16	0.47	Father/daughter	13	0.09	Uncle/niece	6	0.55
Sister/brother	17	0.48	Mother/son	12	0.48	Aunt/nephew	14	0.27
Sister/sister	7	0.58**	Mother/daughter	5	0.39	Aunt/niece	10	0.08
Total	67	0.53	Total	45	0.09	Total	42	0.30

** Significant.

TABLE XXI.   Correlation between Proband and Affected Relatives of Polyp Amount by Type (41)

Proband	Affected relatives		Total
	Profuse	Sparse	
Profuse	24	1	25
Sparse	2	26	28
Total	26	27	53

TABLE XXII.   Correlation between Proband and Affected Relatives of GS (41)

Proband		Parents or offspring		GS in affected relative[a]				Total	
				Siblings		Others			
GS	No. family	n	%	n	%	n	%	n	%
+	28	5/13	38.46	8/22	36.36	7/22	31.80	20/57	35.09
−	87	9/51	17.65	9/72	12.50	8/52	15.38	26/175	14.86
Total	115	14/64	21.88	17/94	18.09	15/74	20.27	46/232	19.83
		0.2026		0.2625		0.1868		0.2184	
r		$0.1 < p < 0.2$		$0.01 < p < 0.05$		$0.1 < p < 0.2$		$p < 0.001$	

[a] Excluding proband.

onset of lesions: early and late onset cases. Our results were less clear regarding this aspect. However, there was a significant correlation in age at death between affected sibs of the same sex (Table XX), suggesting there are some genetic heterogenous subsets related to the progression of the disease.

2) *Polyp amount by type*

The profuse and sparse types of the proband were found in families at a rate of 98.1% (Table XXI) suggesting they are genetically heterogenous.

3) *Gardner stigmata (GS)*

The propositi with GS had GS positive relatives in 35.1%, while the GS negative propositi had positive relatives in 14.9% (Table XXII). This familial concentration of GS was independent of the degree of consanguinity (Table XXII). The evidence indicates that GS may be controlled by a single gene and is not multifactorial.

There was a significant correlation between polyp amount by type and GS type. Nineteen (33.9%) of 56 sparse type cases were associated with GS, while only one of 22 profuse type cases was (Table XXIII). Sparse-GS-positive probands showed a 40% GS positive rate in relatives, which was noticeably higher than that of sparse-GS negative type and profuse type families (Table XXIII).

TABLE XXIII. Correlation between Proband and Relatives
of Gardner and Polyp Amount by Type (41)

Proband				Affected relatives		
Polyp amount by type	GS	No. of family	Total n	GS +		
				n	%	
Sparse	+	19	46	17	37.0	
Sparse	−	37	92	16	17.4	
Profuse	+	1	1	0	—	
Profuse	−	21	43	2	4.65	

HT, hard tumor or osteoma; ST, soft tissue tumor; GS. Gardner stigmata.

There are evidently three major common subtypes of AC, simple familial polyposis with sparse polyps, that with profuse polyps and the GS type with sparse polyps (41).

REFERENCES

1. Alm, T. and Licznerski, G. The intestinal polyposes. *Clin. Gastroenterol.*, **2**, 577–602, (1973).
2. Ashley, D.T.B. Colonic cancer arising in polyposis coli. *J. Med. Genet.*, **6**, 376–378 (1969).
3. Bülow, S., Lauristen, K. B., Johansen, A., Svendsen, L. B., and Søndergaard, J. O. Gastroduodenal polyps in familial polyposis coli. *Dis. Colon Rectum.*, **28**, 90–93 (1985).
4. Burt, R. W., Berenson, M. M., Lee, R. G., Tolman, K. G., Freston, J. W., and Gardner, E. J. Upper gastrointestinal polyps in Gardner's syndrome. *Gastroenterology*, **86**, 295–301 (1984).
5. Bussey, H.J.R. Extracolonic lesion associated with polyposis coli. *Proc. R. Soc. Med.*, **65**, 294 (1972).
6. Bussey, H.J.R. (ed.). "Familial Polyposis Coli," (1975). Johns Hopkins Univ. Press, Baltimore.
7. Designan, G., Wang, M., Dunn, G. D., Halster, S., and Vaughan, S. Intramucosal gastric carcinoma in a patient with familial polyposis coli. *Am. J. Gastroenterol.*, **81**, 19–22 (1986).
8. Fujisawa, A., Yanagisawa, A., Koto, H., and Sugano, H. Malignant potential of adenoma in adenomatosis coli. *Igaku no Ayumi* (*J. Clin. Exp. Med.*), **132**, 442–443 (1985) (in Japanese).
9. Gardner, E. J. A genetic and clinical study of intestinal polyposis, a predisposing factor for carcinoma of the colon and rectum. *Am. J. Hum. Genet.*, **3**, 167–176 (1951).
10. Ida, M., Nakamura, T., and Utsunomiya, J. Osteomatous changes and tooth abnormalities found in the jaws of patients with adenomatosis coli. *Oral Surg.*, **52**, 2–11 (1981).
11. Tatsuta, M., Okuda, S., Tamura, H., and Taniguchi, H. Gastric hamartomatous polyps in the absence of familial polyposis coli. *Cancer*, **45**, 818–823 (1980).
12. Iida, M. and Ohmae, T. Extra-colonic tumor-like lesions in familial polyposis of the colon and in Gardner's syndrome. *Fukuoka Igaku Zasshi*, **69**, 169–200 (1981) (in Japanese).
13. Itoh, H. and Ohsato, K. Turcot syndrome and its characteristic colonic manifestations. *Dis. Colon Rectum*, **28**, 399–402 (1985).
14. Iwama, T., Utsunomiya, J., and Sasaki, J. Epithelial cell kinetics in the crypts of familial polyposis of the colon. *Jpn. J. Surg.*, **7**, 230–234 (1977).
15. Iwama, T. Pathological study on adenomatosis coli. *J. Jpn. Surg. Soc.*, **79**, 10–23 (1978) (in Japanese with English abstract).
16. Jarvinen, H., Nyberg, M., and Peltokallio, P. Upper gastrointestinal tract polyps in familial adenomatosis coli. *Gut*, **24**, 333–339 (1983).

17. Jones, T. R. and Nance, F. C. Periampullary malignancy in Gardner syndrome. *Ann. Surg.*, **185**, 565–573 (1977).

18. Maeda, M., Iwama, T., Utsunomiya, J., Aoki, N., and Suzuki, S. Radiological features of familial polyposis coli: Grouping by polyp profusion. *Br. J. Radiol.*, **57**, 217–227 (1984).

19. Kuroki, T., Utsunomiya, J., and Matsumoto, M. Unpublished data.

20. Miura, O., Inoue, K., Matsuda, S., Adachi, T., Hukutome, A., Soga, K., and Aoki, M. A case of familial polyposis coli associated with hereditary multiple cartilaginous exostosis: So-called Zanca's syndrome. *Naika (Internal Medicine)*, **56**, 592–597 (1985) (in Japanese).

21. Morson, B. C. Precancerous lesions of the colon and rectum. Classification and controversial issues. *JAMA*, **179**, 316–321 (1962).

22. Murphy, E. S., Mireles, M., and Beltran, A. Familial polyposis of the colon and gastric carcinoma. *JAMA*, **179**, 1026–1029 (1962).

23. Murata, M., Utsunomiya, J., Iwama, T., and Tanimura, M. Frequency of adenomatosis coli in Japan. *Jpn. J. Hum. Genet.*, **26**, 19–30 (1981).

24. Murata, M. and Utsunomiya, J. Carcinogenesis in familial polyposis coli and cancer family syndrome. *Rinsho Kagaku (J. Clin. Sci.)*, **19**, 175–181 (1983) (in Japanese).

25. Muto, T., Kamiya, J., Sawada, T., Agawa, S., Morioka, and Utsunomiya, J. Mucin abnormality of colonic mucosa in patients with familial polyposis coli. *Dis. Colon Rectum*, **28**, 147–148 (1985).

26. Nakahara, S., Itoh, H., Iida, M., Iwashita, A., and Ohsato, K. Ileal adenomas in familial polyposis coli: Differences before and after colectomy. *Dis. Colon Rectum*, **28**, 875–877 (1985).

27. Nishimura, M., Hirota, T., Itabashi, M., Ushio, K., Yamada, T., and Oguro, Y. A clinical and histochemical study of gastric polyps in familial polyposis coli. *Am. J. Gastroenterol.*, **79**, 98–103 (1984).

28. Ohsato, K., Yao, T., Watanabe, H., Iida, M., and Itoh, H. Small-intestinal involvement in familial polyposis diagnosed by operative intestinal fiberscopy. *Dis. Colon Rectum*, **20**, 414–420 (1977).

29. Pauli, R. M., Pauli, M. E., and Hall, J. G. Gardner syndrome and periampullary malignancy. *Am. J. Med. Genet.*, **6**, 205–219 (1980).

30. Ranzi, T., Castagnone, D., Velio, P., Bianchi, P., and Polli, E. E. Gastric and duodenal polyps in familial polyposis coli. *Gut*, **22**, 363–367 (1981).

31. Reed, T. E. and Neel, J. V. A genetic study of multiple polyposis of the colon (with an appendix deriving a method of estimating relative fitness). *Am. J. Hum. Genet.*, **7**, 236–263 (1955).

32. Shemesh, E., Pines, A., and Bat, U. Spectrum of extracolonic gastrointestinal tract involvement in Gardner syndrome. *Israel Med. Sci.*, **21**, 973–976 (1985).

33. Schurig, W. Multiple Karzinome des Magen-Darm-Traktes. *Zbl. F. Chir.*, **44**, 1538–1543 (1968).

34. Smiddy, F. G. and Goligher, J. C. Results of surgery in the treatment of cancer of the large intestine. *Br. Med. J.*, **1**, 793–796 (1957).

35. Stryker, S. J., Carney, J. A., and Dozois, R. R. Multiple adenomatous polyps arising in a continent reservoir ileostomy. *Int. J. Colorectal Dis.*, **2**, 43–45 (1987).

36. Turcot, J., Desperes, J. P., and St. Pierre, F. Malignant tumors of the central nervous system associated with familial polyposis of the colon: Report of two cases. *Dis. Colon Rectum.*, **2**, 465–468 (1959).

37. Tanaka, K., Utsunomiya, J., Tanimura, M., and Iwama, T. Genetic analysis of adenomatosis coli; on affection of parents of the affected (1978) (unpublished article).

38. Tanimura, M. and Utsunomiya, J. A new coding method for "Working pedigree". *Jpn. J. Hum. Genet.*, **26**, 148 (1981) (in Japanese).

39. Tanimura, M. and Utsunomiya, J. Genetic heterogeneity in adenomatosis coli. *Jpn. J. Hum. Genet.*, **28**, 147 (1982) (in Japanese).

40. Tanimura, M., Utsunomiya, J., Iwama, T., and Komatsu, I. Sporadic cases of adenomatosis coli. *Jpn. J. Hum. Genet.*, **27**, 178 (1982) (in Japanese).

41. Tanimura, M. Study on genetic heterogeneity of adenomatosis coli. *Ochanomizu Med. J.*, **33**, 83–94 (1985) (in Japanese).

42. Tonelli, F., Nardi, F., Bechi, P., Taddei, G., Gozzo, P., and Romagnoli, P. Extracolonic polyps in familial polyposis coli and Gardner's syndrome. *Dis. Colon Rectum*, **86**, 295–301 (1985).

43. Ushio, K., Sasagawa, M., Doi, H., Yamada, T., Ichikawa, H., Hojo, K., Koyama, Y., and Sano, R. Lesions associated with familial polyposis coli: Studies of lesions of the stomach, duodenum, bones and teeth. *Gastrointest. Radiol.*, **1**, 67–80 (1976).

44. Utsunomiya, J., Maki, T., Iwama, T., Matsunaga, Y., Ichikawa, T., Shimomura, T., Hamaguchi, E., and Aoki, N. Gastric lesions of familial polyposis coli. *Cancer*, **34**, 745–754 (1974).

45. Utsunomiya, J., Iwama, T., Suzuki, H., Hamaguchi, H., Tonomura, A., Sasaki, M., Tanaka, K., Mori, W., Nakamura, T., and Komatsu, I. Genetics of adenomatosis coli. *I to Cho (Stomach and Intestine)*, **9**, 1146–1156 (1974) (in Japanese with English abstract).

46. Utsunomiya, J. and Nakamura, T. The occult osteomatous changes in the mandible in patients with familial polyposis coli. *Br. J. Surg.*, **62**, 45–51 (1975).

47. Utsunomiya, J., Iwama, T., Suzuki, H., Tanaka, T., Tonomura, A., Sasaki, M., Nakamura, T., Hamaguchi, H., Mori, W., and Komatsu, I. Clinical and genetic studies on familial polyposis coli; Sex ratio. *Jpn. J. Hum. Genet.*, **20**, 283 (1976) (in Japanese).

48. Utsunomiya, J. Present status of adenomatosis coli in Japan. *In* "Pathophysiology of Carcinogenesis in Digestive Organs," ed. E. Farber *et al.*, pp. 305–321 (1977). Japan Sci. Soc. Press, Tokyo.

49. Utsunomiya, J. and Iwama, T. Studies of hereditary gastrointestinal polyposes. *Asian Med. J.*, **21**, 76–96 (1978).

50. Utsunomiya, J., Tanimura, M., Iwama, T., Tanaka, K., and Tonomura, A. Clinical genetic study of familial polyposis coli: Correlation of the age at onset of cancer between relatives. *Jpn. J. Hum. Genet.*, **24**, 202–203 (1979) (in Japanese).

51. Utsunomiya, J. and Iwama, T. Adenomatosis coli in Japan. *In* "Colorectal Cancer: Prevention, Epidemiology, and Screening," ed. S. Winawer, D. Schottenfeld, and P. Sherlock, pp. 83–95 (1980). Raven Press, New York.

52. Utsunomiya, J., Tanimura, M., Iwama, T., and Murata, M. Natural history of adenomatosis coli. *Cancer Chemother.*, **7** (Suppl.), 16–38 (1980) (in Japanese with English abstract).

53. Utsunomiya, J. and Iwama, T. Clinical and population genetics of the hereditary gastrointestinal polyposis. *In* "Heterogeneity and Genetics of Common Gastrointestinal Disorders," ed. J. I. Rother, I. M. Samloff, and D. L. Rimoin, pp. 351–416 (1980). Academic Press, New York.

54. Utsunomiya, J., Murata, M., and Tanimura, M. An analysis of the age distribution of colon cancer in adenomatosis coli. *Cancer*, **45**, 198–205 (1980).

55. Utsunomiya, J. Hereditary gastrointestinal polyposis. *Nihon Iji Shinppo*, **3044**, 126–128 (1982) (in Japanese).

56. Utsunomiya, J. Polyp and polyposis of the large bowel. *Shindan to Chiryo (Diagnosis and Therapy)*, **73**, 67–76 (1985) (in Japanese).

57. Veale, A.M.O. "Intestinal Polyposis" (1965). Cambridge Univ. Press, Cambridge.

58. Watne, A. L., Core, S. K., and Carrier, J. M. Gardner's syndrome. *Surg. Gynecol. Obstet.*, **141**, 53–56 (1975).

59. Watanabe, H., Enjoji, M., Yao, T., and Ohsato, K. Gastric lesions in familial adenomatosis coli. *Hum. Pathol.*, **9**, 269–283 (1978).

60. Zanca, P. Multiple hereditary cartilaginous exostosis with polyposis of the colon. *US Armed Forces Med. J.*, **6**, 116–122 (1953).

GENETIC ASPECT OF NEUROBLASTOMA: EPIDEMIOLOGY, FAMILIAL NEUROBLASTOMA, AND CYTOGENETIC STUDIES

Michio Kaneko and Shigenori Sawaguchi

Department of Pediatric Surgery, Institute of Clinical Medicine, University of Tsukuba*

Neuroblastoma is estimated to occur in 150 to 200 individuals annually with the occurrence rate of 1 to 10,000 neonates. Prognosis depends mainly on the age of the patient. Patients with advanced disease can survive if treated during infancy. Familial neuroblastoma is very rare compared with other childhood malignant tumors. We find information on only 2 pairs of familial neuroblastoma in Japan. Chromosomal abnormality characteristics of human neuroblastoma cells are 1) double minutes (DMs), 2) homogeneously staining regions (HSRs), and 3) deletion of the short arm of chromosome 1. The *N-myc* oncogene is frequently amplified or overexpressed in neuroblastoma and retinoblastoma. Using an *in situ* hybridization technique amplified *N-myc* is found in HSRs or DMs. *N-myc* amplification is closely related to the tumor progression and is associated with poor prognosis.

Epidemiology

Neuroblastoma is the most frequent malignant solid tumor in childhood. In 1983 the Japanese Registry on Pediatric Solid Tumors of The Committee on Malignant Tumor, The Japanese Society of Pediatric Surgeons collected data on approximately 600 solid malignant neoplasms (*4*). One hundred fifty one were neuroblastomas, which accounted for 25% of the solid childhood neoplasms. The occurrence rate of neuroblastoma per neonate is estimated at 1: 8,000–10,000. Age at diagnosis and the stage of the disease is closely related to the prognosis as shown in Table I (*11*).

Interestingly, patients with advanced disease, even with distant metastasis can survive if treated before the age of 1. Neuroblastoma extending beyond the midline is almost always impossible to completely remove surgically. Five out of 6 patients with stage III disease and under the age of 1 are long-term survivors as shown in Table I. If the distant metastases are confined to liver, skin or bone marrow, the patients are classified in stage IVS, a special category of stage IV. Seven out of 13 stage IVS patients are also long-term survivors. Special attention should be paid to the fact that the long-term survivors of advanced neuroblastomas are limited to those diagnosed before the age of 1.

For the purpose of improving the treatment results of neuroblastoma, mass screening of neuroblastoma by measuring urinary catecholamine metabolite (VMA) was started in 1971 by T. Sawada (*10*). This mass screening system is now performed all over Japan

---

* 1-1-1, Tennodai, Tsukuba, Ibaraki 305, Japan (金子道夫, 澤口重徳).

TABLE I.   Stage, Age, and the Prognosis of Neuroblastomas

Age	Stage						Total
	I	II	III	IVA	IVB	IVS	
Under 1	1/2	11/11	5/6	1/9	2/3	7/13	27/44
1	4/4	1/2	6/16	1/21	0/1	0/0	12/44
Above 2	5/7	3/4	3/19	1/70	0/7	0/0	12/107
Total	10/13	15/17	14/41	3/100	2/11	7/13	51/195

and is partially supported by the Japanese Ministry of Health and Welfare. In 1985, 52 infants were found to have neuroblastoma by this screening system. Of the 90 patients found by the VMA mass screening system, only 2 have died (unpublished data).

Some of the screening centers adopted the use of high performance liquid chromatography and found 29 infants with neuroblastoma out of 183,875 screened, a detection rate of 1: 6,000 (unpublished data). More than 10% of the neuroblastomas are non catecholamine secreters. If the detection rate of 1: 6,000 is true, neuroblastoma is expected to occur in 1 out of 5,000 neonates, which is higher than the number estimated by the tumor registry. Neuroblastoma is known by its characters of spontaneous regression or tumor maturation, as pointed out by Beckwith et al. (1) who found neuroblastoma in situ in neonates 40 times more frequently than expected. Infantile neuroblastoma has completely distinct biological characters from neuroblastoma in the older child, and further basic research is required.

Familial Neuroblastoma

The occurrence of neuroblastoma in more than one member of the same family is rarely reported, in contrast to other malignant solid neoplasms in childhood. Kushner et al. (8) reported half-brother cases with neuroblastoma in 1986 and collected information on familial neuroblastoma in English literature. Their report with its broad literature review brought to 23 the total number of familial aggregations of neuroblastoma and/or ganglioneuroblastoma (Table II). Relationships of the affected subjects included siblings, monozygotic twins, half-siblings, cousins, and parent-child. In three families, parental involvement was strongly suspected. One of the parents of all affected children had an asymptomatic posterior mediastinal tumor, assumed to be a ganglioneuroma which had matured from a (ganglio)neuroblastoma.

The median age of the familial neuroblastoma was 9 months, which was much younger than the ordinary sporadic cases. Sixty percent of the familial neuroblastomas have been diagnosed before the age of 1 year in comparison with only one fourth in unselected neuroblastomas.

Multiple primaries and early onset of disease appear to be the characters of familial or genetic neoplasms. Kushner et al. in their collected data on 55 cases with familial neuroblastoma distributed among 23 families that multiple primaries were found in 11 cases.

There was no statistical differences in prognosis between unselected and familial cases with neuroblastoma. All of the surviving cases with advanced (beyond stage III) disease were diagnosed under the age of one which was considered to be a good prognostic sign even though the disease was advanced.

TABLE II-A. Familial Cases of Neuroblastoma with Multiple Primary Sites

Patient no.	Age of DX (yr)	Sex	Relationship	Stage	Multiple primaries	Urinary catechol	Outcome (age/yr)
1	Birth	M	Proband	IV	+	−	Stillborn
2	2/12	M	Identical twin	IVS	−	+	Died (1)
3	Birth	M	Proband	IV	+	−	Died (1 day)
4	2	F	Sibling	I	−	−	Alive (5)
5	Birth	M	Distant cousin	III	−	−	Died (1 day)
6	26 days	M	Proband	in situ	−	−	Died (1/12)
7	1 3/12	F	Sibling	IV	+	+	Died (2, 4/12)
8	4/12	F	Sibling	I	+	+	Died (1 1/12)
9	5/12	F	Sibling	IV	−	+	Alive (8)
10	28	F	Mother	I	−	+	Alive (37)
11	8/12	NS	Proband	I	+	+	Alive (3)
12	5/12	F	Sibling	IIIU	−	+	Alive (1 3/12)
13	9/12	M	Proband	I	+	+	Alive (5)
14	4 6/12	M	Sibling	I	+	+	Alive (8)
15	9/12	M	Proband	IV	+	−	Died (11/12)
16	1 5/12	F	Sibling	IIIU	−	−	Died (1 6/12)
17	1 9/12	M	Proband	IV	+	−	Died (2 8/12)
18	1 3/12	F	Half sibling	IV	+	−	Died (1 6/12)
19	10	M	Father	I	−	−	Alive (41)
20	2 6/12	F	Proband	IV	−	+	Died (2 9/12)
21	2 days	F	Sibling	in situ	+	−	Died (2 days)

TABLE II-B. Familial Cases of Neuroblastoma with Single Primary Sites
Proband Younger than 1 Year of Age at Diagnosis

Patient no.	Age at DX (yr)	Sex	Relationship	Stage	Urinary catechol	Outcome (age/yr)
22	Birth	F	Proband	IVS	+	Alive (8)
23	4	F	Half sibling (paternal)	IV	NS	Died (5)
24	Birth	M	Half sibling (maternal)	I	−	Died (1 day)
25	Birth	F	Niece of case 23	Metastatic	NS	NS
26	13 days	M	Proband	NS	NS	Died (NS)
27	1 4/12	M	Twin	NS	NS	Died (NS)
28	Infancy	NS	Proband	NS	NS	NS
29	Infancy	NS	Identical twin	NS	NS	NS
30	NS	F	Proband	IV	−	Died (9/12)
31	NS	F	Identical twin	IV	−	Died (11/12)
32	4/12	M	Proband	IV	−	Died (8/12)
33	4/12	M	Identical twin	IV	−	Alive (1 8/12)
34	6/12	M	Proband	IIIU	+	Alive (1 6/12)
35	9/12	M	Father	IIIU	−	Alive (27)
36	6/12	M	Proband	IV	+	Died (9/12)
37	4	F	Sibling	II	−	Alive (NS)
38	9/12	M	1st cousin	NS	−	Died (1 10/12)
39	8/12	F	Proband	IV	−	Died (1 3/12)
40	Birth	F	Sibling	IVS	+	Alive (14)
41	15	F	Sibling	I	+	Alive (15)
42	10/12	M	Proband	IV	−	Alive (5)
43	6	M	Half sibling	IV	+	Alive (6)

TABLE II-C.   Familial Cases of Neuroblastoma with Single Primary Sites:
Proband Over 1 Year of Age at Diagnosis

Patient no.	Age at DX (yr)	Sex	Relationship	Stage	Urinary catechol	Outcome (age/yr)
44	2	F	Proband	IV	—	Died (2 6/12)
45	NS	F	Sibling	IV	—	Died (NS)
46	2 6/12	M	Proband	NS	NS	NS
47	3 4/12	F	2nd cousin	NS	NS	NS
48	3	M	Proband	IV	+	Died (3)
49	NS	F	Mother	I	—	Alive (NS)
50	3 6/12	F	Proband	IV	—	Died (3 8/12)
51	9 6/12	M	Sibling	IV	—	Died (9 9/12)
52	4	F	Proband	IIIU	—	Died (4)
53	7/12	F	Sibling	IV	—	Died (NS)
54	13	M	Proband	IV	—	Died (13)
55	NS	NS	Sibling	IV	—	Died (NS)

Reproduced and revised from ref. 7.

TABLE III.   Familial Cases of Neuroblastoma in Japan

Patient no.	Age of DX (yr)	Sex	Relationship	Stage	Urinary catechol	Outcome
1	1 1/12	F	Proband	III	+	Alive
2	2 3/12	M	Sibling	III	+	Alive
3	0 4/12	M	Monozygotic			Alive
4	0 4/12	M	Twin			Alive

Cases 1, 2: personal communication with Drs. N. Naganawa and N. Sasaki, 2nd Department of Surgery, Medical School, Nagoya City University. Cases 3, 4: personal communication with Dr. K. Okinaga, Department of Surgery, Teikyo University.

No familial cases of neuroblastoma could be found in the literature in Japan. However, we know by personal communication of two such cases which occurred in Japan (Table III). One familial neuroblastoma occurred in siblings and the other in monozygotic twins.

Patients 1 and 2 are sibling cases with stage III neuroblastoma. Cerebellar ataxia and opsomyoclonus associated with mental retardation was noticed at 10 months of age in patient 1. Both patients were subjected to urinary VMA mass screening which failed to find the neuroblastoma though both of the resected tumors were actually catecholamine secreters.

Cases 3 and 4 were monozygotic twins and their neuroblastomas were found almost simultaneously. They are now disease-free and doing well. The cases will soon be published.

Chromosome Analysis of Neuroblastoma

Although there are technical difficulties in obtaining and processing tumor tissues, extensive chromosomal analysis of solid tumors has recently been done. With the banding technique, disease-specific chromosomal abnormalities are becoming recognizable.

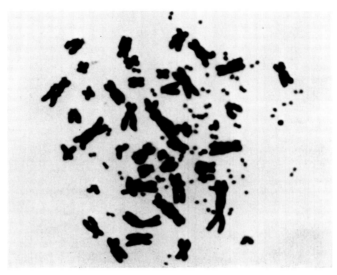

FIG. 1.   Metaphase spread of cultured neuroblastoma cell line newly established
from liver metastasis by one of the authors (MK)
Approximately 40 pairs of DMs can be clearly seen.

Brodeur *et al.* (2) pointed out three major cytogenetic abnormalities noted in human neuroblastoma cells: (1) double minutes (DMs) (Fig. 1). (2) Giant marker chromosomes with homogeneously stained regions (HSRs). DMs and HSRs can occur in other tumor or cell lines and are not necessarily neuroblastoma-specific. (3) Structural abnormalities of the short arm of chromosome 1 have occasionally been reported in primary neuroblastoma and neuroblastoma cell lines. Brodeur *et al.* analyzed 10 primary tumors and 14 neuroblastoma cell lines and found that the short arm of chromosome 1 was preferentially involved in structural rearrangements in 14 cases. The common abnormality of chromosome 1 included deletion of bands 1p32—1pter, rendering the cells partially monosomic. DMs were found in tumors and in cell lines, but HSRs were observed exclusively in cell lines. Either DMs or HSRs were found in 16 of the 24 neuroblastomas. DMs and HSRs were supposed to have the same origin and were alternative manifestations of the same phenomenon. *In situ* hybridization technique revealed that the amplified N-*myc* oncogenes were located in either the HSRs or DMs.

Kaneko *et al.* (7) successfully analyzed the banded karyotype of 8 human neuroblastoma xenografts to nude mice. They found abnormal 1p in 6 cases with the deletion of the terminal portions of 1p, 1pter—1p34 in common consistent with cell line studies. Since the HSRs were exclusively found in the cell line or nude mouse xenograft, they were previously thought to be an artifact of growth, but Balaban and Gilbert (5) and their colleagues showed the HSRs in direct preparations from human neuroblastomas. HSRs and DMs are usually found in advanced neuroblastoma and are thought to be an ominous sign for the prognosis.

N-myc Amplification in Neuroblastoma

N-*myc* oncogene, which was mapped to 2p23, frequently amplified or overexpressed in neuroblastoma and retinoblastoma (Fig. 2). Using an *in situ* hybridization technique amplified N-*myc* gene was frequently found in HSRs or DMs.

Brodeur *et al.* (*3*) and Seeger *et al.* (*12*) reported that N-*myc* amplification was found in stage III or IV advanced neuroblastoma and was closely related to the tumor progression and poor prognosis of the disease.

Seeger *et al.* (*13*) reported the results of N-*myc* amplification assay in 215 patients with neuroblastoma and 7 with ganglioneuroma (Table IV). Less than 10% of the patients with confined disease (stages I, II) had tumors with amplified N-*myc*, while approximately 40% with advanced disease had tumors with markedly amplified N-*myc* oncogene. More than half of the progressive neuroblastomas, however, had a single copy and the expression of N-*myc* in such tumors is not overexpressed by Northern blotting analysis.

Nakagawara *et al.* (*9*) analyzed N-*myc* amplification in 13 infant neuroblastomas and 25 cases of over 1 year of age. The number of dead patients was: 4 of 12 (33%) in the low amplified N-*myc* group ($\leq$10 copies) and 12 of 13 (92%) in the highly amplified group (10 copies), while those less than 1-year-old were only 8% (1/13). They also found

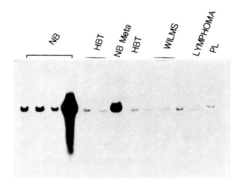

FIG. 2. N-*myc* amplification in primary neuroblastomas by Southern blotting analysis

In lanes No. 4 and 7 from the left N-*myc* was amplified more than 50 fold as compared with placenta DNA. Both patients had stage IV disease and died within 6 months after the removal of the primary tumors.

TABLE IV. N-*myc* Amplification in Neuroblastoma

Clinical stage	No. of patients	% amplification of N-*myc*
I	19	0
II	46	10
III	52	39
IV	80	38
IVS	18	6
Total	215	30
(ganglioneuroma)	7	0

that the low amplified group showed prompt response to therapy, and in the highly amplified group the tumor showed a tendency to progress rapidly, catecholamine metabolism being immature.

Kanda *et al.* (6) isolated amplified DNA sequences from an IMR-32 human neuroblastoma cell line with HSRs in 1p chromosome by fluorescence activated flow sorting. Sequences homologous to all cloned HSR DNA segments were mapped in the short arm of chromosome 2 which carries the *N-myc* gene. Thus, the amplified sequences may be involved in transposition from chromosome 2.

REFERENCES

1. Beckwith, J. B. and Perrcin, E. V. *In situ* neuroblastomas: A contribution to the natural history of neural crest tumor. *Am. J. Pathol.*, **43**, 1089–1104 (1963).
2. Brodeur, G. M., Green, A. A., Hayes, F. A., Williams, K. J., Williams, D. L., and Tsiatis, A. A. Cytogenetic features of human neuroblastoma cell lines. *Cancer Res.*, **41**, 4678–4686 (1981).
3. Brodeur, G. C., Seeger, R. C., and Schwab, M. Amplification of *N-myc* in untreated human neuroblastoma correlates with advanced disease stage. *Science*, **224**, 1121–1124 (1984).
4. The Committee on Malignant Tumor, The Japanese Society of Pediatric Surgeons: Japanese tumor registry on pediatric solid tumors in 1983. *J. Jpn. Soc. Pediatr. Surg.*, **21**, 117–152 (1985).
5. Gilbert, F., Feder, M., Balaban, G., Brangman, D., Lurie, D. K., Podolsky, R., Rinaldt, V., Vinikoor, N., and Weisband, J. Human neuroblastomas and abnormalities of chromosomes 1 and 17. *Cancer Res.*, **44**, 5444–5449 (1984).
6. Kanda, N., Schreck, R., Alt, F., Bruns, G., Baltimore, D., and Latt, S. Isolation of amplified DNA sequences from IMR-32 human neuroblastoma cells: Facilitation by fluorescence-activated flow sorting of metaphase chromosomes. *Proc. Natl. Acad. Sci. U.S.A.*, **80**, 4069–4073 (1983).
7. Kaneko, Y., Tsuchida, Y., Maseki, N., Takasaki, N., Sakurai, M., and Saito, S. Chromosome findings in human neuroblastomas xenografted in nude mice. *Jpn. J. Cancer Res.*, **76**, 359–364 (1985).
8. Kushner, B. H., Gilbert, F., and Helson, L. Familial neuroblastoma. Case reports, literature review and etiologic considerations. *Cancer*, **57**, 1887–1893 (1986).
9. Nakagawara, A., Ikeda, K., Tsuda, T., and Higashi, K. Biological characteristics of *N-myc* amplified neuroblastoma of over one-year-old patients. *In* "Advances in Neuroblastoma Research," pp. 31–39 (1988). Alan R. Liss, New York.
10. Sawada, T. and others. Mass screening for early and immediate detection of neuroblastoma in childhood. *Acta Pediatr. Jpn.*, **20**, 55–61 (1978).
11. Sawaguchi, S. and Kaneko, M. An analysis of prognosis of the registered neuroblastoma patients. *J. Jpn. Soc. Pediatr. Surg.*, submitted.
12. Seeger, R. C., Brodeur, G. M., and Sather, H. Association of multiple copies of the *N-myc* oncogene with rapid progression of neuroblastoma. *N. Engl. J. Med.*, **313**, 1111–1116 (1985).
13. Seeger, R. C., Moss, T. J., Bjork, R. L., Feig, A., Brodeur, G. M., Sousa, L., and Slamon, D. Expression of *N-myc* by neuroblastomas with one or multiple copies of the oncogene, *In* "Advances in Neuroblastoma Research," pp. 41–49 (1988). Alan R. Liss, New York.

EPIDEMIOLOGY OF WILMS' TUMOR IN JAPAN WITH EMPHASIS ON ONCOTERATOLOGICAL ASPECTS

Yoshiyuki Hanawa

*First Department of Pediatrics, Toho University School of Medicine**

Wilms' tumor accounted for 848 of the total of 19,853 cases of cancer and allied disorders which were registered in the Children's Cancer Registry during the 16-year period from 1969 to 1984. Excluding benign neoplasms and allied disorders, the relative frequency of Wilms' tumor was 4.5% among all types of cancer in the Registry; bilateral Wilms' tumor was reported in 25 cases. Incidence was calculated based on the results of the Kanagawa Children's Cancer Registry, which is maintained on a population base: the estimated annual incidence was calculated as being 0.38 per 100,000 children under 15 years of age. In the 86 cases of Wilms' tumor appearing in the Japan Children's Cancer Registry (JCCR), one or more type(s) of anomalies was registered. Excluding the 97 cases without information on the presence or absence of anomalies, the rate of congenital anomalies associated with Wilms' tumor was 11.5%. In the group with congenital anomalies, 27.9% of the cases were less than one year of age, whereas in another group without congenital anomalies the figure was 24.3%. The most frequent congenital anomalies were those of the central nervous system (CNS). In 22 cases (2.9%) CNS anomalies such as macrocephalus, microcephalus, hydrocephalus, and other anomalies were noted. In 18 cases (2.4%), eye anomalies such as aniridia, congenital cataracts and others were reported. Genital anomalies (cryptorchidism, hypospadias) were observed in 23 cases (3.1%).

Hemihypertrophy was observed in 7 cases. Congenital anomalies in the urinary tract, heart, ear, and the skeletal system were also registered. Two cases of Beckwith-Wiedemann syndrome and one case of Marfan syndrome were registered. No cases of Down syndrome were registered. Wilms' tumor occurred in both members of one pair of twins and in two siblings. No other familial occurrence was registered.

In children whose mother was 35–39 years of age at delivery, the rate of congenital anomalies was 26.9%, which was more than twice the overall rate; other rates were 12.6% (20–24 years), 8.6% (25–29 years), and 14.8% (30–34 years).

Wilms' tumor is one of the typical malignant neoplasms observed almost exclusively during early childhood. Also called nephroblastoma, it arises from the kidney and is seen as an abdominal mass without any pathognomonic signs. The mass is not rarely noticed coincidentally during a routine health check. Sometimes children with Wilms' tumor have additional symptoms of abdominal pain, vomiting or hematuria. The mass varies in size from 5–10 cm or more in diameter and is generally smooth and firm. Metastasis to the liver as well as to the lung is very common. Wilms' tumor was first described by

* 6-11-1, Omori Nishi, Ota-ku, Tokyo 143, Japan (塙　嘉之).

Race in 1814, and later a surgeon, Max Wilms, identified the lesion accurately in 1899 as of mixed embryonal nature. The success of actinomycin D in the improved survival of children with Wilms' tumor opened the door for a new era of cancer chemotherapy. In 1935 survival rate with Wilms' tumor was 30% by operation. But in 1985 the survival rate was reported as 90% by operation and chemotherapy combined with or without radiation (7). In addition to this progress in clinical pediatric oncology, the association of several kinds of congenital anomalies with Wilms' tumor has been noticed and the interest of pediatric oncology focused on the teratological aspect. Miller *et al.* (25) reported aniridia, hemihypertrophy and other congenital anomalies associated with Wilms' tumor in 1964. Pendergrass (29) and Breslow and Beckwith (2) also reported close association between congenital anomalies and Wilms' tumor. Familial occurrence of Wilms' tumor is also recognized. Meadows (23) reported Wilms' tumor in three siblings in one family; Juberg *et al.* (11) reported two cases among 3 siblings; Cordero *et al.* (6) reported occurrence in five cousins. As for the etiology of retinoblastoma, which is an embryonal cancer like Wilms' tumor, Knudson (14) proposed a two-step mutational process. Later he hypothesized that Wilms' tumor may also be attributed to a two-mutational model (15). Based on the occurrence of Wilms' tumor in two pairs of monozygous twins, Maurer *et al.* (21) also supported the hypothesis that the development of Wilms' tumor requires the occurrence of two successive mutational events.

These findings further confirm the hypothesis that genetic factors may play a major role in the etiology of Wilms' tumor. Matsunaga (20) analysed the published data on this type of tumor and showed the mode of inheritance of familial cases. Nakagome *et al.* (26) found 11p deletion in the phenotypically normal mother of a child with aniridia-Wilms' tumor association.

The present study was made to ascertain both the incidence of Wilms' tumor and the rate of congenital anomalies among afflicted children in Japan and to compare these results with those of other countries.

Children's Cancer Registry and Birth Defect Monitoring

1)   Most of the data in this study were obtained from the Japan Children's Cancer Registry (JCCR) (N. Kobayashi, Director of the National Children's Hospitl, Representative of the Registry) (3–5). This registration program was formulated by the Children's Cancer Association of Japan and is supported by the Cancer Committee of both the Japan Pediatric Society and the Pediatric Surgeon's Society of Japan. The Committee of Pediatric Ophthalmologists also supports this nationwide, hospital based registry. Information has been compiled since 1969, and as of 1984 a total of 18,900 cases of children's cancer and 953 cases of allied diseases diagnosed in those under 15 years of age were registered. Information concerning the presence or absence of associated congenital anomalies was also registered in most cases. These latter have already been partly reported by Kobayashi (13).

2)   The Children's Cancer Registry covers Japan in its entirety. However, as this registration is hospital-based it is not possible to calculate the incidence rate of cancer in children in Japan.

In Kanagawa Prefecture a children's cancer registry has been conducted in parallel with the JCCR. In this registry all types of malignant solid tumors and all leukemias are included, as in the JCCR: this registry is compiled by the Kanagawa Children's

Medical Center and is called the Kanagawa Children's Cancer Registry (KCCR). The registry has been able to collect almost 100% information on cases of children's cancer occurring in Kanagawa with the support of the governments of Kanagawa Prefecture and Yokohama City, which is located in the Prefecture. This data was kindly made available to the author by H. Nishihira (Chief of the Department of Oncology, Kanagawa Chidlren's Medical Center, Director of the Registry) (27).

3) To compare the incidence rate of congenital anomalies in Wilms' tumor with that of the general population in Japan, data was used from the Kanagawa Birth Defect Monitoring Program (KAMP), generously made available to the author by Y. Kuroki (Chief of the Department of Genetics, Kanagawa Children's Medical Center, Director of the Program) (18). KAMP has been in operation since October, 1981 as the first population-based system in Japan to monitor selected congenital anomalies diagnosed during the early neonatal period. It covers about 50% of the total births in Kanagawa Prefecture, about 47,000 births annually. From October 1981 to December, 1983, the total monitored number of births including stillbirths was 106,043.

Incidence of Wilms' Tumor and Associated Congenital Anomalies

1. Relative frequency of Wilms' tumor among children's cancers

Among the 18,900 cases of cancer registered nationwide during the 16-year period from 1969 to 1984, a total of 5,445 cases of malignant tumors were registered from 1969 to 1973, 5,665 cases from 1974 to 1978 and 6,407 cases from 1979 to 1983. In 1984 another 1,383 cases were registered. In Table I distribution of all types of cancer in each 5-year period is shown, excluding those cases occurring in 1984. The most common type of children's cancer in each of the 5-year periods was leukemia, accounting for 47.6% (1969–1973), 44.7% (1974–1978), and 43.4% (1979–1983) of all types of cancer.

TABLE I.   Distribution of Childhood Malignancy
Japan Children's Cancer Registry (1979–1983)

Diagnosis	1969–1973	1974–1978	1979–1983	1969–1983
Leukemia	2,592	2,535	2,784	7,911
Malignant lymphoma	391	435	640	1,466
Brain and spinal cord tumor	639	487	571	1,697
Neuroblastoma	562	598	714	1,874
Retinoblastoma	218	601	517	1,336
Wilms' tumor	259	274	273	806
Hepatoblastoma and liver cell carcinoma	126	131	151	408
Malignant neoplasms				
bone	87	58	117	262
testis	111	98	57	266
ovary	40	47	75	162
soft part	100	159	228	487
the thyroid and adrenal glands	22	28	41	91
Malignant teratoma[a]	21	33	52	106
Letterer-Siwe disease	55	41	33	129
Other malignant neoplasms	222	140	154	516
Total	5,445	5,665	6,407	17,517

[a] Retroperitoneal, mediastinal sacrococcygeal, and others except gonad and brain.

Wilms' tumor was the 5th or 6th most common cancer in each 5-year period, at 4.8%
(both 1969–1973 and 1974–1978) and 4.3% (1979–1983).

2. *Frequency by age, sex, bilaterality, and familial occurrence*

Table II summarizes the age distribution of Wilms' tumor for each 5-year registration period. There were no significant changes in the age distributions among the three
periods. Cases under one year of age including 0 year of age. were from 21.6 to 28.2%
of the total, while cases under 5 years of age were 82–87% of the total. The male to
female ratio was 0.85 in the period from 1969 to 1973, 1.34 (1974–1978), 1.08 (1979–
1983), and overall 1.08 (1969–1983). Bilateral Wilms' tumor was reported in 25 cases.
Mean age at diagnosis was 31.1 ± 27.5 mos. in unilateral cases and 20.7 ± 18.2 mos. in
bilateral cases excluding one case of unknown age ($p<0.05$). Two cases of extrarenal

TABLE II.   Age Distribution of Wilms' Tumor
Japan Children's Cancer Registry

Age (yr.)	1969–1973		1974–1978		1979–1983		Total	
	No.	%	No.	%	No.	%	No.	%
0	73	28.2	64	23.4	59	21.6	196	24.3
1	58	22.4	73	26.6	62	22.7	193	23.3
2	41	15.8	51	18.6	37	13.6	129	16.0
3	37	14.3	31	11.3	34	12.5	102	12.7
4	15	5.8	19	6.9	31	11.4	65	8.1
0–4	224	86.5	238	86.9	223	81.7	685	85.0
5	13	5.0	11	4.0	13	4.8	37	4.6
6	6	2.3	7	2.6	10	3.7	23	2.9
7	1	0.4	7	2.6	11	4.0	19	2.4
8	3	1.2	2	0.7	2	0.7	7	0.9
9	4	1.5	1	0.4	3	1.1	8	1.0
10	2	0.8	0	0	1	0.4	3	0.4
11	0	0	1	0.4	2	0.7	3	0.4
12	1	0.4	1	0.4	—	—	2	0.2
13	0	0	1	0.4	—	—	1	0.1
14	0	0	0	0	1	0.4	1	0.1
Unknown	5	1.9	5	1.8	7	2.6	17	2.1
Total	259	100	274	100	273	100	806	100

TABLE III.   Children's Cancer and Wilms' Tumor in the Kanagawa Children's
Cancer Registry (Jan. 1, 1979–Dec. 31, 1982)

Year	Number of children under 15 years of age[a] ($\times10^3$)	Children's cancer		Wilms' tumor	
		Total number	Rate per 100,000	Total number	Rate per 100,000
1979	1,714.3	213	12.4	9	0.52
1980	1,703.1	190	11.2	2	0.12
1981	1,698.1	210	12.4	5	0.29
1982	1,704.8	214	12.6	10	0.59
1979–1982	6,820.3	827	12.1	26	0.38

[a] Population in Kanagawa Prefecture on January 1st of each year.

Wilms' tumor were reported, and the disease occurred in both members of one pair of twins and in two siblings. No other familial occurrences were reported.

TABLE IV. Congenital Anomalies Associated with Wilms' Tumor
Japan Children's Cancer Registry (1969–1984)

No.	Organ(s)	ICD-9	Congenital anomalies (number of diseases)	No. of cases[a]	Rate[b] (%)
1	Central nervous system	742.1	Microcephalus (5)	22	2.9
		742.3	Hydrocephalus (6)		
		742.4	Cerebellar cyst (1), Moya-moya disease (1)		
		742.9	Macrocephalus (9)		
2	Eye	743.1	Microphthalmia (2)	18	2.4
		743.2	Glaucoma (2)		
		743.3	Congenital cataracts (4)		
		743.4	Aniridia (11), persistent of the pupillary membrane (1)		
		743.9	Anomaly of the eye (NOS) (1)		
3	Heart and great vessels	745.2	Tetratogy of Fallot (1)	9	1.2
		745.4	Ventricular septal defect (3)		
		745.5	Atrial septal defect (1)		
		746.9	CHD (NOS) (3)		
		747.0	Patent ductus arteriosus (1)		
4	Genital organs	752.5	Cryptorchidism (17)	23	3.1[c]
		752.6	Hypospadias (12)		
		752.8	Micropenis (1)		
5	Urinary tract	753.1	Polycystic kidney (1)	8	1.1
		753.3	Horseshoe kidney (3), double kidney (1)		
		753.7	Urachal rest (1)		
		753.8	Rectovesical fistula (1)		
		753.9	Renal anomalies (NOS) (1)		
6	Skeletal system	Extremities		14	1.9
		754.5	Pes varus (1)		
		754.6	Pes valgus (2)		
		Thorax			
		754.8	Funnel chest (4), pigeon chest (1)		
		Finger and toe			
		755.0	Polydactyly (5)		
		755.1	Syndactyly (2)		
		Spine and rib			
		756.1	Short neck (1)		
		756.3	Rib defect (1)		
7	Spleen	759.0	Accessory spleen (1)	1	—
8	Others	759.8	Marfan syndrome (1), Beckwith-Wiedemann syndrome (2)	3	0.4
		759.8	Hemihypertrophy (7)	7	0.9

[a] Total number of this column exceeds the actual number of Wilms' tumors associated with congenital anomalies.
[b] Rate per total cases ($N=751$) of Wilms' tumor in which information concerning congenital anomalies was registered.
[c] 5.9% in male group.

3. Annual incidence rate

The Kanagawa Children's Cancer Registry, which is supported by the government of Kanagawa Prefecture, is regarded as a population-based registry. As shown in Table III, each year from 1979 to 1982 the total number of children's cancers was between 190 to 214, and the rate of occurrence was between 11.2 to 12.6 per 100,000 children under 15 years of age. For Wilms' tumor the average incidence during the same period was calculated to be 0.38 per 100,000.

4. Congenital anomalies associated with Wilms' tumor

The total number of Wilms' tumor cases registered from 1969 to 1984 was 848, and in 751 cases information concerning the presence or absence of congenital anomalies was included. The anomalies were classified according to ICD-9 categories 741–759, as shown in Table IV. In this table minor anomalies such as DuBois' sign, simian line, and congenital fistula of the ear were excluded even if they were noted. In 86 cases of Wilms' tumor, one or more types of anomaly were registered. Excluding those without anomaly information, the rate of congenital anomalies was 11.5%. The most frequent were those of the central nervous system (CNS). In 22 cases (2.9%), macrocephalus, microcephalus, hydrocephalus, and other anomalies of the CNS were registered. In 18 cases (2.4%), eye anomalies including aniridia, congenital cataracts and others were reported. Genital anomalies (cryptorchidism, hypospadias) were observed in 23 cases (3.1%). Hemihypertrophy was observed in 7 cases (0.9%). Congenital anomalies in the urinary tract, heart, ear, and skeletal system were also noted. Two cases of Beckwith-Wiedemann syndrome and one case of Marfan syndrome were registered; no cases of Down syndrome were recorded.

TABLE V. Multiple Anomalies Associated with Wilms' Tumor
Japan Children's Cancer Registry (1969–1984)

Registration no.	Congenital anomalies
284068	Microcephalus+congenital cataracta, retinitis pigmentosa (infantile spasm)
775098	Hydrocephalus+polydactyly (mental retardation)
376298	Macrocephalus+pes varus
376143	Macrocephalus+pes varus+cryptorchidism (low set ear, small auricle, mental retardation, short stature)
373160	Aniridia+hypospadia
373241	Microphthalmos+microcephalus+funnel chest (hyperterolism, simian line, Dubois' sign, mental retardation)
371350	Microphthalmos+short neck
383124	Aniridia, congenital cataracta+polydactyly
384294	Aniridia+cryptorchidism (inguinal hernia)
680009	Aniridia+congenital heart disease (VSD)+microcephalus (high arched palate, mental retardation, short stature)
482109	Aniridia+cryptorchidism (strabismus, blephalophimosis, malformed head)
183001	Congenital heart disease (VSD)+micropenis (accessory ear)
376322	Cryptorchidism+hemihypertrophy (congenital fistula of ear)
574109	Urachal rest+hemihypertrophy
670086	Funnel chest+hemihypertrophy
371278	Marfan syndrome (high arched palate, Dubois' sign)
379399	Beckwith-Wiedemann syndrome
675098	Beckwith-Wiedemann syndrome+hemihypertrophy

TABLE VI. Aniridia-Wilms' Tumor Association
Japan Children's Cancer Registry (1969–1984)

Registra-tion no.	Sex	Age at diagnosis (mos.)	Laterality	Associated anomalies and diseases
671017	F	?	L	Glaucoma, cataract
373160	M	16	R	Hypospadia
673068	M	22	R	
477114	F	55	R	
680009	M	? (1y)	R	CHD, microcephalus, high arched palate, short stature, mental retardation
382137	F	31	L	Cataract, mental retardation
482109	M	19	R	Strabismus, cryptorchism
383124	F	26	R	Cataract, polydactyly
384294	M	11	L	Cryptorchism, inguinal hernia
684004	F	11	L	
784019	F	14	L	

TABLE VII. Age at Diagnosis by Sex and Presence or Absence of Congenital Anomalies (mos.)
Japan Children's Cancer Registry (1969–1984)

| | All registered cases | | | Laterality | | Congenital anomalies | | | |
| | | | | | | Present | | Absent | |
	Total	Male	Female	Uni.	Bi.	Male	Female	Male	Female
N	786	412	374	760	24	52	28	317	313
MIN	0	0	0	0	0	0	0	0	0
MAX	172	157	172	172	64	118	150	157	172
M	30.9	28.7	33.2	31.1	20.7	21.9	45.2	30.5	32.3
SD	27.4	26.1	28.7	27.5	18.2	21.2	36.8	27.0	27.7

Uni., unilateral; Bi., bilateral.

In addition to the congenital anomalies coded according to the ICD-9 categories 741–759, several kinds of diseases were also registered: 17 cases with inguinal hernia, 6 with various types of hemangioma, 3 with short stature and 2 with infantile spasm. It is noteworthy that 15 cases were complicated by mental retardation; one case of Wilms' tumor was associated with mediastinal neuroblastoma.

Of the 25 cases of bilateral Wilms' tumor, information on congenital anomalies was shown in 24 cases, 3 of which (12.5%) indicated their presence.

In Table V shows multiple anomalies, those occurring in two or more organs (tissues). Aniridia-Wilms' tumor association was reported in 11 cases, as shown in Table VI. The average age of these cases at diagnosis was 22.7 mos. excluding cases of unknown age.

Age distribution in the presence or absence of congenital anomalies was examined. The frequency of cases under one year of age with congenital anomalies was 27.9%, whereas it was 24.4% among those without such anomalies. This difference was not significant statistically. The age at diagnosis, however, was different between male and female in the presence or absence of congenital anomalies (Table VII). The mean age at diagnosis was lowest in the male group: of the 22 cases having CNS anomalies, 10 (45.5%) were under one year of age. Similarly, of the 23 cases having genital anomalies,

TABLE VIII.   Rates of Congenital Anomalies by Mother's Age at Delivery

Mother's age (yrs.)	Total registered cases	Cases including information on congenital anomalies (A)	Cases with congenital anomalies (B)	Cases without congenital anomalies	Rate of congenital anomalies (B/A %)
<20	6	6	0	6	0
20–24	110	103	13	90	12.6
25–29	316	292	25	267	8.6
30–34	135	122	18	104	14.8
35–39	27	26	7	19	26.9
>40	3	3	0	3	0
Unknown	251	199	23	176	11.6
Total	848	751	86	665	11.5

7 (30.4%) were under one year of age, and 18 (78.3%) were under 2 years of age. The mother's age at delivery of children with Wilms' tumor is shown in Table VIII. In afflicted children whose mother was 35–39 years of age at delivery, the rate of congenital anomalies was 26.9%, twice that of the overall rate. The rate was 12.6% in children whose mother was 20–24 years of age at birth, and in the other two groups it was 8.6% (25–29 years) and 14.8% (30–34 years).

International Comparison of Wilms' Tumor Epidemiology

Wilms' tumor accounted for 4.5% of the registered cases of children's cancer in

TABLE IX.   Distribution of Malignant Neoplasms

	Japan, 1969–1983		U.S.A., 1969–1971			
	Japan Children's Cancer Registry (3–5)		3rd National Cancer Survey (32)			
			Whites		Blacks	
	No.	%	No.	%	No.	%
Leukemia	7,911	45.2	651	33.8	56	24.9
CNS tumor	1,697	9.7	370	19.2	55	24.4
Malignant lymphoma Histiocytosis	1,466	8.4	204	10.6	32	14.2
Neuroblastoma	1,874	10.7	146	7.6	16	7.1
Wilms' tumor	806	4.6	117	6.1	18	8.0
Primary malignant bone tumor	262	1.5	86	4.5	11	4.9
Hepatoblastoma, hepatocarcinoma	408	2.3	26	1.4	1	0.5
Retinoblastoma	1,336	7.6	52	2.7	7	3.1
Malignant soft tumor Teratoma	487	2.8	130	6.7	9	4.0
Malignant ovarial tumor	162	0.9	17	0.9	5	2.2
Malignant testicular tumor	266	1.5	16	0.8	1	0.5
Others	842	4.8	110	5.7	14	6.2
Total	17,517	100	1,925	100	225	100

[a] Histionzytosen.
[b] Rhabdomyosarcoma.

the JCCR during the 16-year observation period; in KCCR it was 3.2%. The difference between these two registries is most likely due to the fact that the JCCR information is largely from pediatricians, pediatric surgeons and ophthalmologists and a number of cases of bone, brain, and other cancers might not be included in the registry. On the other hand KCCR has registered almost all types of children's cancer using the applications submitted by parents to the local government to defray the cost of medical treatment.

The relative incidence of Wilms' tumor in Japan was compared to data in a number of other countries, as shown in Table IX. Rates in other countries were between 3.0 and 8.0 and there was no remarkable difference on the relative frequency among them. As the scope of children's cancer may differ among these series, however, it is difficult to conclude from these data that no racial variation in incidence exists.

The age-specific incidence rate in Japan was calculated based on the KCCR as described earlier. Overall children's cancer incidence rate was 12.2 per 100,000 annually and that of Wilms' tumor was 0.38 as an average during the years observed. In 1972 the author (9) postulated the annual incidence rate of Wilms' tumor to be 0.54 in Japan, based on data compiled by the Ministry of Health and Welfare.

In other countries reports of the Wilms' tumor incidence rate have for the most part been based on population-based registries, as follows: 0.65 in Great Britain, 1962–1970 (8); 0.66 in Queensland, 1981 (22); 0.41 in South Australia, 1977–1979 (1); 0.65 in Torino, Italy, 1969–1978 (28); and 0.76 among whites and 0.78 among blacks in the U.S.A., 1969–1971 (32).

Racial variation in incidence has been accepted as minimal since Innis (10) reported

in Children, International Comparison

Great Britain, 1954–1977		F.R.G., 1980–1985		Italy, 1967–1978		India, 1964–1972		Africa, 1960–1972	
Manchester and Great Britain		Michaelis, Univ. Mainz (24)		Torino (28)		Greater Bombay (12)		Nigeria Ibadan (31)	
No.	%	No.	%	No.	%	No.	%	No.	%
809	33.1	2,448	36.3	291	33.4	192	20.4	60	4.5
549	22.5	1,058	15.7	179	20.6	71	7.6	29	2.2
198	8.1	795	11.8	92	10.6	122	13.0	180	58.9
		232[a]	3.5						
158	6.5	494	7.3	61	7.0	23	2.4	33	2.5
124	5.1	412	6.1	39	4.5	28	3.0	74	5.6
132	5.4	413	6.1	37[c]	4.2	36	3.8	33	2.5
13	0.5	38	0.6	11	1.3			12	0.9
73	3.0			24	2.8	49	5.2	97	7.3
123	5.0	458	6.8	53	6.1	24	2.5	83[b]	6.3
		228	3.4					19[d]	1.4
								13	1.0
								6	0.5
263	10.8	163	2.4	83	19.5	397	42.1	86	6.4
2,442	100	6,739	100	870	100	942	100	1,325	100

[c] Osteosarcoma, Ewing's sarcoma.
[d] Extragonad.

Wilms' tumor to be a possible index cancer of childhood by analyzing the data from
"Cancer Incidence in Five Continents, 1966 and 1970" published by WHO. Recently,
Kramer *et al.* (*16, 17*) reported that the annual incidence of this tumor is significantly
higher among nonwhites than whites based on data derived from the Greater Delaware
Valley Pediatric Tumor Registry: 0.62 per 100,000 in whites and 1.19 in nonwhites.

Applying the annual Wilms' tumor incidence rate of 0.38 per 100,000 children
under 15 years of age in Kanagawa to all Japan, total annual cases throughout the country would be 102. As in JCCR, the number registered each year has been between 50 to
55 and the registration rate is supposed to be 50–60% of total, so that 102 is reasonably
accepted as the number of children newly diagnosed each year. The incidence rate of
bilateral Wilms' tumor was reported to be 25 cases per 848, or 2.95% in the JCCR,
which is low compared to that of National Wilms' Tumor Study (NWTS) with statistical significance ($p < 0.01$). But in 1980 Tsunoda (*30*) conducted a nationwide survey
and found 36 cases of bilateral Wilms' tumor among 803 cases of this disease, which
were reported from 105 hospitals; this was a ratio of 4.48%. In the U.S.A. bilaterality
was reported by NWTS to be 4.41% at the onset of the disease (*2*), whereas the ratio
increased to 5.41% due to the additional occurrence of contralateral Wilms' tumor during the follow-up period. In the Greater Delaware Valley Pediatric Tumor Registry
(*17*) the frequency of bilateral tumor was reported to be 12.5% in blacks and 7.9% in

TABLE X.   Rate of Congenital Anomalies in Japan Children's Cancer
Registry (JCCR) *versus* Those in NWTS[a] and KAMP[b]

		JCCR	NWTS	KAMP
Years of study		1969–1984	1969–1981	1981. 10. 1–1983. 12. 31
Ages		0–14 yrs.	0–14 yrs.	7 days after birth
No. of		M 388	M 900	M 54,337
cases		F 363	F 1,005	F 51,686
studied		T 751[c]	T 1,905	Unknown 20, T 106,043
ICD-9	Anomalies	Rate per 1,000 cases		
741–742	CNS	29.3	4.7	15.8[d]
743.4	Aniridia	14.6	8.4	0.01
745–747	Heart and great vessels	12.0 ⎫	15.2	—
748	Respiratory organ	0.0 ⎭		
752.5[e]	Cryptorchidism	43.8	27.8	—
752.6[e]	Hypospadias	30.9	17.8	0.39
753.3	Horseshoe kidney	4.0	3.7	—
755.0	Polydactyly	6.7	—	0.96
755.1	Syndactyly	2.7	—	0.74
758.0	Down syndrome	0.0	0.5	0.63
759.0	Accessory spleen	1.3	6.3	—
759.8	Beckwith-Wiedemann syndrome	2.6	2.1	—
	Marfan syndrome	1.3	0.0	—
	Hemihypertrophy	9.3	24.7	—

[a] National Wilms' Tumor Study.

[b] Kanagawa Birth Defect Monitoring Program.

[c] Excluded 97 cases which had no information about congenital anomalies.

[d] Anencephaly (0.67), encephalocele (0.07), microcephaly (0.16), hydrocephaly (0.36), and spina bifida
(0.32).

[e] Rate for males.

whites. The low JCCR incidence might be due to the lack of additional data concerning the late onset of contralateral tumor.

Male-to-female Wilms' tumor sex ratio in JCCR was 1.8 between 1969 and 1983. As the sex ratio at the time of birth in Japan has been 1.05 to 1.06, both sexes have equal susceptibility to this disease.

Age distribution of the JCCR differed from that of NWTS. In the latter, the incidence peak existed between the 2nd and 4th year of life with the mean age 42.1±32.7 months in male and 46.1±33.7 months in female. In the JCCR, the incidence peak was at under one year (1969–1973) or at one year of age (1974–1978; 1979–1983). Mean age at diagnosis was 28.7±26.1 months in male and 33.2±28.7 months in female. Wilms' tumor seems to reveal its clinical manifestations at an earlier age in Japan than in the U.S.A. In both countries male cases have a tendency to be diagnosed several months earlier than female.

In Table X the rates of congenital anomalies among the series reported in the JCCR were compared with those from NWTS (2). In 22 JCCR cases CNS anomalies were registered (29.3 per 1,000), whereas in NWTS series these anomalies were observed in 9 out of 1,905 cases (4.7 per 1,000). Besides CNS anomalies, 15 cases were associated with mental retardation in JCCR, but only 5 were accompanied by head anomalies.

Aniridia-Wilms' tumor association was registered in 11 of 751 JCCR cases of Wilms' tumor providing information on associated congenital anomalies. Thus, the incidence rate was calculated to be 1.46%, which is higher than the rate of 0.84% in the NWTS series, but this difference was not significant statistically. The average age at diagnosis in the JCCR was 22.7 months, which was close to that of 24.4 months in NWTS. As for additional congenital anomalies in aniridia-Wilms' tumor association, 12 out of 16 aniridia-Wilms' tumor association showed multiple congenital anomalies outside of the eye, in the NWTS series. In the JCCR series only 6 out of 11 cases reported additional congenital anomalies existing outside of the eye. However, in 1983 Matsuoka (19) reviewed 8 case reports from the Japanese literature and found that in 5 of these cases multiple congenital anomalies were described. The additional association of congenital anomalies actually occurs almost equally in both races.

Besides aniridia-Wilms' tumor association, genital anomalies such as cryptorchidism and hypospadias occur almost twice as frequently as those of NWTS, but this difference was also not significant. However, contrary to the above results, hemihypertrophy occurred less frequently in the JCCR than in the NWTS series, although the low rate in JCCR might be due to diagnostic difficulty.

As for racial differences in the association rate of congenital anomalies in Wilms' tumor, Kramer et al. (17) reported that sporadic aniridia, genito-urinary anomalies and hemihypertrophy were associated more frequently in black cases than in white. The true rate of congenital anomalies in the Japanese series might reflect the exclusion of obscure cases, in which such information was not registered.

The rate of congenital anomalies in Wilms' tumor in Japan was compared to the rate among the country's general population, that is, the data from KAMP. Because selected surface malformations in newborns under 7 days of age, including stillborns, are registered by KAMP, the comparison between JCCR and KAMP figures may not be relevant. However, genital anomalies such as hypospadias, polydactyly and syndactyly should be noted equally both in children with Wilms' tumor and each newborn. The differences in these incidences are considered remarkable.

CONCLUSION

1) Relative frequency of Wilms' tumor among children's cancer in Japan was 4.6% during the period observed, which is similar to that in most counties.

2) Wilms' tumor occurred at a younger age in Japan than in the U.S.A. or Great Britain.

3) The annual incidence rate of Wilms' tumor in Japan was 0.38 per 100,000 under 15 years of age, which was lower than that of other countries.

4) The overall rate of congenital anomalies associated with Wilms' tumor was almost the same between Japan and the U.S.A. In JCCR, the rate of congenital anomalies increased among children whose mother's age was over 35 years at delivery.

5) CNS anomalies occurred more frequently in Japan whereas hemihypertrophy occurred less frequently compared to the data from NWTS.

6) Further study is needed to draw a definite conclusion concerning racial differences in the incidence of Wilms' tumor as well as the rate of congenital anomalies among afflicted children.

REFERENCES

1. Bonett, A. Incidence of childhood cancers in South Australia. *Med. J. Aust.*, **1**, 21–22 (1982).
2. Breslow, N. E. and Beckwith, J. B. Epidemiological features of Wilms' tumor: results of the national Wilms' tumor study. *J. Natl. Cancer Inst.*, **68**, 429–436 (1982).
3. Children's Cancer Association of Japan. All Japan Children's Cancer Registration, 1969–1973, Vol. I (1975).
4. Children's Cancer Association of Japan. All Japan Children's Cancer Registration, 1974–1978, Vol. II (1982).
5. Children's Cancer Association of Japan. Japan Children's Cancer Registry, 1979–1983, Vol. III (1986).
6. Cordero, J. F., Li, F. P., Holmes, L. B., and Geraled, P. S. Wilms' tumor in five cousins. *Pediatrics*, **66**, 716–719 (1980).
7. D'Angio, G. J. Oncology seen through the prism of Wilms' tumor. *Med. Pediat. Oncol.*, **13**, 53–58 (1985).
8. Draper, G. J., Birch, J. M., Bithell, J. F., Kinnier Wilson, L. M., Leck, I., Marsden, H. B., Morris Jones, P. H., Stiller, C. A., and Swindell, R. Childhood cancer in Britain. Studies on Medical and Population Subjects No. 37 (1982). Her Majesty's Stationery, London.
9. Hanawa, Y. Childhood cancer registry. *Sougou Rinsho*, **23**, 2037–2044 (1974) (in Japanese).
10. Innis, M. D. Nephroblastoma: possible index cancer of childhood. *Med. J. Aust.*, **1**, 18–20 (1972).
11. Juberg, R. C., St. Martin, E. C., and Hundley, J. R. Familial occurrence of Wilms' tumor: nephroblastoma in one of monozygous twins and another sibling. *Am. J Hum. Genet.*, **27**, 155–164 (1975).
12. Jussawalla, D. J., Yeole B. B., and Natekar, M. V. Cancer in children in Greater Bombay (1964–72), a comparative study. *Indian J. Cancer*, **12**, 135–143 (1975).
13. Kobayashi, N. (Committee of Children's Cancer Registry of Japan). Children's Cancer Registration in Japan, with special reference to prenatal factors. XVIII International Congress of Pediatrics, Honolulu, Hawaii, 1986.
14. Knudson, A. G., Jr. Mutation and cancer: statistical study of retinoblastoma. *Proc. Natl.*

Acad. Sci. U.S.A., **68**, 820–823 (1971).

15. Knudson, A. G., Jr. and Strong, L. C. Mutation and cancer: a model for Wilms' tumor of the kidney. *J. Natl. Cancer Inst.*, **48**, 313–324 (1972).

16. Kramer, S., Meadows, A. T., and Evans, J. P. The incidence of childhood cancer: experience of a decade in a population-based registry. *J. Natl. Cancer Inst.*, **70**, 49–55 (1983).

17. Kramer, S., Meadows, A. T., and Jarrett, P. Racial variation in incidence of Wilms' tumor: relationship to congenital anomalies. *Med. Pediat. Oncol.*, **12**, 401–405 (1984).

18. Kuroki, Y. and Konishi, H. Current status and perspectives in the Kanagawa Birth Defects Monitoring Program (KAMP). *Congenital Anomalies*, **24**, 385–393 (1984).

19. Matsuoka, K. The aniridia-Wilms' tumor syndrome, report of a case and interstitial deletion of 11p13. *Jpn. J. Pediatr. Surg.*, **19**, 97–107 (1983) (in Japanese with English abstract).

20. Matsunaga, E. Genetics of Wilms' tumor. *Hum. Genet.*, **57**, 231–246 (1981).

21. Maurer, H. S., Pendergrass, T. W., Borges, W., and Honig, G. R. The role of genetic factors in the etiology of Wilms' tumor. *Cancer*, **43**, 205–208 (1979).

22. McWhirter, W. R. Queensland Childhood Malignancy Registry, Fourth annual report 1983, Queensland Cancer Fund.

23. Meadows, A. T. Wilms' tumor in three children of a woman with congenital hemihypertrophy. *N. Engl. J. Med.*, **291**, 23–25 (1974).

24. Michaelis, J. (Projektgruppe Pädiatrische Onkologie) IMSD-Techinischer 1/86, Klinikum der Johannes Gutenberg-Universität, Mainz, Juni (1986).

25. Miller, R. W., Fraumeni, J. F., Jr., and Manning, M. D. Association of Wilms' tumor with aniridia, hemihypertrophy and other congenital malformations. *N. Engl. J. Med.*, **270**, 922–927 (1964).

26. Nakagome, Y., Ise, T., Sakurai, M., Nakajo, T., Okamoto, E., Takano, T., Nakahori, Y., Tsuchida, Y., Nagahara, N., Takada, Y., Ohsawa, Y., Sawaguchi, S., Toyosaka, A., Kobayashi, N., Matsunaga, E., and Saito, S. High-resolution studies in patients with aniridia-Wilms' tumor association, Wilms' tumor or related congenital abnormalities. *Hum. Genet.*, **67**, 245–248 (1984).

27. Nishihira, H. Children's cancer in Kanagawa Prefecture in 1981. *Child. Med. Center J.*, **12**, 62–63 (1983) (in Japanese).

28. Pastore, G., Magnai, C., Zanetti, R., and Terracini, B. Incidence of cancer in children in the province of Torino (Italy) 1967–1978. *Eur. J. Cancer Oncol.*, **17**, 1337–1341 (1981).

29. Pendergrass, T. W. Congenital anomalies in children with Wilms' tumor. *Cancer* **37**, 403–408 (1976).

30. Tsunoda, A., Nishi, H., Sasaki, Y., and Misugi, K. Bilateral Wilms' tumor (2nd report), nationwide survey. *Shouni Geka*, **13**, 1517–1524 (1981) (in Japanese).

31. Williams, A. O. Tumors of childhood in Ibadan, Nigeria. *Cancer*, **36**, 370–378 (1975).

32. Young, J. L. and Miller, R. W. Incidence of malignant tumors in U. S. children. *J. Pediat.*, **86**, 254–258 (1975).

NEUROFIBROMATOSIS

Kintomo TAKAKURA

*Department of Neurosurgery, University of Tokyo Hospital**

Statistical analysis, clinical manifestations and the outcome of treatment of intracranial neurofibromatosis of Recklinghausen disease in Japan are summarized based on the Japanese Brain Tumor Registry and our own clinical cases. The risk factor for development of various neoplasia in the central nervous system such as bilateral acoustic neurinoma, optic nerve glioma and multiple meningiomas is greater than in the ordinary population. The outcome of surgical treatment for acoustic neurofibromatosis has greatly improved recently due to microsurgical techniques and the development of imaging diagnosis such as computerized tomographic scan and magnetic resonance imaging. Further studies are required, however, to elucidate the genesis and to establish the essential therapeutic modalities for this disastrous intracranial neurofibromatosis.

Various hereditary tumors of the central nervous system are included in a group of disorders called neurocutaneous syndrome. Since this syndrome contains a variety of different disorders, Cairns (*1*) classified it into four groups: phakomatosis, developmental disorders, chromosomal disorders, and acquired systemic disorders. Many hereditary brain tumors are closely related to phakomatosis.

The term phakomatosis was initially introduced by van der Hoeve (*19*) in 1923 and its concept has been modified by several investigators since then. Kawamura (*8*) recently proposed the definition of phakomatosis as a disorder in which multiple naevus-like pathological changes (histological anomaly often showing a growth tendency) develop both on the skin and other organs and demonstrate an independent clinical features of

TABLE I. Phakomatosis and Related Fetal Cells (Based on Kawamura's Classification (*8*))

A. Generalized phakomatosis
  1. Bourneville-Pringle disease (tuberous sclerosis, epiloia) (M)
  2. Recklinghausen disease (neurofibromatosis) (NC)
  3. Hippel-Lindau syndrome (M)
  4. Angiomatosis (M)
  5. Neurocutaneous melanosis (mélanoses neurocutanées) (NC)
  6. Pentz-Jeghers syndrome (?)
  7. Pigmented vascular naevus (?)
  8. Basal cell naevus syndrome (Gorlin-Golts syndrome) (?)
B. Localized phakomatosis
  1. Sturge-Weber syndrome (M)
  2. Klippel-Weber syndrome (M)
  3. Oculo-maxillar pigmented naevus (Naevus Ohta) (NC)

M, mesodermal origin speculated; NC, neural crest origin speculated; ?, unknown origin.

* 7-3-1, Hongo, Bunkyo-ku, Tokyo 113, Japan (高倉公朋).

the disease. Although the genesis of phakomatosis is generally considered to be by genetic mutation of the cells during the fetal period, the pathological changes which appear should be considered differently for cellular systems developed by mutation (cells playing an initiative role in phakomatosis) and histological changes induced by those cells. Kawamura (9) classified various diseases of phakomatosis and postulated the original cells (phakomatoblast) involved in each disorder (Table I).

Tumors of the central nervous system frequently observed in neurosurgical clinics are neurofibromatosis in Recklinghausen disease, hemangioblastoma in Hippel-Lindau syndrome and astrocytoma in tuberous sclerosis (Bourneville-Pringle disease). Sturge-Weber syndrome and neurocutaneous melanosis sometimes require neurosurgical treatment. In this paper, clinical characteristics of the neurofibromatosis accompanying phakomatosis are presented.

Neurofibromatosis (Recklinghausen disease)

Recklinghausen disease is a hereditary disorder involving various symptoms including pigmented skin lesions, multiple neurofibromatosis, various tumors of the central nervous system and osteogenic changes. Cutaneous multiple fibromatosis was originally reported by Tilesius (18) in 1793, and a case demonstrating multiple tumors in the central nervous system was first reported by Wishart (20) in 1822. The precise clinicopathological features of generalized fibromatosis were presented by von Recklinghausen (11) in 1882, who clarified that the tumors in skin and nervous system originated from the connective tissue of Schwann cells. He, however, neglected a famous symptom of café-au-lait spots in this disease and thought that tumors in the central nervous system rarely accompanied the disease. Cutaneous pigmentation, however, soon attracted the attention of many physicians and, since introduction of van der Hoeve's concept of phakomatosis (19) this disease has been considered as a syndrome origi-

TABLE II.   Neurological Disorders of Recklinghausen Disease (Canale and Bebin (2))

I.   Tumors of peripheral nerves
   Neurofibroma, plexiform neurofibroma, dermal nodules, ganglioneuroma, malignant neurofibroma and schwannoma
II.   Spinal tumors
   A.   Extra-medullary tumors
   Schwannoma, neurofibroma, ganglioneuroma, meningioma
   B.   Intra-medullary tumors
   Astrocytoma, ependymoma, hamartomatous lesions
III.   Intra-cranial tumors
   A.   Cerebral, cerebellar, and brain stem tumors
   Astrocytoma, grade I-IV, polar-spongioblastoma, optic nerve glioma, diffuse gliomas (gliomatosis), hamartomatous lesions
   B.   Tumors of cranial nerves
   Neurofibroma, schwannoma, ganglioneuroma, retinoblastoma
   C.   Tumors of meninges
   Meningioma, hamartomatous lesions
IV.   Hamartomatous lesions (Russell and Rubinstein)
   Schwannosis, meningiomatosis, angiomatosis, glial heterotopias
V.   Miscellaneous lesions
   Meningoceles, spinal cord anomalies, syringomyelia, hydrocephalus, myelopathy associated with skeletal defects

nating from developmental abnormality of the ectodermal cellular system. Since Schwann cells are originated from the neural crest, this disease has recently been considered a developmental disorder of the neural crest.

Horton (6) classified Recklinghausen disease in three forms in 1976: peripheral form, central form, and mixed variety. A number of pathological changes are found in the central nervous system in this disease. Canale and Bebin (2) described various tumors appearing in the nervous system (Table II). In peripheral nerves, multiple neurofibromatoses are generally present and neurinoma (schwannoma, neurilemoma) occasionally develops; sometimes demonstrating malignant transformation. In the spinal cord, neurinoma, neurofibroma as well as meningioma and intramedullary astrocytoma or ependymoma frequently develop. Various tumors also develop intracranially, in which neurofibroma, meningioma, and astrocytoma are often encountered. The incidence of tumors accompanying Recklinghausen disease has been reported by several investigators: 2.7% (4/150 cases by Niimura (10)), 11.3% (188/1,657 cases, Japanese cases (10)), and 5–10% (by Riccardi (12)). In autopsied cases, a higher incidence of intracranial tumors accompanying Recklinghausen disease has been reported: 44% (45/102 cases, Japanese autopsied cases (10)) and 47% (35/74 by Horie et al. (5)).

General Statistics of Neurofibromatosis (Recklinghausen disease) in Japan

A study group on neurocutaneous syndrome was organized with research funds from the Ministry of Health and Welfare, and recently reported its preliminary results on the epidemiology of Recklinghausen disease in Japan (14). Out of 936 cases of the disease, 483 cases (51.6%) were reported by dermatologists, 94 cases (10.4%) by pediatricians, 91 cases (9.7%) by plastic surgeons, 86 cases (9.2%) by orthopedists and 84 cases (9.0%) by neurosurgeons. There was no sex difference of incidence (male: female 453: 478). The diagnosis of Recklinghausen disease was established in 21% of patients under 5 years of age, in 25% from 5 to 15 years and in 25% between 15 and 30 years. Familial incidence of Recklinghausen disease was proved in 35.6% of these patients, and familial marriage of the parents was noted in 1.4%.

From dermatological points of view, café-au-lait spots were observed in 80% of the patients and cutaneous neurofibromatosis in 58%. The deformity was present in 5.0% of the patients in the skull, 14.4% in the spine and thoracic bones and 4.5% in their extremities. Neurological examinations revealed neurological symptoms in 13.1%, epileptic seizure in 6.0% and mental retardation in 8.8% of the patients. Regarding tumors of the central nervous system, brain tumors (mainly acoustic neurofibromatosis) were found in 8.5%, spinal cord tumors in 5.6% and optic nerve glioma in 1.7%. Accompanying disorders included hypertension, which was noted in 4.6%, cardiovascular diseases in 2.4%, renal failures in 1.1%, cerebrovascular disease in 1.3%, hepatic diseases in 0.9%, and diabetes mellitus in 0.2% of the patients. During this survey, 12 patients (6 of each sex) died, the direct cause of death being neoplasm in 7 patients and unknown in 2 of them.

Intracranial Neurofibromatosis

Neurofibromatosis is the most frequently observed intracranial neoplasm involved with phakomatosis, and constitutes more than half of the brain tumors accompanying

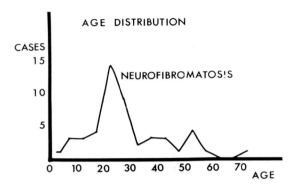

FIG. 1. Age distribution of the onset of intracranial neurofibromatosis

Recklinghausen disease. Neurofibromatosis generally develops in sensory nerves, usually in the acoustic nerves and, to a lesser degree in trigeminal or lower cranial nerves.
The prominent feature of acoustic tumors which accompany Recklinghausen disease
is the bilateral development of the tumor (75%, Japanese registry (10)). General incidences of bilateral acoustic tumors have been reported to be 4.9% (18/369 cases, Shimizu et al. (13)), and 3.9% (4/103 cases, Kasantikul et al. (7)); these bilateral acoustic
tumors were only found in cases of Recklinghausen disease. On the other hand, it is
interesting to note that patients carrying bilateral acoustic neurofibromatosis rarely
demonstrate café-au-lait spots or marked cutaneous neurofibromatosis (22).

The clinical characteristics of intracranial neurofibromatosis are as follows:

1)   No sexual difference of incidence: General acoustic neurinoma develops more
often in female than male: the sex ratio is 1: 1.6 (male: female, 504: 807 cases from the
All Japanese Brain Tumor Registry (17)), and 1: 1.3 (our cases (15)). However, No sex
difference was found in acoustic tumors in Recklinghausen disease (36: 39 from the
Japanese Brain Tumor Registry (37)).

2)   Onset of symptoms at young age: although the peak incidence of general neurinoma
appears at between 40 and 50 years of age, the peak of neurofibromatosis in Recklinghausen disease is found at between 20 and 30 years (Fig. 1). Eldridge (3) reported that
the average age of onset of bilateral acoustic tumors (50 cases) was 20.4 years, and 51%
(112/220 cases) of the cases appearing in the literature had developed initial symptoms
before the age of 25.

3)   Familial incidence: all cases of bilateral acoustic neurofibromatosis were found in
Recklinghausen disease and all had hereditary backgrounds.

4)   Frequent incidence of multiple tumors: multiple meningiomas are also often encountered in Recklinghausen disease.

5)   Impairment of auditory acuity as an initial symptom: the most frequent initial
symptom is an impairment of auditory acuity, especially bilateral dysfunction. Eldridge
(3) reported that more than half of the initial symptoms were bilateral disturbance of
auditory acuity and only one fifth of the patients complained of impaired auditory acuity
on one side. It is not rare, however, that neurofibroma develops only on one side of the
acoustic nerves. When acoustic tumors are found in patients under 20 years old, Recklinghausen disease should be the first consideration.

TABLE III. Familial Incidence of Brain Tumors (Japanese Brain Tumor Registry (16))

Familial incidence, 56 families/total number of brain tumors, 19,580 cases	
Phakomatosis	26
Hippel-Lindau syndrome	17
Recklinghausen disease	8
Bourneville-Pringle disease	1
Concordant cases	14
Medulloblastoma	4
Astrocytoma	4
Meningioma	3
Pituitary adenoma	2
Pineal teratoma	1
Discordant cases	16
Astrocytoma+others	6
Pituitary adenoma+others	3
Glioblastoma+others	2
Ependymoma+others	2
Others	2

TABLE IV. Multiple Tumors in Brain Tumor Patients (Japanese Brain Tumor Registry (17))

	Number of primary brain tumors	Neurinoma	Neurofibro-matosis
Total number of cases	10,215	765	50
Multiple tumors in nervous system	37 (0.4%)	6 (0.8%)	3 (6.0%)
Multiple tumors in other organs	179 (1.8)	16 (2.1)	5 (10.0)

1. Familial incidence of intracranial neurofibromatosis and other brain tumors

Intracranial neurinoma constitutes 7.5% (1,314 cases) and neurofibromatosis of Recklinghausen disease constitutes 0.5% (75 cases) of the 15,839 verified brain tumors listed in the Japan Brain Tumor Registry (17). The term neurinoma in this report is applied to a tumor with no relationship to Recklinghausen disease. Neurinoma is a synonym of schwannoma or neurilemoma. The term neurofibromatosis is applied to multiple tumors associated with Recklinghausen disease. It is generally difficult to differentiate neurinoma and neurofibromatosis by histological or electron microscopical findings.

The familial incidence of brain tumors was also studied statistically by the All Japan Brain Tumor Registry (16). Out of 19,580 brain tumors, 56 families had multiple brain tumor patients among their members (Table III), such as two families with brothers suffering from medulloblastoma.

The genesis of neural crest tumors including neurofibromatosis is thought to be mutation of a gene during the development of neural crest, and the development of multi-focal (centric) or multiple tumors (different histological types of tumor) is known to be more frequent in patients with neural crest tumors than in the ordinary population. The frequency of multi-focal or multiple tumors in the central nervous system and multiple tumors in various organs is shown in Table IV. From 10,215 cases of primary brain tumors, 37 multi-focal brain tumors (0.4%) and 179 multiple tumors (1.8%) in various organs (e.g., astrocytoma in brain and lung adenocarcinoma) were found. Out of 765 cases of intracranial neurinomas, there were 6 multi-focal brain tumors

(0.8%) and 16 cases of multiple tumors (2.1%). On the other hand, out of 50 cases of intracranial neurofibromatosis, 3 multi-focal brain tumors (6.0%) and 5 cases of multiple tumors (10.0%) were encountered. Our 369 cases of acoustic tumors revealed 15 cases of bilateral acoustic neurofibromatosis. Among those patients, 9 cases of spinal cord tumors, 4 cases of neurofibromatosis in lower cranial nerves (IX, X, XI, and XII), 2 cases of meningiomas and one case of intracranial arterio-venous malformation coexisted. Six cases had familial history of Recklinghausen disease. It is generally recognized that patients of neurofibromatosis often develop gliomas and meningiomas in the brain and spinal cord. Glushien *et al.* (*4*) reported that 5% of their patients with neurofibromatosis had pheochromocytoma. This combined evidence suggests that patients carrying intracranial neurofibromatosis have genetically high risk factors to develop various tumors.

2. *Clinical aspects of intracranial neurofibromatosis*

The clinical manifestations of neurofibromatosis may be divided into four groups (*21*). 1) Central neurofibromatosis: intradural tumors such as acoustic neurofibroma, optic glioma or meningioma without peripheral manifestations. 2) Peripheral neurofibromatosis: multiple cutaneous and peripheral nerve neurofibromatosis. 3) Visceral neurofibromatosis: neurofibromatosis, ganglioglioma, and neurinoma arising from the visceral autonomic system. 4) Forme fruste: a mild expression of the syndrome.

In this report, the clinical aspects of central neurofibromatosis are summarized. Intracranial neurofibromatosis develops most dominantly in acoustic nerves. Bilateral involvement is quite often encountered. The initial signs and symptoms are tinnitus and lowering of auditory acuity. As a tumor grows, deafness, cerebellar ataxia, nystagmus, and headaches develop. The widening and destruction of the internal acoustic meatus is visualized by a simple or tomographic X-ray examination of the skull. The auditory evoked potential (AEP) is able to detect a minor dysfunction of the acoustic nerve by revealing an abnormally low amplitude of the first wave corresponding to the

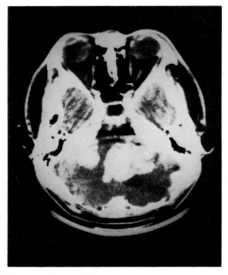

FIG. 2. CT-scan of neurofibromatosis in bilateral acoustic nerves

function of cochlear nerve and an extended interpeak latency between the first to third waves. AEP is the most sensitive examination for detecting small neurofibromatosis of the acoustic nerve, but the abnormal finding is not specific to this tumor. The morphological diagnosis must be established by computerized tomographic scans or magnetic resonance imaging (MRI). Figure 2 demonstrates a CT-scan of bilateral acoustic neurofibromatosis found in a patient of Recklinghausen disease. Intracranial neurofibromatosis often involves lower cranial nerves other than an acoustic nerve.

The only method of treatment for intracranial neurofibromatosis is surgical removal of the tumor. There are, however, several problems in deciding whether surgical treatment is appropriate. When a tumor is small in size, the preservation of auditory acuity might be possible, but when a tumor is quite large or has invaded the cochlear nerve, auditory acuity remains impaired after surgery. When a tumor involves lower cranial nerves, the possibility of swallowing and speech disturbance or the risk of developing pneumonia increases post-operatively. Those problems are not so serious in cases of acoustic neurinoma at only one side. Due to such post-operative complications, the long-term outcome of patients having bilateral neurofibromatosis was previously extremely poor compared to neurinomas. However, surgical techniques greatly improved after introduction of a microscope for neurosurgery in the middle of the 1970s. The 5-year survival rate of patients with bilateral neurofibromatosis increased dramatically. Long-term results of surgical treatment for patients with neurinoma and neurofibromatosis accompanying Recklinghausen disease (17) are summarized in Fig. 3. The 5-year survival rate of neurofibromatosis patients treated during the 5 years from 1969 to 1973 was 34.4%, while for those treated between 1974 and 1978 it improved to 77.0%. The main causes of this improvement were the introduction of microsurgery and CT-scan for precise morphological diagnosis. During the same periods, the 5-year survival rate of neurinoma patients improved from 78.6% to 90.0%. Radiotherapy or chemotherapy have not yet been proved effective in curing intracranial neurofibromatosis, and further basic research on neurofibromatosis is required to establish a new way of treating those afflicted with this condition. Besides acoustic neurofibromatosis, meningioma or glioma often develops in patients of Recklinghausen disease; Fig. 4 demonstrates CT-scans of intracranial meningiomatosis (multiple meningiomas) found in a 26-year old female patient. Meningiomatosis or neurofibromatosis develops not only intracranially but also in the spinal canal. Congenital optic nerve gliomas also some-

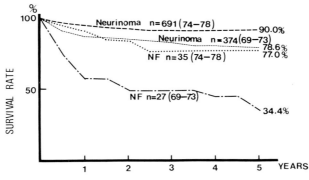

Fig. 3.   Historical improvement in 5-year survival rates of intracranial neurinoma and neurofibromatosis (NF)

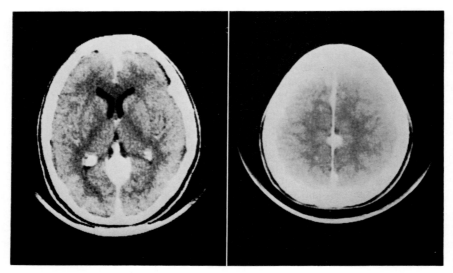

FIG. 4.   CT-scans of meningiomatosis (multiple meningioma) in a patient with Recklinghausen disease

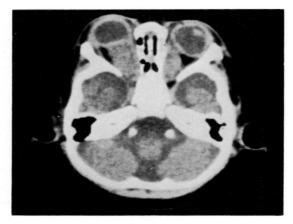

FIG. 5.   CT-scan of bilateral optic nerve glioma in a 2-year old girl accompanying Recklinghausen disease

times develop in patients of Recklinghausen disease; Fig. 5 shows a CT-scan of a 2-year old girl. There are clinically two types of optic nerve glioma. A benign type can be successfully treated by radiotherapy with or without partial resection of the tumor, while a malignant type has low sensitivity to radiation and grows rapidly like other malignant astrocytomas and requires adjuvant chemotherapy treatment. The long-term outcome of optic nerve glioma patients is generally favorable except those with the malignant type.

3.   Bony deformity of neurofibromatosis

Bony deformity of skull, spine, and extremities is a disastrous manifestation of neurofibromatosis, and its cause is not well known. Since the tumor cells do not usually

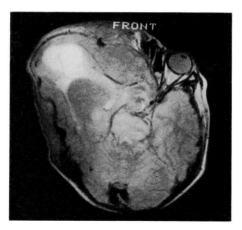

FIG. 6. Magnetic resonance image of a skull deformity with exophthalmos accompanying Recklinghausen disease in a 9-year old boy

invade the affected bone, the genesis of the deformity is thought to be a genetic defect. Deformity of the skull and face is often encountered in patients of Recklinghausen disease. Exophthalmos due to a defect in the orbital roof is not as common but is a well-known manifestation of Recklinghausen disease. The reason for treatment of the skull deformity is not only cosmetic but also to save visual acuity. Figure 6 shows a MRI of the skull deformity in a 9-year-old boy with Recklinghausen disease. His mother also has this disease. This patient had severe right exophthalmos and a marked bulging of his right temporal bone. Various bony anomalies including defects in the sphenoid wing, other parts of the skull, orbital deformity, kyphoscoliosis and generalized café-au-lait spots were also present. CT-scan and MRI revealed a marked non-communicating asymmetrical hydrocephalus with small fourth ventricle and prominent meningoencephalocele protruding into his right orbit and temporal region. Walter E. Dandy (1886–1946) performed the first successful surgical treatment of such a skull deformity, reconstructing the defective orbital roof with an autologous bone graft. Many successful surgical treatments have since been reported with minor modification in cranioplastic materials and operative approach. We performed reconstructive surgery on this boy to repair his fronto-temporo-orbital bony defect which accompanied the severe exophthalmos. The material used for the reconstruction was a coarse stainless steel mesh reinforced with acrylic, and proved satisfactory in reconstructing the large complicated bony defect fairly well in the desired shape.

There is controversy regarding reconstructive surgery for bony defects of the skull in patients of Recklinghausen disease as to when to operate and what kind of materials should be used. Early operation seems advocated because the herniation of the brain into the orbit gradually progresses, resulting in more severe exophthalmos or craniofacial deformity. In very young patients, however, the decision on when to operate might be difficult. The materials which have been used are autologous bone graft, tantalum mesh, acrylic with mesh, and other foreign materials. Among these, autologous bone graft seems to be preferable an advantage over others. However, if the bony defect is large, it is not always possible to get a sufficient amount of autologous bone graft. Using stainless steel mesh as a framework for the cranioplasty and coating it with acrylic for fortification, a time saving reconstruction could be performed with good strength and cosmetically satisfactory outcome.

CONCLUSION

Statistical analysis of intracranial neurofibromatosis is summarized in this report, based on the large number of cases listed in the Japanese Brain Tumor Registry and our own cases. The risk factor for developing various neoplasms in the central nervous system and other organs in patients of neurofibromatosis is greater than in the ordinary population. Clinical aspects of intracranial neurofibromatosis and the outcome of surgical treatment were reported. Although much progress has recently been achieved in the survival rate for intracranial neurofibromatosis, further studies are required to elucidate the genesis of neurofibromatosis and to establish the essential therapeutic modalities for this disastrous disease.

Acknowledgments
This work was partly supported by the Cancer Research Fund of the Ministry of Health and Welfare of Japan, and the Research Fund for the study of neurocutaneous syndrome from the same Ministry. The assistance of Mrs. Haruko Sano in preparing the manuscript is also gratefully acknowledged.

REFERENCE

1. Cairns, R. J. The skin and nervous system. *In* "Textbook of Dermatology," ed. A. Rook *et al.*, pp. 1791–1818 (1972). Blackwell, Oxford.
2. Canale, D. J. and Bebin, J. von Recklinghausen disease of the nervous system. *In* "Handbook of Clinical Neurology," ed. P. J. Vinken and G. W. Bruyn, Vol. 14, pp. 132–162 (1972). North-Holland, Amsterdam.
3. Eldridge, R. Central neurofibromatosis with bilateral acoustic neuroma. *Adv. Neurol.*, **29**, 57–65 (1981).
4. Glushien, A. S., Mansuy, M. M., and Littman, D. S. Pheochromocytoma. *Am. J. Med.*, **14**, 317–327 (1953).
5. Horie, A., Shigemi, U., Fukushima, T., and Tanaka, K. Neurofibromatosis complicated by intracranial tumors. *Acta Pathol. Jpn.*, **24**, 705–716 (1974).
6. Horton, W. A. Genetics of central nervous system tumors. *Birth Defects*, **12** 91–97 (1976).
7. Kasantikul, V., Netsky, M. G., Glasscock, M. E., and Hays, J. W. Acoustic neurilemmoma, clinicoanatomical study of 103 patients. *J. Neurosurg.*, **52**, 28–35 (1980).
8. Kawamura, T. Neurocutaneous syndrome. *Brain Nerve*, **26**, 145–159 (1974).
9. Kawamura, T. Tumors of melanocyte system. *In* "Modern Dermatology," ed. Y. Yamamura *et al.*, Vol. 11, pp. 143–158 (1982). Nakayama Shoten, Tokyo.
10. Niimura, N. Recklinghausen disease. *Clin. Dermatol.*, **15**, 973–982 (1973).
11. von Recklinghausen, F. "Über die multipler Fibrome der Haut und ihre Beziehung zu den multiplen Nueromen," (1882) Hirschwàld, Berlin.
12. Riccardi, V. M. Von Recklinghausen neurofibromatosis. *N. Engl. J. Med.*, **305**, 1617–1627 (1981).
13. Shimizu, H., Masuzawa, H., and Sano, K. Bilateral acoustic tumor: Its clinical features and surgical treatment. *Neurol. Med. Chir.*, **19**, 623–627 (1979).
14. Takagi, H., Inaba, Y., Takahashi, T., Niimura, N., and Nakauchi, Y. Intermediate report of Second All Japan Epidemiological Study. Reported by the Study Group Meeting on

Neurocutaneous Syndrome. Ministry of Health and Welfare, Tokyo (1987).

15. Teramoto, A., Manaka, S., and Takakura, K. Sex difference of primary brain tumors. *Brain Nerve*, **35**, 869–875 (1983).

16. The Committee of Brain Tumor Registry in Japan. "Brain Tumor Registry in Japan," Vol. 5 (1984).

17. The Committee of Brain Tumor Registry in Japan. "Brain Tumor Registry in Japan," Vol. 3 (1981). National Cancer Center, Tokyo.

18. Tilesius, W. G. "Historia Pathologia Singularis Cutis Turpitudinis," Leipzig (1793).

19. van der Hoeve, J. Eye disease in tuberous sclerosis of the brain and in Recklinghausen's disease. *Trans. Ophthal. Soc. U. K.*, **43**, 534–541 (1923).

20. Wishart, J. Case of tumors of the skull, dura mater and brain. *Edinb. Med. J.*, **18**, 393–397 (1822).

21. Youmans, J. R. and Ishida, W. Y. Tumors of peripheral and sympathetic nerves. *In* "Neurological Surgery," ed. J. R. Youmans, 2nd ed., pp. 3299–3315 (1982). W. B. Saunders, Philadelphia.

22. Young, D. F., Eldridge, R., and Gardner, W. J. Bilateral acoustic neuroma in a large kindred. *JAMA*, **214**, 347–353 (1970).

CANCER-PRONE HEREDITARY DISEASES AND FAMILIAL CANCER

XERODERMA PIGMENTOSUM: DNA REPAIR DEFICIENCY AND THE CURRENT STATUS OF CELLULAR AND MOLECULAR APPROACHES*

Yoshisada FUJIWARA

*Department of Radiation Biophysics, Kobe University School of Medicine**

Xeroderma pigmentosum (XP) A and variant groups are the major groups in 92 assigned XP patients in Japan, despite recent increase in numbers in other rare groups. The cancer incidence is very high, in accordance with the higher mutagenic effects of both pyrimidine dimers and (6–4) photoproducts in XP cells. XP-A and D, but not XP-C, patients have neurologic defects, though Japanese XP-D cases lack severe neurologic defects. In the XP groups overall, greater defective dimer excision from the DNA correlates with greater UV hypersensitivity of XP cells. XP-A and G cells are almost completely defective, while XP-C cells can perform domain-limited repair, in contrast to the dispersed residual repair in XP-D cells. XP-E and F cells have leaky repair, and the latter may lack only the early rapid repair response. Upon fusion, XP-C and D factors are slow-complementing. Studies on the cell-free extract for dimer excision and repair restoration by microinjection into XP cells suggest, though they do not prove, that XP factors rather than UV endonuclease(s) may be defective. Any definite statement is premature about human repair genes, mutations in multiple XP genes, and the direct or indirect role of XP products (UV nucleases or regulating factors?) in molecular DNA repair.

Xeroderma pigmentosum (XP) is a rare autosomal recessive, UV-sensitive and cancer-susceptible disorder. Some XP patients have progressive neurologic defects. Since Cleaver's first discovery in 1968 of defective nucleotide excision repair in XP cells (5), great progress has been made in understanding the basic cellular and molecular mechanisms of DNA repair and the defects of these in XP. Many excellent reviews on XP have appeared (6, 9, 15, 16, 31, 32, 46). This report primarily updates the XP data gathered between 1983 and 1986.

Compilation of Japanese XP Patients, Carcinogenesis, and Neurologic Defects

XP consists currently of the 9 excision-defective complementation groups (A through I) identified by the complementation analysis in the fused heterokaryons, and one excision-proficient XP variant group. Table I contains the January 1987 compilation of 92 definitely identified XP cases from Japan. Worldwide, groups A, C, D, and variant are more common, groups E and F are rare, and groups B, G, H, and I are very rare (20, 31, 32, 50). Compared with the major groups C, A, D, and variant in the U.S./Europe/Egypt (31, 32, 50), the current characteristic status in Japan, is a 69% preva-

---

* 7-5-1, Kusunoki-cho, Chuo-ku, Kobe 650, Japan (藤原美定).

TABLE I. DNA Repair, Cell Sensitivity, Clinical Phenotype, and Frequency in Japan of the XP Groups

Complementation groups	DNA repair deficiency			UV sensitivity[d]			Clinical phenotype			Assigned cases in Japan[e]	Intra-group heterogenous strains (representative)
	% UDS[a]	% breaks induced by araC/HU[b]	% ESS loss[c]	n	D_0 (J/m²)	$\frac{D_0(N)}{D_0(XP)}$	Skin sympt.	Neurologic defect	Skin cancers		
A	<5	5	0	1.0	0.3–0.5	15	Severe	+ (−)	+	32	XP8LO (36% UDS), XP1BE (15% UDS)
B XP11BE[f] (XP/Cockaye)	3–7	5[g]					Severe	+	+	0	
C	10–20	10–20	10	1.0	1.0	5	Severe	− (+)	+	5	XP5RO (30% UDS), XP8MA (43% UDS)
D	20–50	10–20	0–15	1.0	0.7	7	Severe	+	+	5	
E	40–60	40–60	40–60	1.4	2.2–2.4	2	Mild/moderate	−	+	6	
F	10–15	10–20	60	1.2	1.7	3	Mild	−	+	12	
G XP2BI, XP3BR	<5	0	0	1.0	0.6	8	Severe	+	+	1	XP38KO (25% UDS)
H GM3248 (XP/Cockaye)	30			1.0	0.3	15	Severe	+	+	0	XP31KO (25% UDS)
I[h]	15–25						Severe	+	+	0	
Variant	75–100	140–200	100	1.5	2.4–4.5	2	Mild	−	+	31	
Normals	100	100	100	1.5	5.0					(Total 92)	

a Autoradiographic UDS after a 3 hr [³H]thymidine labeling following 10 J/m², relative to normal.

b Alkaline sucrose single-strand breaks accumulated during a 4 hr incubation of 10 μM araC-plus-2.5 mM HU, relative to normal.

c Disappearance of T4 endonuclease-susceptible sites 24 hr after 10 J/m², relative to normal.

d From Fig. 1, except for D_0 of XP-I cited from ref. 14.

e Compiled from Takebe, Satoh, and our recent assignments. XP-A contains 2 recent prenatal XP44KO and XP51KO cases (Fujiwara et al., unpublished data). XP-C: XP2KA, XP3KA, XP40OS, XP40KO, XP21SE; XP-D: XP10TO, XP58TO, XP59TO, XP43KO, XP77TO; XP-E: XP24KO, XP26KO, XP70TO, XP80TO, XP81TO, XP82TO; XP-F: XP23OS, XP2YO, XP3YO, XP101OS, XP25KO, XP27KO, XP28KO, XP41KO, XP38KO, XP46KO, XP13NA, XP7KA; XP-G: XP31KO. The final number of assigned Japanese cases in each group was kindly made available by Dr. Y. Satoh, Department of Dermatology, Tokyo Medical and Dental University.

f From ref. 32.

g From ref. 59.

h From ref. 14.

i Most XP variants worldwide show a normal level of UDS, while 5 out of 8 XP variants in the Mannheim series exhibit low levels of 40–70% UDS (27b).

TABLE II. Characteristics of XP-D Patients in Japan

Patient[a]	Age at assignment and sex	Neurologic manifestation	Skin symptoms	Skin neoplasms	DNA repair phenotype as XP-D	Source
XP10TO	51 M	None	Mild	SCC (41 yr)	Typical	Takebe, H.
XP58TO	8 M	Borderline loss of hearing	Mild	None	Typical	Satoh, Y.
XP59TO	6, F	None	Mild	None	Typical	Satoh, Y.
XP43KO	31 F	None	Mild	BCE (31 yr)	Typical	Ichihashi, M.
XP77TO	66 M	Slight loss of hearing	Mild	BCE, SCC (65 yr)	Typical	Satoh, Y.

[a] All other than XP10TO were assigned by the systematic complementation test (Y. Fujiwara).

lence of groups A (32/92=35%) and variant (31/92=34%), a relatively high incidence of group F (12/92=13%), still rare occurrences of groups C and D (5 each/92=5% each), and so far no incidence of groups B, H, and I. Despite recently increasing identification of cases of rare groups (C, D, E), these trends in Japan have not much changed from the previous status in 1978 (50) and 1985 (20). Total cases and clinical details are presented in another chapter by Satoh.

Incidence of skin cancers was abnormally high at 45% of the total cases: 33.5% basal epithelioma, 19.7% squamous cell carcinoma and 6.7% malignant melanoma (20). The highest skin oncogenesis in XP-A and XP-C patients occurred at the average age of about 10 years (20). A similarly high, delayed oncogenesis was observed in XP variants at the higher average age of about 40 years (20). The 3 out of 5 XP-D cases showed delayed tumorigenesis found at 31, 41, and 65 years, due presumably to unexpectedly mild skin lesions (Table II). Clinically mild Japanese XP-E, F, and G patients with higher residual repair also showed a lower delayed oncogenesis between 37 and 64 years. Thus, there is a good correlation between the extents of repair defect and carcinogenesis.

A variety of neurological abnormalities are associated with XP-A, B, D, G, H, and I (Table I). Such manifestation occurs by 7 years in XP-A (1, 32, 38, 45) and usually between 7 and 12 years in XP-D (delay to the second decade in some) (1, 35, 45), but not in XP-C (9, 20, 32). Robbins (45) has shown a good correlation between neurologic defects and greater fibroblast hypersensitivity in XP-A, B, D, and G. Among only 5 Japanese XP-D cases, however, 7-year-old XP58TO and 66-year-old XP77TO had slight hearing loss, but the others had no apparent complications between 6 and 51 years of age (Table II). Thus, unlike the U.S. / European cases, Japanese XP-D patients have a phenotypic deviation showing the absence, slightness or extremely delayed onset of neurologic manifestation, although the defective repair phenotype is similar. Heterogenous group G XP31KO (Table I) had no neurologic defect at age 37.

Recently Developed Mechanism for Excision Repair in Human Cells

Prokaryotic excision repair is fully understood, but the eukaryotic mechanism is still obscure in spite of extensive research. Cleaver (7) has recently studied the repair of excision gaps in detail by means of specific enzymatic digestion and polymerization/ligation. He has implied that the dimer excision mechanism in normal human cells is not the "patch and cut" mode (nick translation or strand displacement), but involves either oligonucleotide excision to leave a single-strand gap or widening of the gap to a size 10–25 bases long by the 5′–3′ exonuclease action. Such a gap is also a suitable substrate for DNA polymerase-α that is predominantly engaged in repair synthesis. Weinfeld et al. (56) have studied excised fragments from normal fibroblasts 24 hr after UV irradiation that were extracted in a 5% acid-soluble fraction. Such excision fragments were heterogenous in size, but 3.7 bases long on average, the photoreversal of which produced free thymidine (dT) and dTMP. The results led them to postulate that the initial step of the multistep excision repair in human cells may involve a cleavage of the intradimer phosphodiester linkage presumably by dimer phosphodiesterase (the enzyme not proven), followed by oligonucleotide excision. However, a possibility that such cleavage and shortening may occur in the post-excision fragments within cells cannot be excluded. This situation contrasts with the finding that no photoreleasable T is present in the dimer-containing excision fragments by Escherichia coli UVRABC complex (47a).

Correlation of Repair Defect with UV Hypersensitivity in XP

1)   XP repair defects

For heterogenous repair defects in XP (9, 20, 32, 50), we measured UV-induced unscheduled DNA synthesis (UDS) and loss of T4 endonuclease V-sensitive sites (ESS). Table I summarizes our results with others. Regarding the ESS loss (dimer exision) during a 24 hr period after 10 J/m², groups A, B, C, D, and G cells had extremely low rates of ESS loss at 0–15% of normal cells, as described previously (19, 20, 59). Groups A, B, C, and G cells showed correspondingly low levels of 1–20% UDS during the initial 3 hr period, except for a higher residual level of 20–50% UDS in XP-D cells. Heterogenous XP strains within the same groups which show higher residual levels of UDS are, for example, group A XP8LO (36% UDS) and XP1BE (15% UDS), group C XP5RO (30% UDS), group F XP38KO (25% UDS), and group G XP31KO (25% UDS) (Table I). XP-E cells had comparable levels of 60% dimer excision (ESS loss) in 24 hr and 40–60% UDS in 3–4 hr (22, 24, 58), showing a leaky excision activity. XP-F cells had a low level of 10–15% UDS during the initial 3 hr, but a disproportionately higher level of 60% ESS loss in 24 hr (21, 24, 58). Such a characteristic phenotype of group F arises only from the normal slow repair in the specific absence of the early rapid repair phase (21, 24, 59). XP-H GM3248 (41) and XP-I XP3MA (14) showed higher residual UDS (15–30%). Therefore, group A through I cells have defective incision, as supported by evidence that introduced T4 or Micrococcus luteus UV endonuclease catalyzed incision and restored otherwise defective UDS in groups A through I (11, 51). Mitchell et al. (39) have shown by using the polyclonal antibody specific to (6-4)photoproducts that XP-A, C, and D cells have negligible repair of Pyr(6-4)Pyo, although normal cells remove 75% within 4 hr at a rate faster than that for cyclobutane dimers. Complete monomerization of dimers in the pSV2catSVgpt still left 30% lethal hits in the cat gene of the plasmid grown in XP-A cells, but no hit when grown in normal cells (43), also indicating the defective Pyr(6-4)Pyo repair in XP-A cells.

1-β-D-Arabinofuranosyl cytosine (araC)-plus-hydroxyurea (HU) present after UV-irradiation inhibits the filling by polymerization/ligation of excision gaps and accumulates single-strand breaks (13). With this method, the less early-time UDS and 24 hr-ESS loss correlate with the lower accumulation of such excision breaks in XP cells,

despite exceptions in XP-D and F (Table I). XP variants show excessive 140–200%
accumulations of breaks in the presence of araC/HU (26) (Table I), which have been
ascribed to defective post-incision resynthesis and ligation (13).

2) Hypersensitive response to the lethal effect of 254 nm UV
   In exponentially growing conditions, the typical strains of XP-A, D, G, and H
exhibited 7–15 times more hypersensitivity to UV killing than did normal human cells,
based on the mean lethal dose (*Do*) comparison (Fig. 1, Table I). Surprisingly, XP-H
GM3248 strain, an XP/CS double mutant (41), displayed an extremely UV-hypersensi-
tive phenotype (Fig. 1), suggesting that GM3248 cells may be almost completely defective in dimer excision (not tested) despite having 30% UDS. Another XP/CS double
mutant, XP-B XP11BE, has been reported to be very UV-sensitive (46). Most of the
XP-C strains exhibited less hypersensitivity (*n*=1, *Do*=1.0 J/m²) than most group
A strains (Fig. 1, Table I). Sensitivity of XP-I XP3MA cells resembles that of XP-C
cells (14). XP-E and F cells with leaky repair are only 2 and 3 times more sensitive,
respectively, than normal (Fig. 1, Table I). In the various XP groups generally, greater
defective repair of ESS (dimers) correlates well with greater UV hypersensitivity.
   In non-dividing cells, survival curves of dye-excluded cells have shown that XP-A
and D cells are also very UV-sensitive (29), as found in the clonogenic survival curves

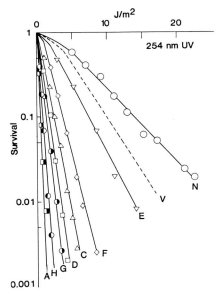

FIG. 1. Clonogenic 254 nm UV survival of log-growth phase fibroblasts of all XP
groups except groups B and I
   The method has been described (21). The strains used were: ○ N (normals):
NHSF3, NHSF6, NHSF46, NHSF63, NHSFAS; ■ XP-A: XP6KO and 15 other
strains; △ XP-C: XP2KA, XP3KA, XP40KO, XP21SE; □ XP-D: XP6BE,
XP58TO, XP59TO, XP43KO, XP77TO; ▽ XP-E: XP2RO, XP24KO, XP26KO,
XP70KO; ◇ XP-F: XP25KO, XP27KO, XP28KO, XP2YO, XP3YO, XP46KO;
◗ XP-G: XP2BI; ◖ XP-H: GM3248; ---- XP variant: XP5TO and 10 other
strains. Each point was mean of repeats for all strains in a group. The *n* and *Do*
values are listed in Table I.

of exponentially growing cells (Fig. 1). However, non-dividing XP-C cells become more resistant (29) than those in log-growth phase (Fig. 1). The more effective recovery in XP-C cells than in XP-D cells in confluent or non-dividing state arises from the selective domain-limited repair in the former (see below).

Heterogeneity in DNA Damage Processing

1) Intragenomic repair heterogeneity in XP-C

Confluent XP-C cells (10–40% UDS) can perform preferential clustered repair at the normal rate only in some limited domains, but no apparent repair in bulk DNA, as first demonstrated by Mansbridge and Hanawalt (37) and confirmed later by others (30, 42). Such preferential repair is evidenced by the selective reduction in the T4 endonuclease V sensitivity of post-UV repaired domains. Mullenders et al. (42) have shown that domain-limited repair in XP-C is associated with attachment sites to the nuclear matrix, implying that such domains may include actively transcribing regions of DNA. However, XP-C cells remove little or no cyclobutane dimers from the active single-copy dihydrofolate reductase (DHFR) gene, while normal human cells remove 70–80% of the dimers from the gene in 24 hr (2). Thus, efficiently reparable domains of XP-C DNA may not include the essential DHFR gene, thus explaining the XP-C hypersensitivity, since UV survival of mammalian cells correlates with efficient repair of the vital gene (2). Further, in XP-C cells a dramatic change occurs from clustered repair at confluent phase to randomly dispersed repair at the proliferative phase (8). Such repair

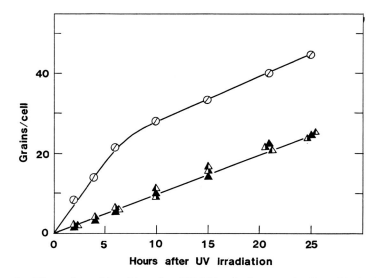

FIG. 2. The early rapid and late slow UDS kinetics in normal cells and lack of the early phase in XP-F strains

Log-phase cells were continuously labeled with [³H]thymidine of a relatively low specific activity and sampled at the indicated times for measurement of UDS (21). Normal cells (⊘) showed the early rapid repair until 6–8 hr, followed by the late, 4 times slower repair phase. XP-F cells lacked the former and showed only the latter (21). XP-F: ▲ XP25KO; ▲ XP27KO; ▲ XP28KO.

clustering in confluent XP-C cells facilitates more efficient recovery of post-UV RNA-synthesis and thus more efficient cellular recovery than does the randomly dispersed residual repair in XP-D cells (37). However, whether the XP-C gene mutation is structural or regulatory to result in a low-level repair or domain-limited accessibility, and which of the vital genes in XP-C cells are repaired preferentially remain to be elucidated. In CHO cells, 80% of the dimers are removed from the active DHFR gene, while only 10% are removed from an inactive DNA 30 kb upstream in 26 hr (2, 3). Altogether, change in the mammalian chromatin structure and gene expression will determine the accessibility of particular genomic regions to repair enzymes.

2) Kinetic heterogeneity in XP-F

In normal human cells, excision repair itself is inherently processive and non-random (10), and the repair kinetics shows the early rapid and late slow phases (21, 59). In the rapid phase with nucleosomal rearrangement that involves about 70% repair, excisions and subsequent repair incorporations are more enahnced in linker DNA and in both core-DNA ends than in the central core regions (34). The rapid phase may be controlled by nucleosomal constraint at an early time, and the slow phase by randomization via slow nucleosomal movement at a later time.

XP-F cells show a 10–15% low UDS in 3 hr, but a disproportionately higher level of about 60% dimer removal in 24 hr (21, 24, 58) (Table I). This arises from the particular repair kinetics of only normal slow repair due to the specific lack of early rapid repair (Fig. 2) (21, 58). Such a leaky repair differs from the proportionately 40%-lower repair throughout the early rapid and late slow phases in XP-E cells (21). Correction of UV-induced UDS in XP-F fibroblasts by introduction of UV endonucleases reaches 50% at most (11, 24). An XP-F gene product may be a specific regulator for the early rapid accessibility of damaged chromatin to the repair system.

DNA Repair in Chromatin by Cell-free Extracts

Some or all of the multiple XP gene products may form a complex to incise DNA or to render damaged chromatin accessible to catalytically active nucleases for uncleotide excision repair. Mortelmans et al. (40), Friedberg et al. (17) and we (18, 28) showed that cell-free extracts of XP fibroblasts catalyzed thymine dimer excision from the exogenous DNA, but not from the DNA present in endogenous cell sonicates and that catalysis required Mg^{2+}. Further, we analyzed the dimer excision from various chromatin preparations of XP cells by their own cell-free extracts under the previously described conditions (18, 28). Table III shows the result by thin layer chromatography (TLC) analysis of dimer excision. Extracts of normal fibroblasts excised about 40% of dimers from all substrates (nuclear sonicate, native chromatin, nonhistone-depleted (0.35 M NaCl-treated) chromatin, and native DNA) during a 30-min incubation at 37°C (18, 28). However, extracts of XP-A, C, and G cells failed to excise thymine dimers from their own endogenous nuclear sonicates and native chromatin, but catalyzed them normally from nonhistone-deprived chromatin and naked DNA (18, 20, 28). Curiously, however, XP-D extract excised dimers normally from all such substrates, as indicated previously (17, 28). As far as the in vitro assay is concerned, therefore, XP groups A, C, D, and G cells may not be deficient in the activity of incision and dimer excision.

TABLE III. Catalysis of Thymine Dimer Excision from XP Chromatin by Cell-free Extracts

Substrate containing 5 μg DNA	Cell-free extract, mg/assay	% thymine dimer excised
NHSF6 and NHSF46 (normal)		
Nuclear sonicate	0.5	36
Native chromatin	0.4–0.6	25–40
DNA	0.4–0.6	30–45
XP6KO and XP2OS (group A)		
Nuclear sonicate	0.4–0.6	0–5
Native chromatin	0.4	5
Non-histone depleted chromatin	0.4–0.6	15–25
DNA	0.4	25–30
XP2KA (group C)		
Native chromatin	0.4	0
Non-histone depleted chromatin	0.4	25
DNA	0.4	30
XP2BI (group G)		
Native chromatin	0.4	0
Non-histone depleted chromatin	0.4	25
DNA	0.4	40

The *in vitro* combination of chromatin or DNA and cell-free extracts was incubated for 30 min at 37°C under standard conditions (*18, 28*) to assay for thymine dimers by thin layer chromatography.

Rather, XP-A, C, and G cells may be defective in "XP factors" to make damaged sites in chromatin accessible to repair enzymes. These factors can complement each other (*28*).

On the other hand, XP-A or XP-C extract is deficient in incising UV-irradiated circular DNA under Mg^{2+}-free conditions not optimal for dimer excision, but extract combination can complement for such incision (*25, 53*). Such an activity may differ from that for specific dimer excision, since the former can also incise γ-irradiated and osmium tetraoxide-treated DNA (*25*).

Characteristics of Complementing XP Factors by Fusion and Microinjection

In fused heterokaryons, allelic dose, gene expression and stability or turnover of gene products will affect the complementing effect. Giannelli *et al.* (*23*) have revealed the following characteristics in XP-A, C, and D: (i) XP-A factor is fast-complementing within 6 hr after fusion even in the absence of protein synthesis, in a 30-fold abundance in non-XP A cells, and moves freely from and to the nucleus or turns over rapidly. (ii) XP-C and D factors cause slow complementation which requires 16 hr and more than 24 hr, respectively, and is prevented by inhibition of protein synthesis. These two factors are in small amounts and do not move freely, but persist in the nucleus. We have also often observed slow and incomplete elevation of UDS in the XP-C/XP-D heterodikaryon (*22*) (Fujiwara, unpublished data).

Microinjection of wild-type HeLa and placenta extracts or complementing XP extracts into XP fibroblasts can restore UDS in all of the 9 XP groups (A through I), although elevated UDS levels vary greatly, depending on the XP sources used (*12, 55*). Partially purified XP-A factor is active in probably multimeric forms of 90 and 160 kD protein(s) (*57*). All XP factors in cell-free extracts are stable on storage and freezing

(12, 18, 55, 57), differing from the storage/freezing-sensitive mammalian UV endonuclease activity. Legerski *et al. (33)* have presented the first evidence that microinjection of HeLa polyA+ mRNA can complement XP-A cells (with 11S mRNA=700 bases) and XP-G cells (with 12S mRNA=900 bases), but not XP-D and F cells. They suggest that XP-A and G factors are present in a 30-fold excess, but XP-D and F factors may be limited in amount. In this regard, interestingly, the cytoplasmic and nuclear microinjections of *E. coli* UVRABCD nuclease complex have no effect on elevation of UV-induced UDS in XP-A and C cells *(60)*, although a normal level of UDS is attained by microinjection of UV-endonuclease into all XP groups *(51, 60)*.

Interspecies genetic complementation occurs between XP (A through I) and UV-sensitive CHO mutants *(48, 54)*. Thus, each gene defective in such CHO mutants differs from each of the XP genes. The recently cloned human ERCC-1 gene that complements the CHO 43-3B mutant cannot confer UV resistance on its transfected XP-A and F cells (van Duin, personal communication).

Recently, it has been shown that only XP-D cells do not complement the fibroblasts (~10% UDS) from some patients with autosomal recessive trichothiodystrophy with photosensitivity, which manifests brittle hair with low sulfur content, peculiar face, ichthyosis, and mental/physical retardations *(47b)*. This suggests that trichothiodystrophy is often associated with the XP-D gene defect: the two genes being in close proximity or the same gene being mutated at different sites to cause either or both, although the latter is far less likely.

Besides the unusual behavior of the cell-free excision system *(28)*, another curiosity is also seen in XP-D. A clone derived from UV-resistant HeLa/XP-D hybrids displayed the XP-D phenotype for its own cellular sensitivity and DNA repair, but retained

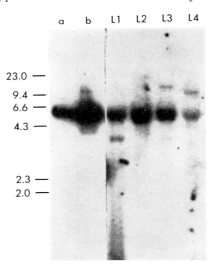

FIG. 3. Southern blot analysis of integrated pSV2neo sequence in XP2OS(SV) neo[r] transformants

Genomic DNA (10 μg/lane) purified after 28 divisions of more resistant large neo[r] clones (L1–L4) was restricted to completion with *Eco*RI (which cuts pSV2neo once), electrophoresed on agarose gel, and hybridized to the pSV2neo probe. All clones had 4–25 tandemly amplified copies of the 5.6 kb plasmids per cell at 2–3 different integration sites. Copy markers are 5 plasmid copies/cell (lane a) and 50 copies/cell (lane b). Uehara and Fujiwara, unpublished data.

normal hcr activity for UV-irradiated adenovirus 2 (*27a*). Such a complexity may arise either from dissociation of linkage of 2 XP-D genes by chromosome segregation, from differential activity of XP-D factor for sufficient support of only viral hcr (but not for cellular repair), or from different accessibility of viral DNA and cell chromatin.

DNA-mediated Gene Transfer to XP Cells

Only one study succeeded in conferring UV resistance (UV^r) on XP cells (*49*), while many extensive trials proved unfruitful. On the other hand, transfection of pSV2neo DNA to SV40-immortalized group A XP20S(SV) cells by the calcium precipitation method produced neo-resistant (neo^r) transformants at a fairly high frequency of ~5×10^{-4}/cell/μg DNA. Southern blot analysis of genomic DNA of XP20S(SV)neo^r cells revealed the integration of 2–25 tandemly amplified repeats of full-length pSV2neo DNA per cell at 1–3 different chromosomal sites (Uehara and Fujiwara, unpublished data), as shown in Fig. 3. However, only a single copy integration gave a very weak neo^r phenotype to XP20S(SV), suggesting a limited expression of the cloned gene under control of the SV40 promoter/enhancer in semipermissive human cells.

With the same strategy, we transfected a constructed human fibroblast cDNA library to XP20S(SV) cells and obtained several clones with partial UV^r after UV selection. The two phage clones of the library of genomic fragments from a UV^r XP20S(SV) transformant also conferred similar partial resistance on the parental line (*36*). Molecular study to identify this cDNA is now under way.

UV-induced Mutation in XP Cells

XP cells have been well documented to be hypermutable to UV. There have been arguments about the mutagenicity of cyclobutane dimer and Pyr(6-4)Pyo. UV-induced mutational spectrum has recently been determined by base sequencing of the 150 bp *supF* tRNA gene in the pZ189 shuttle vector plasmid, that confers the ability to suppress *amber* mutation in *E. coli* β-galactosidase gene (*4*). After UV-irradiated plasmids were propagated in normal human and XP-A cells, recovered plasmids were selected for mutants, which form white and light blue colonies in the presence of Xgal. XP-A cells yielded a higher mutation frequency, and 93% and 73% base substitutions at hot spots of the gene propagated in XP-A and normal cells respectively were G: C → A: T transitions. Such base-change mutations occurred at C 3′ to T or C (5′-T$\underline{C}$-3′, 5′-C$\underline{C}$-3′) (*4*), in agreement with the preferential "A insertion" rule. Role of cyclobutane dimer and Pyr(6-4)Pyo in UV mutagenesis of pZ189 was also distinguished using *E. coli* photolyase. A 90% removal of dimers by photolyase reduced the vector killing by 75% and UV mutagenesis by 80% (*44*). Thus, cyclobutane dimer is the principal premutagenic lesion in mammalian cells (*44*), even though Pyr(6-4)Pyo has a much more mutagenic potential in *E. coli* than does cyclobutane dimer (*52*). UV mutagenesis is therefore strongly related to the high UV carcinogenesis in XP.

Acknowledgments

This work was supported in part by Grants-in-Aid from the Ministry of Education, Science and Culture, Japan. I thank Drs. Y. Satoh, H. Takebe, and M. Ichihashi for information on some unpublished XP patients.

REFERENCES

1. Andrews, A. D., Barrett, S. F., and Robbins, J. H. Xeroderma pigmentosum neurological abnormalities correlate with colony-forming ability after ultraviolet irradiation. *Proc. Natl. Acad. Sci. U.S.A.*, **75**, 1984–1988 (1978).

2. Bohr, V. A., Okumoto, D. S., and Hanawalt, P. C. Survival of UV-irradiated mammalian cells correlates with efficient DNA repair in an essential gene. *Proc. Natl. Acad. Sci. U.S.A.*, **83**, 3830–3833 (1986).

3. Bohr, V. A., Smith, C. A., Okumoto, D. S., and Hanawalt, P. C. DNA repair in an active gene: removal of pyrimidine dimers from the DHFR gene of CHO cells is much more efficient than in the genome overall. *Cell*, **40**, 359–369 (1985).

4. Bredberg, A., Kraemer, K. H., and Seidman, M. M. Restricted ultraviolet mutational spectrum in a shuttle vector propagated in xeroderma pigmentosum cells. *Proc. Natl. Acad. Sci. U.S.A.*, **83**, 8273–8277 (1986).

5. Cleaver, J. E. Defective repair replication in xeroderma pigmentosum. *Nature*, **218**, 652–656 (1968).

6. Cleaver, J. E. Xeroderma pigmentosum. *In* "The Metabolic Basis of Inherited Disease," ed. J. B. Stanbury, J. B. Wyngaarden, and D. S. Fredericksen, pp. 1227–1248 (1983). McGraw-Hill, New York.

7. Cleaver, J. E. Completion of excision repair patches in human cell preparations: identification of a probable mode of excision and resynthesis. *Carcinogenesis*, **5**, 325–330 (1984).

8. Cleaver, J. E. DNA repair in human xeroderma pigmentosum group C cells involves a different distribution of damaged sites in confluent and growing cells. *Nucleic Acids Res.*, **14**, 8155–8165 (1986).

9. Cleaver, J. E. and Bootsma, D. Xeroderma pigmentosum-biochemical and genetic characteristics. *Annu. Rev. Genet.*, **9**, 19–38 (1975).

10. Cohn, S. M. and Liberman, M. W. The distribution of DNA excision-repair sites in human diploid fibroblasts following ultraviolet irradiation. *J. Biol. Chem.*, **259**, 12463–12469 (1984).

11. de Jonge, A.J.R., Vermeulen, W., Keijzer, W., Hoeijmakers, J.H.J., and Bootsma, D. Microinjection of *Micrococcus luteus* UV-endonuclease restores UV-induced unscheduled DNA synthesis in cells of 9 xeroderma pigmentosum complementation groups. *Mutat. Res.*, **150**, 99–105 (1985).

12. de Jonge, A.J.R., Vermeulen, W., Klein, B., and Hoeijmakers, J.H.J. Microinjection of human cell extracts corrects xeroderma pigmentosum defect. *EMBO J.*, **150**, 637–641 (1983).

13. Dunn, W. C. and Regan, J. D. Inhibition of DNA excision repair in human cells by arabinofuranosyl cytosine, effect on normal and xeroderma pigmentosum cells. *Mol. Pharmacol.*, **15**, 367–374 (1979).

14. Fischer, E., Keijzer, W., Thielmann, H. W., Popanda, O., Bohnert, E., Edler, L., Jung, E. G., and Bootsma, D. A ninth complementation group in xeroderma pigmentosum, XP I. *Mutat. Res.*, **145**, 217–225 (1985).

15. Friedberg, E. C. "DNA Repair" (1984). W. H. Freeman and Co., New York.

16. Friedberg, E. C., Ehmann, U. K., and Williams, J. I., Jr. Human diseases associated with defective DNA repair. *Adv. Radiat. Biol.*, **8**, 85–174 (1979).

17. Friedberg, E. C., Rüde, J. M., Cook, K. H., Ehmann, U. K., Mortelmans, K., Cleaver, J. E., and Slor, H. Excision repair in mammalian cells and the current status of xeroderma pigmentosum. *In* "DNA Repair Processes," ed. W. W. Nichols and P. G. Murphy, pp. 21–36 (1977). Symposia Specialist, Miami.

18. Fujiwara, Y. and Kano, Y. Characteristics of thymine dimer excision from xeroderma pigmentosum chromatin. *In* "Cellular Responses to DNA Damage," ed. E. C. Friedberg

and B. A. Bridges, pp. 215–224 (1983). Alan R. Liss, Inc., New York.

19. Fujiwara, Y., Kano, Y., Paul, P., Goto, K., Yamamoto, K., and Miyazaki. N. Excision and cross-link repair of DNA and sister chromatid exchanges in cultured human fibroblasts with different repair capacities. *Gann. Monogr. Cancer Res.*, **27**, 33–44 (1981).

20. Fujiwara, Y., Matsumoto, A., Ichihashi, M., and Satoh, Y. Heritable disorders of DNA repair: xeroderma pigmentosum and Fanconi's anemia. *Curr. Top. Dermatol.*, **17**, 182–198 (1987).

21. Fujiwara, Y., Uehara, Y., Ichihashi, M., and Nishioka, K. Xeroderma pigmentosum complementation group F: more assignments and repair characteristics. *Photochem. Photobiol.*, **31**, 629–634 (1985).

22. Fujiwara, Y., Uehara, Y., Ichihashi, M., Yamamoto, Y., and Nishioka, K. Assignment of 2 patients with xeroderma pigmentosum to complementation group E. *Mutat. Res.*, **145**, 55–61 (1985).

23. Giannelli, F., Pawsey, S. A., and Avery, J. A. Differences in patterns of complementation of the more common groups of xeroderma pigmentosum: possible implications. *Cell*, **26**, 451–458 (1982).

24. Hayakawa, H., Ishizaki, K., Inoue, M., Yagi, T., Sekiguchi, M., and Takebe, H. Repair of ultraviolet radiation damage in xeroderma pigmentosum cells belonging to complementation group F. *Mutat. Res.*, **80**, 381–386 (1981).

25. Helland, D., Kleppe, R., Lillehang, J. R., and Kleppe, K. Xeroderma pigmentosum: *in vitro* complementation of DNA repair endonuclease. *Carcinogenesis*, **5**, 833–836 (1984).

26. Ichihashi, M. and Fujiwara, Y. Clinical and photobiologic characteristics of Japanese xeroderma pigmentosum variant. *Br. J. Dermatol.*, **105**, 1–12 (1981).

27a. Johnson, R. T., Squires, S., Elliott, G. C., Rainbow, A. J., Kock, G.L.E., and Smith, M. Analysis of DNA repair in XP-HeLa hybrids; lack of correlation between excision repair of UV damage and adenovirus reactivation in an XP(D)-like cell line. *Carcinogenesis*, **7**, 1733–1738 (1986).

27b. Jung, E. G., Bohnert, E., and Fischer, E. Heterogeneity of xeroderma pigmentosum (XP): variability and stability within and between the complementation groups C, D, E, I, and variants. *Photodermatology*, **3**, 125–132 (1986).

28. Kano, Y. and Fujiwara, Y. Defective thymine dimer excision from xeroderma pigmentosum chromatin and its characteristic catalysis by cell-free extracts. *Carcinogenesis*, **4**, 1419–1424 (1983).

29. Kantor, G. L. and Hull, D. R. The rate of removal of pyrimidine dimers in quiescent cultures of normal human and xeroderma pigmentosum cells. *Mutat. Res.*, **132**, 21–31 (1984).

30. Karentz, D. and Cleaver, J. E. Excision repair in xeroderma pigmentosum group C but not group D is clustered in a small fraction of the total genome. *Mutat. Res.*, **165**, 165–174 (1986).

31. Kraemer, K. H. Xeroderma pigmentosum. *In* "Clinical Dermatology," ed. K. J. Demis, R. L. Dobson, and J. McGuire, Vol. 4, pp. 1–13 (1980). Harper and Row, Hagerstown.

32. Kraemer, K. H. and Slor, H. Xeroderma pigmentosum. *Clin. Dermatol.*, **3**, 33–60 (1985).

33. Legerski, R. J., Brown, D. B., Peterson, C. A., and Robberson, D. L. Transient complementation of xeroderma pigmentosum cells by microinjection of poly(A)+ RNA. *Proc. Natl. Acad. Sci. U.S.A.*, **81**, 5676–5679 (1984).

34. Lan, S. Y. and Smerdon, M. J. A nonuniform distribution of excision repair synthesis in nucleosome core DNA. *Biochemistry*, **24**, 7771–7783 (1985).

35. Mansbridge, J. N. and Hanawalt, P. C. Domain-limited repair of DNA in ultraviolet-irradiated fibroblasts from xeroderma pigmentosum complementation group C. *In* "Cellular Responses to DNA Damage," ed. E. C. Friedberg and B. A. Bridges, pp. 195–207 (1983). Alan R. Liss, Inc., New York.

36. Matsumoto, A. and Fujiwara, Y. A search for cDNA conferring UV resistance on xeroderma pigmentosum group A. *J. Radiat. Res.*, **28**, 93 (1987).

37. Mayne, L. V. and Lehmann, A. R. Failure of RNA synthesis to recover after UV irradiation: an early defect in cells from individuals with Cockayne's syndrome and xeroderma pigmentosum. *Cancer Res.*, **42**, 1473–1478 (1982).

38. Mimaki, T., Itoh, N., Abe, J., Tagawa, T., Sato, K., Yabuuchi, H., and Takebe, H. Neurological manifestations in xeroderma pigmentosum. *Ann. Neurol.*, **20**, 70–75 (1986).

39. Mitchell, D. L., Haipek, C. A., and Clarkson, J. M. (6-4) Photoproducts are removed from the DNA of UV-irradiated mammalian cells more efficiently than cyclobutane pyrimidine dimers. *Mutat. Res.*, **143**, 109–112 (1985).

40. Mortelmans, K., Friedberg, E. C., Slor, H., Thomas, G., and Cleaver, J. E. Defective thymine dimer excision by cell-free extracts of xeroderma pigmentosum cells. *Proc. Natl. Acad. Sci. U.S.A.*, **73**, 2757–2761 (1976).

41. Moshell, A. N., Ganges, M. R., Lutzner, M. A., Coon, H. G., Barrett, S. F., Dupay, J. M., and Robbins, J. H. A new patient with both xeroderma pigmentosum and Cockayne syndrome comprises the new xeroderma pigmentosum group H. *In* "Cellular Responses to DNA Damage," ed. E. C. Friedberg and B. A. Bridges, pp. 209–213 (1983). Alan R. Liss, Inc., New York.

42. Mullenders, L.H.F., van Kesteren, A. C., Bussmann, C.J.M., van Zeeland, A. A., and Natarajan, A. T. Preferential repair of nuclear matrix associated DNA in xeroderma pigmentosum complementation group C. *Mutat. Res.*, **141**, 75–82 (1984).

43. Protić-Sabljić, M. and Kraemer, K. H. Reduced repair of non-dimer photoproducts in a gene transfected into xeroderma pigmentosum cells. *Photochem. Photobiol.*, **43**, 509–513 (1986).

44. Protić-Sabljić, M., Tuteja, N., Munson, P. T., Hauser, J., Kraemer, K. H., and Dixon, K. UV light-induced cyclobutane pyrimidine dimers are mutagenic in mammalian cells. *Mol. Cell. Biol.*, **6**, 3349–3356 (1986).

45. Robbins, J. H. Hypersensitivity to DNA damaging agents in primary degenerations of excitable tissue. *In* "Cellular Responses to DNA Damage," ed. E. C. Friedberg and B. A. Bridges, pp. 671–700 (1983). Alan R. Liss, Inc., New York.

46. Robbins, J. H., Kraemer, K. H., Lutzner, M. A., Festoff, B. W., and Coon, H. G. Xeroderma pigmentosum. An inherited disease with sun sensitivity, multiple cutaneous neoplasms, and abnormal DNA repair. *Ann. Intern. Med.*, **80**, 225–248 (1974).

47a. Sancar, A. and Rupp, W. D. A novel repair enzyme: UVRABC endonuclease from *E. coli* cuts a DNA strand on both sides of the damaged region. *Cell*, **33**, 249–260 (1983).

47b. Stefanini, M., Lagomarsini, P., Arlett, C. F., Marinoni, S., Borrone, C., Crovato, F., Trerisan, G., Cordone, G., and Nuzzo, F. Xeroderma pigmentosum (complementation group D) mutation is present in patients affected by trichothiodystrophy with photosensitivity. *Hum. Genet.*, **74**, 107–112 (1986).

48. Stefanini, M., Keijzer, W., Westerveld, A., and Bootsma, D. Interspecies complementation analysis of xeroderma pigmentosum and UV-sensitive Chinese hamster cells. *Exp. Cell Res.*, **161**, 373–380 (1985).

49. Takano, T., Noda, M., and Tamura, T. Transfection of cells from a xeroderma pigmentosum patient with normal human DNA confers UV resistance. *Nature*, **296**, 269–270 (1982).

50. Takebe, H., Fujiwara, Y., Sasaki, M. S., Satoh, Y., Kozuka, T., Nikaido, O., Ishizaki, K., Arase, S., and Ikenaga, M. DNA repair and clinical characteristics in xeroderma pigmentosum patients in Japan. *In* "DNA Repair Mechanisms," ed. P. C. Hanawalt, E. C. Friedberg, and C. F. Fox, pp. 617–620 (1978). Academic Press, New York.

51. Tanaka, K., Sekiguchi, M., and Okada, Y. Restoration of ultraviolet-induced unscheduled DNA synthesis of xeroderma pigmentosum cells by the concomitant treatment with bac-

teriophage T4 endonuclease V and HVJ (Sendai virus). *Proc. Natl. Acad. Sci. U.S.A.*, **72**, 4071–4075 (1975).

52. Tang, M-S., Hrncir, J., Mitchell. D., Ross, J., and Clarkson, J. The relative cytotoxicity and mutagenicity of cyclobutane pyrimidine dimers and (6-4) photoproducts in *Escherichia coli* cells. *Mutat. Res.*, **161**, 9–17 (1986).

53. Thielmann, H. W. and Georgiades, A. Correlation of post-UV colony forming ability of xeroderma pigmentosum fibroblasts with DNA incision reaction catalyzed by cell-free extracts. *In* "Chromosome Damage and Repair," ed. E. Seeberg and K. Kleppe, pp. 321–328 (1981). Plenum Press, New York.

54. Thompson, L. H., Mooney, C. L., and Brookman, K. W. Genetic complementation between UV-sensitive CHO mutants and xeroderma pigmentosum fibroblasts. *Mutat. Res.*, **150**, 423–429 (1985).

55. Vermeulen, W., Osseweijer, P., de Jonge, A.J.R., and Hoeijmakers, J.H.J. Transient correction of excision repair defects in fibroblasts of 9 xeroderma pigmentosum complementation groups by microinjection of crude human cell extracts. *Mutat. Res.*, **165**, 199–206 (1986).

56. Weinfeld, M., Gentner, N. E., Johnson, L. D., and Paterson, M. C. Photoreversal-dependent release of thymidine and thymidine monophosphate from pyrimidine dimer-containing DNA excision fragments isolated from ultraviolet-damaged human fibroblasts. *Biochemistry*, **25**, 2656–2664 (1986).

57. Yamaizumi, M., Sugano, T., Asahina, H., Okada, Y., and Uchida, T. Microinjection of partially purified protein factor restores DNA damage specifically in group A of xeroderma pigmentosum cells. *Proc. Natl. Acad. Sci. U.S.A.*, **83**, 1476–1479 (1986).

58. Zelle, B., Behrends, F., and Lohman, P.H.M. Repair of damage by ultraviolet radiation in xeroderma pigmentosum cell strains of complementation groups E and F. *Mutat. Res.*, **73**, 157–169 (1980).

59. Zelle, B. and Lohman, P.H.M. Repair of UV-endonuclease-susceptible sites in the 7 complementation groups of xeroderma pigmentosum A through G. *Mutat. Res.*, **62**, 363–368 (1979).

60. Zwetsloot, J.C.M., Barbeiro, A. P., Vermeulen, W., Arthur, H. M., Hoeijmakers, J.H.J., and Backendorf, C. Microinjection of *Escherichia coli* UvrA, B, C, and D proteins into fibroblasts of xeroderma pigmentosum complementation groups A and C does not result in restoration of UV-induced unscheduled DNA synthesis. *Mutat. Res.*, **166**, 89–98 (1986).

XERODERMA PIGMENTOSUM: CLINICAL ASPECTS

Yoshiaki Satoh[*1] and Chikako Nishigori[*2]

Department of Dermatology, Tokyo Women's Medical College, Dai-Ni Hospital,[*1] *Department of Experimental Radiology, Faculty of Medicine, Kyoto University*[*2]

Clinical characteristics of 272 xeroderma pigmentosum (XP) patients in Japan are recorded. Clinical symptoms appear to be related to the level of DNA repair deficiency which is controlled by XP genes. There were nine genetic complementation groups of excision repair deficient type of XP and a variant type whose cells showed normal excision repair capacity. Distribution of genetic complementation groups in XP patients in Japan is considerably different from that in other countries: complementation group A and the variant are far more frequent in Japan than in other countries. Complementation group F was originally found in Japan and has been limited to that country except for one case. Skin cancers in XP patients in Japan are less frequent than in patients elsewhere presumably due to difference in skin color and possible difference in response to ultraviolet light (UV). Basal cell epithelomas were most common followed by squamous cell carcinoma and malignant melanoma. Malignant melanoma in XP patients developed mostly in areas exposed to sunlight, contrary to such melanomas in Japanese non-XP sufferers. Prevention and treatment of the clinical symptoms in XP patients have improved recently. Early diagnosis by a sun sensitivity test and a DNA repair test helps to warn susceptible individuals of the dangers of sunlight exposure during their early years of life when the skin is particularly sensitive. Although photoprotection and treatment of skin lesions reduces the skin manifestations, neurological abnormalities associated with some of the complementation groups cannot be prevented.

Xeroderma pigmentosum (XP) is a rare disease of autosomal recessive inheritance. One hundred and twenty-five years have passed since Kaposi first recognized XP in his patients, and twenty-five years thereafter he termed the disease xeroderma pigmentosum (*16*). Twenty years ago Cleaver reported his discovery that the cells of XP patients were defective in repairing damage to DNA caused by ultraviolet light (UV) (*5*). The high incidence of skin cancer in XP patients is well known, and because of this cancer proneness, XP has received much attention from many investigators who have tried to elucidate the role of DNA repair in the mechanisms of carcinogenesis.

A joint research group for basic and clinical studies on XP was organized in Japan in 1975 as one of the projects under Grants-in-Aid for Cancer Research. This report is based primarily on the results of the studies carried out by this group, which was organ-

---

[*1] 2-1-10, Nishioku, Arakawa-ku, Tokyo 116, Japan (佐藤吉昭).
[*2] Yoshida-konoecho, Sakyo-ku, Kyoto 606, Japan (錦織千佳子).

ized by H. Takebe (one of the editors of this volume) and participated in by many cell biologists and dermatologists in Japan (49–53).

More than 300 XP patients were examined by this study group, but those whose clinical and DNA repair data were insufficient were excluded from these results. Skin cancer in relation to DNA repair capacity is the main topic to be discussed in this chapter.

Prevention and management of skin symptoms in XP patients have been successful in recent years mainly by avoiding or reducing patient sunlight exposure and by early surgical treatment or removal of the tumors (45). Some of the XP patients develop neurological abnormalities of which no mechanisms are known. Avoidance of exposure to sunlight and subsequent delay in the development of skin lesions appear unrelated to the development of these neurological abnormalities (43).

XP Patients in Japan

XP patients have been recorded in essentially all populations in the world. Some countries appear to have higher frequencies presumably due to the high consanguinity (6, 10, 56). In Japan, frequency of XP in newborn babies is believed to be approximately 1/100,000 or less (27, 37, 53). The frequency in a neighbouring country, Korea, is estimated to be 1/183,000 (21). Frequency of the first cousin marriage in parents of Japanese XP patients is approximately 30% (50), while no consanguineous marriage was recorded among the Korean XP families where first cousin marriages are prohibited (53).

Table I shows the comparison of genetic complementation groups in XP patients in different populations (11, 12, 26, 53). An XP patient belonging to complementation group F was identified first in Japan in 1979 (2). Patients belonging to other minor groups were recorded recently: D (14), E (17, 20), F (15), and G (18). When the genetic groups of XP patients in Japan are compared with those in other countries, the following differing characteristics are apparent: 1) the number of patients in group A and variant (4) are large in Japan; 2) number of patients in group C, which is the most common group in other countries, is small in Japan, and 3) patients in group F have been found mainly in Japan, except one (3, 57).

In other countries, one group B patient was known in the U.S.A. who was also affected by Cockayne syndrome, another rare genetic disorder; the number of patients in groups C and D are large in the U.S.A. and in Europe. There were reports of two group E patients in a family in the Netherlands, two group G patients in U. K., one French group H patient who also had Cockayne syndrome (32), and two group I patients in a

TABLE I.   Genetic Complementation Groups of XP Patients

Complementation group	A	B	C	D	E	F	G	H	I	Va	Total
Japan	32	0	5	5	6	12	1	0	0	31[a]	92
Other countries	28	1	38	18	5	1	2	1	2	21	118

The number of patients in other countries was quoted from refs. *13, 14,* but the number of patients in group A was quoted from ref. *26.*
Va, variants.
[a] From Dr. Y. Fujiwara.

family in Germany (*13*). In Korea, 23 XP patients were recorded, and none of these had neuormental abnormalities (*21, 53*).

Clinical Symptoms and Diagnosis of XP Patients

1. Symptoms and diagnosis of XP patients in each complementation group

XP is the most typical photodermatosis and is characterized by severe photosensitivity after first exposure to sunlight in perinatal period or early infancy. At birth, the skin of the individual appears normal. Infants of group A usually begin expressing XP symptoms with severe sunburn, with or without blistering, and photophobia within a year after birth. Continued exposure to sunlight yields dry ("xero-"), scaly, pigmented ("pigmentosum") skin ("-derma"), multiple freckles, hypopigmented maculae, telangiectases, and skin (especially epidermal) atrophy (Kaposi was the first to classify it as such). Later cutaneous manifestations are verrucous papules, keratoses, keratoacanthomas, angiomas, and premature development of skin malignancies, including epithelial neoplasms and melanomas.

Figure 1 is a diagram of diagnostic procedures for XP routinely performed by the authors. The approach begins with confirmation of clinical hypersensitivity to sunlight

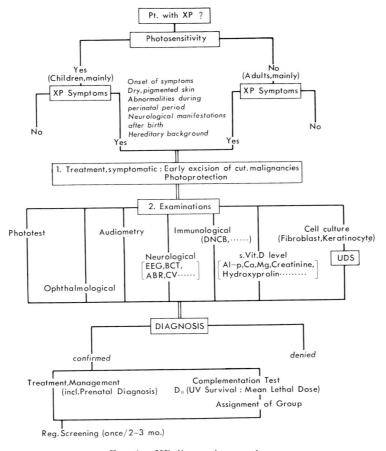

FIG. 1. XP diagnostic procedure

and skin manifestations followed by various examinations. The photosensitivity of XP patients, especially group A patients, is characterized by markedly lowered minimal erythema doses (MEDs) at various wavelengths (UVB and UVA), a delayed erythemal reaction peak at 72 hr after irradiation, prolonged persistent erythema, and response other than erythema (*36, 41, 43*). Figure 2 shows the MEDs in group A patients, and Fig. 3 shows the erythema action spectra of patients in group A and variant, based on results using monochromatic UV (*42*). Diagnosis of XP is also made based on DNA repair capacity, which is usually measured by relative amounts of unscheduled DNA synthesis (UDS) after UV irradiation of cultured fibroblast (or keratinocytes (*23*)) from the skin of patients. Finally, in certain cases, a test is performed to determine the genetic complementation group to which the patient belongs.

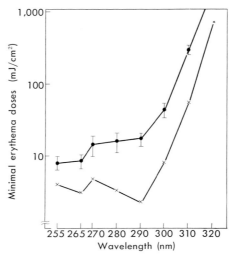

FIG. 2.   MEDs in XP group A

● mean MEDs and standard deviation in normal controls, measured at 24 hr after irradiation; × MEDs in XP group A patients, measured at 72 hr after irradiation.

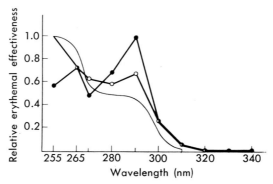

FIG. 3.   Erythema action spectrum in XP group A and XP variant

— normal controls, observed at 24 hr; ● XP group A patients observed at 72 hr; ○ XP variant patients, observed at 24 hr, after irradiation.

TABLE II.   Clinical Characteristics of XP Patients in Japan

Group	Acute sunburn in infancy	Photosensitivity			Manifestation		
		MED	Peak of erythema	UVA-hyper-sensitivity	Skin	Ocular	Neurologic
A and less than 5% UDS	+++	Markedly lowered	72 hr[b]	+	Severe (Inf)[a]	Severe	Severe (Mild)[b]
D	++	Lowered	72 hr	+	Mild (Inf-Ch)	Mild	−/ Borderline
E	++	Lowered	24 or 48 or 72 hr	?	Mild/ Moderate (early Ch)	Mild	−
F	+	Normal/ lowered	24 hr	−	Mild (early Ch)	−	−
G	+	Normal	24 hr	−	Mild (10 yr)	−	−
Variants and over 60% UDS	−/(+)[b]	Normal (lowered)[b]	24 hr	−	Mild/ Moderate (5–6 yr)	Mild	−

+, present; −, absent.

[a] ( ): age (years) or period of onset. Inf, infancy; Ch, childhood.

[b] A small number of exceptions.

The clinical symptoms of XP often vary characteristically according to genetic complementation group (Photos 1–7). Table II summarizes these clinical characteristics of each group (the characteristics of group C patients in Japan have not been established). Characteristics shown here were obtained by our direct observation of each individual patient, and reports from other countries were not considered. For instance, some reports have stated that neurological manifestations were present in group D patients (26, 39), but in Japan we have encountered little definite manifestation of neurological disorder so far, and we therefore have shown "none / borderline" in Table II. The number of our group D patients, however, admittedly may not be sufficient to generalize our observations.

Diagnosis of group A patients is generally easy, but there were a few in this group with very slight neurological symptoms, both Japanese (29) and Caucasian (38), and the authors had an opportunity to observe one of them (a 24-year-old male). In these patients, skin symptoms are usually mild and the neurological symptoms appear to be in parallel. In other rare examples in group A patients, symptoms, including UDS levels, differed between a brother and a sister (47).

2.   XP and neurological manifestations

Progressive neurological abnormalities have been reported in approximately 40% of XP patients (24, 27). The most severely affected have been termed de Sanctis-Cacchione syndrome (xerodermic idiocy) (7, 37); however, the complete form of de Sanctis-Cacchione syndrome has been recognized in very few patients (27). The mechanism of neurological manifestations in XP is still unknown. Group A is the most common type in Japan with neurological symptoms, and clinical treatment is difficult since no effective therapeutic or prophylactic method is known at present.

There has been a set pattern in the appearance of the neurological symptoms in group A patients, as well as in the mode of subsequent progress (30). Some symptoms, such as speech and hearing impairment and clumsy gait with Parkinsonian posture appear by around age 5 and progress with increasing age; other symptoms are then gradually manifested. The weakness of the extremities begins in the lower limbs, extends ascendingly, and muscular atrophy develops soon after age 10; thereafter a patient may not be able to walk. Occasions requiring emergency treatment may often take place in daily life caused by urinary retention, dyspnea due to swallowing, or the inability to remove sputum. These clinical symptoms can be detected much earlier through various examinations: 1) mental retardation as shown by a decrease in score of intelligence quotient (IQ) or development quotient (DQ) test, 2) diminution or disappearance of alpha rhythms, with increase of theta activity on the electroencephalogram, 3) moderate dilatation of ventricles and sulci, and cranial bone thickening observed in a brain computed tomogram, 4) disappearance of auditory brainstem response around 8 years of age, 5) decrease in hearing level to around 90 dB at about age 13, 6) delay of conduction velocity of peripheral sensory and motor nerves with increasing age (30). Thus, XP is a disease typified by the chronic progressive degenerative status of the nervous system.

These neurological symptoms would develop even if individuals were completely protected from sunlight. Occasional perinatal abnormalities (e.g., episodes of decreased fetal movements, vomiting, retarded growth, etc.) have been reported in some patients (30). Abnormalities in the development of the nervous system may be present even in the fetus. Possible involvement of environmental factors causing damage to neuron cells during development also cannot be excluded.

Dermatologists alone are unable to treat these various neurological symptoms in XP patients, and the authors organized a joint team of pediatricians, otorhinolaryngologists, ophthalmologists, and orthopedists (43, 45). We recently encountered a new case, a boy of group A with delayed awakening from general anesthesia during dental therapy. When the time required for awakening from general anesthesia was compared with his past record, we noticed that it had become longer with his age. In addition, when the patient had to be in bed for some period, his motility rapidly decreased and a long period was required for rehabilitation. Since it is suggested that the entity of this disease is systemic, physicians participating from various departments must work in close cooperation.

3. XP and ocular manifestations

Ocular abnormalities are often reported, and the cells of the conjunctiva in XP patients are also defective in DNA repair of UV damage (8, 34, 43, 55). Although the degree of symptom severity varies, it is worst in group A patients, and some of them may lose their sight (43). Symptoms are: diffuse superficial keratitis, conjunctivitis with photophobia, lacrimation, teleangiectasia, pigmentation of bulbar conjunctiva, ectropium palpebrae, loss of cilia, malignant tumors of conjunctiva, cornea and lower lid, and blindness.

Malignant Tumors in XP

The incidence of malignant skin tumors of sun-exposed areas in XP patients under 20 years of age is reportedly over 1,000-fold higher than that in the control group (19, 27, 28). This implies that UV, a potent mutagen in the environment, constitutes the primary cause.

TABLE III.   Skin Tumors in XP Patients

Group	Number of patients	Patients with skin tumor			
		Total[a]	BCE	SCC	MM
A and less than 5% UDS	117	41	35	20	5
C	5	4	4	3	2
D	5	3	2	2	0
E	6	2	2	0	0
F	12	3	2	1	0
G	1	1	1	0	0
Other intermediate UDS	37	24	11	11	2
Variants and over 60% UDS	89	41	30	14	9
Total	272	119	87	51	18

[a] The reason for disagreement between the total number and the total of the number of tumor types is because some patients had multiple tumors (see Table V).

TABLE IV.   Age Distribution and Age of Onset of Skin Tumors

Group	Number of patients	Average age (years)	Average age of onset (years)		
			BCE	SCC	MM
A and less than 5% UDS	117 (41)[a]	7.8	9.3	8.2	7.5
C	5 (4)	7.2	14.8	8.3	11
D	5 (3)	31.4	31	42.5	—
E	6 (2)	27.0	43.5	—	—
F	12 (3)	28.3	45.5	64	—
G	1 (1)	32	32	—	—
Other intermediate UDS	37 (24)	29.2	45.4	37.7	14.0
Variants and over 60% UDS	89 (41)	38.1	40.8	42.0	46.8

[a] Number in parentheses: patients with skin tumors.

The authors carried out a statistical observation on types of skin tumors in different groups of 272 XP patients (Table III), and Table IV gives average age of patients at the onset of each tumor. Development of skin tumors appears to be related to the level of DNA repair capacity, the lower this capacity is, the earlier the symptom and skin tumor may develop. The relative incidence of XP patients who developed tumor in all XP patients in Japan was 43.8% (119 in 272 patients). The most frequent tumor was basal cell epithelioma (BCE) (87 cases, 32.0%), followed by squamous cell carcinoma (SCC) (51 cases, 18.6%), and malignant melanoma (MM) (18 cases, 6.7%), with multiple types recorded separately. These figures suggest that DNA repair deficiency enhances the susceptibility of the basal cells. The most frequent multiple skin tumors consisting of different histopathological types were 20 cases of BCE and SCC, followed by 7 cases of BCE, SCC and MM, and 2 cases each of BCE and MM, and of SCC and MM, respectively (Table V). One of the most severe cases, a male patient of variant type who died at 51 years of age, had 48 tumors on his body, including 14 BCEs, 2 MMs, 2 lentigo maligna, 1 Bowen's disease, and 6 solar keratoses (40). Much earlier tumor onset was found in two boys who had SCC at the age of 3 and lentigo maligna melanoma at age 7; both were of group A (22). All these skin malignancies occured on so-called XP-skin: the skin with dermatoheliosis ("helio": the sun) early in life, characterized by several histopathological changes, i.e., parakeratosis, epidermal atrophy and budding, pigment anomaly, actinic

TABLE V.   Multiple Skin Tumors of Different Histopathological Types in XP Patients

DNA repair level	Number of patients	BCE+ SCC	BCE+ MM	SCC+ MM	BCE+ SCC+MM	Total
Less than 5% of normal UDS	117 (41)[a]	8	2	1	1	12
Intermediate UDS	66 (37)	6	0	0	3	9
Over 60% of normal UDS	89 (41)	6	0	1	3	10
Total	272 (119)	20	2	2	7	31

[a] Number in parentheses: patients with skin tumors.

TABLE VI.   Non-skin Cancers Observed in XP Patients

Complementation group	Cancer	Age (years)	Sex
A	Died of glioblastoma of brain	9	F
F	Died of bile duct carcinoma	65	F
Va	Died of stomach carcinoma	53	M
	Transitional cell carcinoma of bladder	68	M
	Squamous cell carcinoma of pharynx	56	M
Unknown	Died of uterus carcinoma	51	F
	Died of malignant melanoma of eye	33	F

Va, variants.

elastosis, *etc.* These skin changes are equal to a senile precancerous condition observed on sun-exposed areas reflecting the progress of photoaging. Consequently, the most important point for the prophylaxis of UV-carcinogenesis in XP patients should be a means of preventing the development into dermatoheliosis.

As for MM, the incidences in the U.S.A. and in Europe are very high, accounting for approximately half of all XP patients; in Japan, however, only 18 patients are known (about 7%). It should be noted that most MM in Japanese patients developed in sun-exposed areas, while that in non-XP patients was often found in unexposed areas (54).

The incidence of skin malignancies in Japanese XP patients is, as a whole, very low in comparison with that in Caucasians. A general comparison of skin reactivity between the two groups shows a definite difference in the degree of skin damage caused by UV, revealing a higher risk to Caucasians. This may be due not only to the difference in skin color, but also to difference in photobiological cutaneous responses to UV radiation. It was also found that, unlike Caucasians, the skin color of a Japanese individual and the sensitivity to UV did not always correlate (46). These racial and individual differences may interwine in complex manner, causing normal skin to develop dermatoheliosis, and finally to develop skin cancer.

Systemic defective DNA repair in XP patients could imply that the incidence of cancer in organs other than skin would also be frequent. Cancers in internal organs in XP patients in the U.S.A. were reported (25, 28) at approximately 10 to 20-fold higher frequency than normal controls (28), while in Japan only 7 such cancers have been recorded so far (Table VI). Swift and Chase reported that the incidence of skin tumors was 4-fold higher in XP heterozygotes than in normal controls (48). In Japan, however, we have no data to support this because no parents of XP patients developed skin tumor, presumably reflecting the low incidence of skin cancer in general. Since it has been pointed out that XP cells are sensitive to many mutagens (27), the non-skin and multiple cancers should receive more attention in future.

Prevention and Treatment of XP Symptoms

Early detection of the disease, reduction of instances of exposure to sunlight and treatment of malignant skin tumors (surgical excision, *etc.*) have been the basic strategy for the prevention and treatment of symptoms in XP patients.

1. Photoprotection

In addition to avoiding sunlight, photoprotection by sunscreening agents has been very effective in protecting the skin and eyes from damage by sunlight (*27, 43*). Since the UV action spectrum in XP encompasses the UVB and UVA wavelength regions, the absorber of UVB and the reflector (sunshade, scattering agents) of UVA must be combined "PreSun 15 (Creamy and Facial)" (Westwood Pharmaceuticals Inc., U.S.A.) and "Creme ecran total 10A+B or 15+A+B" (RoC S. A., France) (or "Cover Mark" O'Leary, Japan) have been found effective in our experience. Similar photoprotection for lips has also been applied (*43, 45*).

For eye protection, patients have been advised to wear special eyeglasses with "Nikon SX-13" (Nippon Kogaku K. K., Japan) (*43*) or "CPF" (Corning, U.S.A.) lenses which cut out UV. So-called colored sunglasses did not adequately eliminate UV, and may expand the pupils ("ultraviolet windows" (*1*)).

If these procedures are regularly followed, photoaging of the skin and development of skin malignancies can be prevented, and ocular manifestations will be reduced.

Dermabrasion or skin grafting of sun-damaged areas is occasionally recommended, because it is believed to delay the development of skin malignancies (*9, 33*).

2. Guidance for daily life

As the majority of patients are children, improved therapeutic effect can only be expected by educating their parents, particularly mothers. In practice, patients should be prohibited from being outdoors during the daytime. When they go out, they should wear long sleeves, long trousers, gloves and a broad-brimmed hat and a sunscreen preparation should be topically applied (*27, 43*). If fluorescent lamps are used at home, they should be covered with a shade. Patients are advised to wear the sunglasses described above with side shields, and a hearing aid. Window glass should be covered with an insulating film to reduce UV light. Long hair covering the individuals ears, neck, and forehead may be encouraged.

The authors devised an XP Notebook, similar to the Maternity Passbook used in Japan, in which the progression of the disease is recorded, and have used this to exchange information with families and schoolteachers (*43*).

3. Regular checkups

Patients come to us at least once every 2 or 3 months for a regular checkup, and problems are discussed at that time. Teeth are also checked, because the oral hygienic condition of a patient is invariably poor. When a patient is given a hearing test, he/she should receive conversation training by a speech therapist (*43*).

Thus, children with XP are always expected to avoid exposure to sunlight. Since the IQ is sometimes low and the mental faculties are not strong, and there may be difficulty in swallowing foods, the balance of nutrition tends to be imperfect. These factors, coupled with the reduced sunlight exposure, will inevitably reduce the vitamin D level in the blood (*44*). When a regular checkup is given a patient, not only the vitamin D level in the blood, but various other factors associated with vitamin D should be measured quantitatively. If abnormalities are detected, vitamin D should immediately be given.

4. Miscellaneous

Few data are available on the photoimmunological approach to XP. Recently, Morison *et al.* reported that the development of contact allergy in sun-exposed-skin was markedly impaired in patients with XP, and the degree of this immunological impairment was directly related to the severity of the cutaneous disease (*31*). They concluded that this raised the possibility that sunlight-induced alterations of the immune function might be involved in the marked susceptibility of these patients to the development of nonmelanoma skin cancer.

Prenatal amniotic diagnosis (*36*) can be applied to a mother who has one XP child in the repair defect group and who conceives another child. The treatment, however, involves several difficult ethical problems including the human rights of a fetus.

Physicians should do their utmost to educate those around a patient in what XP is, and to have them to understand to what degree they can help the patient and the family. This can be said of any hereditary disease, and XP may serve as a good example of successful prevention of clinical symptoms through better understanding of the disease by those related to a sufferer.

Acknowledgments

The authors wish to express their deepest appreciation to many dermatologists from the departments of dermatology in universities and hospitals throughout Japan who kindly told them of many valuable cases. Their sincere thanks are also expressed to Prof. Y. Fujiwara, Department of Radiation Biophysics, Kobe University School of Medicine, Kobe, who conducted many of the complementation tests. This work was supported in part by Grants-in-Aid for Cancer Research from the Ministry of Education, Science and Culture of Japan.

REFERENCES

1. Anderson, W. J. and Gebel, R.K.H. Ultraviolet windows in commercial sunglasses. *Appl. Opt.*, **16**, 515–517 (1977).
2. Arase, S., Kozuka, T., Tanaka, K., Ikenaga, M., and Takebe, H. A sixth complementation group of xeroderma pigmentosum. *Mutat. Res.*, **59**, 143–146 (1979).
3. Botcherby, P. K., Magnus, I. A., Marimo, B., and Giannelli, F. Actinic reticuloid—An idiopathic photodermatosis with cellular sensitivity to near ultraviolet radiation. *Photochem. Photobiol.*, **39**, 641–649 (1984).
4. Burk, P. G., Lutzner, M. A., Clark, D. D., and Robbins, J. H. Ultraviolet-stimulated thymidine incorporation in xeroderma pigmentosum lymphocytes. *J. Lab. Clin. Med.*, **77**, 759–767 (1971).
5. Cleaver, J. E. Defective repair replication of DNA in xeroderma pigmentosum. *Nature*, **218**, 652–656 (1968).
6. Cleaver, J. E., Zelle, B., Hashem, N., El-Hefnawi, M. H., and German, J. Xeroderma pigmentosum patients from Egypt: II. Preliminary correlations of epidemiology, clinical symptoms and molecular biology. *J. Invest. Dermatol.*, **77**, 96–101 (1981).
7. De Sanctis, C. and Cacchione, A. L'idiozia xerodermica. *Riv. Sper. Freniat.*, **56**, 269–292 (1932).

8. El-Hefnawi, H. and Mortada, A. Ocular manifestations of xeroderma pigmentosum. *Br. J. Dermatol.*, **77**, 261–276 (1965).

9. Epstein, E. H., Jr., Burk, P. G., Cohen, I. K., and Deckers, P. Dermatome shaving in the treatment of xeroderma pigmentosum. *Arch. Dermatol.*, **105**, 589–590 (1972).

10. Fathy, S. and Khafagy, H. Xeroderma pigmentosum in Qatar. *Cutis*, **37**, 377–379 (1986).

11. Fischer, E., Thielmann, H. W., Neundörfer, B., Rentsch, F. J., Edler, L., and Jung, E. G. Xeroderma pigmentosum patients from Germany: Clinical symptoms and DNA repair characteristics. *Arch. Dermatol. Res.*, **274**, 229–247 (1982).

12. Fischer, E., Schnyder, U. W., and Jung, E. G. Report of three sisters with XP-E, a rare xeroderma pigmentosum complementation group. *Photodermatology*, **1**, 232–236 (1984).

13. Fischer, E., Keijzer, W., Thielmann, H. W., Popanda, O., Bohnert, E., Edler, L., Jung, E. G., and Bootsma, D. A ninth complementation group in xeroderma pigmentosum, XP I. *Mutat. Res.*, **145**, 217–225 (1985).

14. Fujiwara, Y. and Satoh, Y. Assignment of two Japanese xeroderma pigmentosum patients to complementation group D and their characteristics. *Jpn. J. Cancer Res (Gann)*, **76**, 162–166 (1985).

15. Fujiwara, Y., Uehara, Y., Ichihashi, M., and Nishioka, K. Xeroderma pigmentosum complementation group F: more assignments and repair characteristics. *Photochem. Photobiol.*, **31**, 629–634 (1985).

16. Hebra, F. and Kaposi, M. *In* "On Diseases of the Skin Including the Exanthemata," Vol. 3, pp. 252–258 (1874). The New Sydenham Soc., London.

17. Ichihashi, M., Nakanishi, T., Ueda, M., Hayashibe, K., Fujiwara, Y., and Nishioka, K. Clinical and photobiological characteristics of xeroderma pigmentosum complementation group E. *Jpn. J. Dermatol.*, **95**, 721–729 (1985) (in Japanese).

18. Ichihashi, M., Fujiwara, Y., Uehara, Y., and Matsumoto, A. A mild form of xeroderma pigmentosum assigned to complementation group G and its repair heterogeneity. *J. Invest. Dermatol.*, **85**, 284–287 (1985).

19. Jung, E. G., Bohnert, E., and Fischer, E. Heterogeneity of xeroderma pigmentosum (XP); variability and stability within and between the complementation groups C, D, E, I and variants. *Photodermatology*, **3**, 125–132 (1986).

20. Kawada, A., Satoh, Y., and Fujiwara, Y. Xeroderma pigmentosum complementation group E: a case report. *Photodermatology*, **3**, 233–238 (1986).

21. Kim, Y. P. Genodermatoses among Koreans. *Jpn. J. Dermatol.*, **96**, 1307 (1986) (Abstract).

22. Kobayashi, M., Satoh, Y., Irimajiri, T., Mitoh, Y., Kozuka, T., Sato, K., Ichihashi, M., and Nakanishi, T. Skin tumors of xeroderma pigmentosum (1). *J. Dermatol. (Tokyo)*, **9**, 319–322 (1982).

23. Kondo, S., Satoh, Y., and Kuroki, T. Defect in UV-induced unscheduled DNA synthesis in cultured epidermal keratinocytes from xeroderma pigmentosum. *Mutat. Res.*, **183**, 95–101 (1987).

24. Kraemer, K. H. and Slor, H. Xeroderma pigmentosum. *Clin. Dermatol.*, **3**, 33–69 (1985).

25. Kraemer, K. H., Lee, M. M., and Scotto, J. DNA repair protects against cutaneous and internal neoplasia: evidence from xeroderma pigmentosum. *Carcinogenesis*, **5**, 511–514 (1984).

26. Kraemer, K. H. Xeroderma pigmentosum. *In* "Clinical Dermatology," ed. D. J. Demis, R. L. Dobson, J. McGuire, Vol. 4, pp. 1–33 (1980). Harper & Row, Hagerstown.

27. Kraemer, K. H. Xeroderma pigmentosum. *In* "Dermatology in General Medicine," ed. T. B. Fitzpatrick, A. Z. Eisen, K. Wolff, I. M. Freedberg, K. F. Austen, 3rd ed., pp. 1791–1796 (1987). McGraw-Hill, New York.

28. Lambert, W. C. Xeroderma pigmentosum. *In* "Pathogenesis of Skin Disease," ed. B. H. Thiers, pp. 579–599 (1986). Churchill Livingstone, New York.

29. Mimaki, T., Itoh, N., Abe, J., Tagawa, T., Sato, K., Yabuuchi, H., and Takebe, H.

Neurological manifestations in xeroderma pigmentosum. *Ann. Neurol.*, **20**, 70–75 (1986).

30. Mitoh, Y., Kobayashi, M., Satoh, Y., and Iwakawa, Y. Neurological manifestations in XP Group A patients. *Rinsho Derma (Tokyo)*, **25**, 347–352 (1983) (in Japanese).

31. Morison, W. L., Bucana, C., Hashem, N., Kripke, M. L., Cleaver, J. E., and German, J. L. Impaired immune function in patients with xeroderma pigmentosum. *Cancer Res.*, **45**, 3929–3931 (1985).

32. Moshell, A. N., Ganges, M. R., Lutzner, M. A., Coon, H. G., Barrett, S. F., Dupay, J. M., and Robbins, J. H. A new patient with both xeroderma pigmentosum and Cockayne syndrome comprises the new xeroderma pigmentosum group H. *In* "Cellular Responses to DNA Damage," ed. E. C. Friedberg and B. A. Bridges, pp. 209–213 (1983). Alan R. Liss, New York.

33. Mouly, R., Dufourmentel, C., Banzet, P., and Papadopoulos, O. Xeroderma pigmentosum. *Ann. Chir. Plast.*, **25**, 117–125 (1980).

34. Newsome, D. A., Kraemer, K. H., and Robbins, J. H. Repair of DNA in xeroderma pigmentosum conjunctiva. *Arch. Ophthalmol.*, **93**, 660–662 (1975).

35. Okayasu, I., Satoh, Y., Irimajiri, T., and Mitoh, Y. Fetal case of xeroderma pigmentosum. First report of an autopsy case. *Acta Pathol. Jpn.*, **28**, 459–464 (1978).

36. Ramsay, C. A. and Giannelli, F. The erythemal action spectrum and deoxyribonucleic acid repair synthesis in xeroderma pigmentosum. *Br. J. Dermatol.*, **92**, 49–56 (1975).

37. Robbins, J. H., Kraemer, K. H., Lutzner, M. A., Festoff, B. W., and Coon, H. G. Xeroderma pigmentosum. An inherited disease with sun sensitivity, multiple cutaneous neoplasms, and abnormal DNA repair. *Ann. Intern. Med.*, **80**, 221–248 (1974).

38. Robbins, J. H., Polinsky, R. J., and Moshell, A. N. Evidence that lack of deoxyribonucleic acid repair causes death of neurons in xeroderma pigmentosum. *Ann. Neurol.*, **13**, 682–684 (1983).

39. Robbins, J. H. Hypersensitivity to DNA-damaging agents in primary degenerations of excitable tissue. *In* "Cellular Responses to DNA Damage," ed. E. C. Friedberg and B. A. Bridges, pp. 671–700 (1983). Alan R. Liss, New York.

40. Sasaki, A., Esumi, H., and Ikeda, S. Plantar basal cell epithelioma occurring in a xeroderma pigmentosum variant case. *Iyaku no Mon*, **25**, 38–43 (1985) (in Japanese).

41. Satoh, Y., Irimajiri, T., Mitoh, Y., and Takeuchi, I. Photosensitivity and photoprotection in patients with xeroderma pigmentosum. *Jpn. J. Dermatol.*, **87**, 728–731 (1977) (in Japanese).

42. Satoh, Y., Mitoh, Y., and Irimajiri, T. Erythema action spectrum in xeroderma pigmentosum. *Photomed. Photobiol.*, **1**, 189–190 (1979) (in Japanese).

43. Satoh, Y. and Ichihashi, M. Xeroderma pigmentosum. *In* "Photosensitive Dermatoses," ed. Y. Satoh, pp. 113–144 (1983). Kanehara Shuppan, Tokyo (in Japanese).

44. Satoh, Y. Serum levels of vitamin D in xeroderma pigmentosum. Proceedings of The 2nd Kanto Conference on Calcium and Bone Metabolism, pp. 1–19 (1985) (in Japanese).

45. Satoh, Y. Xeroderma pigmentosum. *In* "Dermatology MOOK No. 5," ed. Y. Hori, pp. 167–176 (1986). Kanehara Shuppan, Tokyo (in Japanese).

46. Satoh, Y. and Kawada, A. Action spectrum for melanin pigmentation to ultraviolet light, and Japanese skin typing. *In* "Brown Melanoderma (Biology and Disease of Epidermal Pigmentation)," ed. T. B. Fitzpatrick, M. M. Wick, K. Toda, pp. 87–95 (1986). University of Tokyo Press, Tokyo.

47. Stefanini, M., Keijzer, W., Dalpra, L., Elli, R., Porro, N., Nicoletti, B., and Nuzzo, F. Differences in the levels of UV repair and in clinical symptoms in two sibs affected by xeroderma pigmentosum. *Hum. Genet.*, **54**, 177–182 (1980).

48. Swift, M. and Chase, C. Cancer in families with xeroderma pigmentosum. *J. Natl. Cancer Inst.*, **62**, 1415–1421 (1979).

49. Takebe, H., Fujiwara, Y., Sasaki, M. S., Satoh, Y., Kozuka, T., Nikaido, O., Ishizaki, K,

Arase, S., and Ikenaga, M. DNA repair and clinical characteristics of 96 xeroderma pigmentosum patients in Japan. *In* "DNA Repair Mechanisms," ed. P. C. Hanawalt, E. C. Friedberg, and C. F. Fox, pp. 617–620 (1978). Academic Press, New York.

50. Takebe, H. Xeroderma pigmentosum: DNA repair defects and skin cancer. *Gann Monogr. Cancer Res.*, **24**, 103–117 (1979).

51. Takebe, H., Yagi, T., and Satoh, Y. Cancer-prone hereditary diseases in relation to DNA repair. *In* "Biology of Cancer (1)," ed. E. A. Mirand, W. B. Hutchinson, and E. Mihichi, pp. 267–275 (1983). Alan R. Liss, New York.

52. Takebe, H., Tatsumi, K., and Satoh, Y. DNA repair and its possible involvement in the origin of multiple cancer. *Jpn. J. Clin. Oncol.*, **15** (Suppl. 1), 299–305 (1985).

53. Takebe, H., Nishigori, C., and Satoh, Y. Genetics and skin cancer of xeroderma pigmentosum in Japan. *Jpn. J. Cancer Res. (Gann)*, **78**, 1135–1143 (1987).

54. Takebe, H., Nishigori, C., and Tatsumi, K. Melanoma and other skin cancers in xeroderma pigmentosum patients, and mutation in their cells. *J. Invest. Dermatol.*, in press.

55. Zabel, M., Brandle, I., and Westkott, C. Augenveränderungen beim Xeroderma pigmentosum. *Hautarzt*, **31**, 188–190 (1980).

56. Zghal, M. Le xeroderma pigmentosum. *In* "Explorations Photobiologiques," Thesis, Universite de Tunis, Faculté de Medicine de Tunis, pp. 112–119 (1984).

57. Zwetsloot, J.C.M., Hoeijmakers, J.H.J., Vermeulen, W., Eker, A.P.M., and Bootsma, D. Unscheduled DNA synthesis in xeroderma pigmentosum cells after microinjection of yeast photoreactivating enzyme. *Mutat. Res.*, **165**, 109–115 (1986).

EXPLANATION OF PHOTOS

PHOTO 1. Group A patient, 6-year-old girl (XP13TO).

PHOTO 2. Group C patient, 8-year-old girl (XP21SE) (Courtesy of the late Dr. M. Seiji, Tohoku University).

PHOTO 3. Group D patient, 6-year-old boy (XP58TO).

PHOTO 4. Group E patient, 5-year-old girl (XP70TO).

PHOTO 5. Group F patient, 49-year-old female (XP1010S).

PHOTO 6. Group G patient, 37-year-old female (XP31KO) (Courtesy of Dr. M. Ichihashi, Kobe University).

PHOTO 7. XP-variant patient, 25-year-old female (XP5TO).

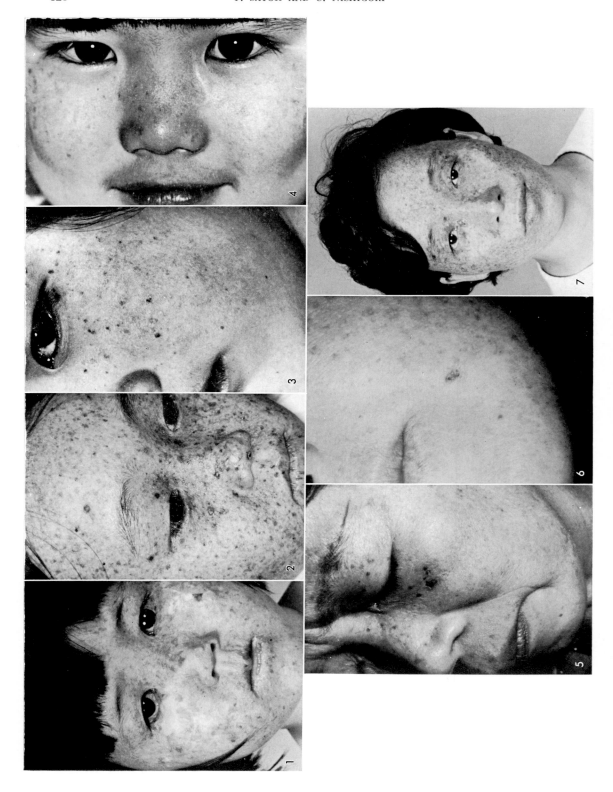

USE OF RETINOBLASTOMA AND WILMS' TUMOR AS SENTINEL PHENOTYPES FOR POPULATION SURVEILLANCE

Ei Matsunaga[*1] and Kensei Minoda[*2]

*National Institute of Genetics[*1] and Teikyo University Ichihara Hospital[*2]*

Retinoblastoma and Wilms' tumor occur in Japan at an approximate frequency of 1 per 16,000 and 1 per 19,000 newborns, respectively. A vast majority of these tumors arise from *de novo* germinal or somatic mutations. Although they are not usually detectable at birth, in countries where systematic registration of childhood malignancies is done, data on the incidence of the two tumors is available for population surveillance of environmental mutagens.

In Japan, the ongoing nationwide registration of all childhood malignancies is supported by a private foundation and maintained by the voluntary cooperation of physicians. Current data are not adequate for population surveillance because of their incomplete ascertainment. However, fairly reliable incidence data at the prefectural level are available in Kanagawa Prefecture, where ascertainment is made by reviewing application forms submitted by patients to the local government to defray the cost of medical treatment. The proposed system of using retinoblastoma and Wilms' tumor as sentinel phenotypes for population surveillance seems workable if the childhood cancer registry is strongly supported by the central government and if the need for surveillance is well recognized by physicians.

Human populations are currently exposed to a variety of environmental mutagens, both natural and man-made, and some of them induce malignant neoplasms in heavily exposed or genetically susceptible individuals. We do not know, however, whether the exposure enhances the rates of germinal mutation. It is therefore desirable to conduct, as economically as possible, a continuous surveillance of newborns, infants, and young children to see if background mutation rates change, and, if a significant rise in the rates occurs, to search for the causal agents. A sentinel phenotype is a marker for that purpose; this refers to certain autosomal dominant or X-linked conditions with early onset of obvious pathologic manifestation, low reproductive fitness, and high penetrance of the gene. Classical examples of sentinel phenotypes include achondroplasia, aniridia, acrocephalosyndactyly (Apert syndrome), and osteogenesis imperfecta (type 1) (*18*). A significant fraction of those conditions occurs as a result of recurrent mutations. Because the number of sentinel phenotypes presently available is limited and their individual frequency is of the order of 10^{-5}, the target population must be sufficiently large to achieve statistically significant results. In other words, the sentinel phenotype approach is not useful for monitoring of a small circumscribed population that has been

---

*1 1111, Yata, Mishima 411, Japan (松永　英).
*2 3426-3, Anesaki, Ichihara 229-01, Japan (箕田健生).

exposed to a known or suspected mutagen, but it may have significance in the surveil-lance of a large population to detect a possible rise in background mutation rates. In this paper we select retinoblastoma and Wilms' tumor, explain the rationale and strategy of using them for population surveillance, and discuss some relevant data from the ongoing registry of childhood cancers in Japan.

Rationale and Strategy

The ICPEMC (International Commission for Protection against Environmental Mutagens and Carcinogens) pointed out that although retinoblastoma is not usually detectable at birth, it has special features that make it a prime candidate for a pilot ef-fort for population surveillance (*10*). To this we would now add Wilms' tumor, which, in the 7th edition of McKusick's catalog (*16*), has finally been enrolled in the group of autosomal dominant conditions with an asterisk. A vast majority of all cases of either tumor occurs sporadically, and all sporadic bilateral cases are hereditary and usually due to a dominant germinal mutation with high penetrance, while most sporadic unila-teral cases are nonhereditary, arising from somatic mutation (*11, 14, 23*). Hence the two tumors can be used for surveillance of both germinal and somatic mutations. A minority of either tumor is associated with constitutional deletion of a specific chromo-some region, usually accompanied by various congenital anomalies and mental retarda-tion, *i.e.*, del(13q14) in retinoblastoma and del(11p13) in aniridia-Wilms' tumor syn-drome (*5, 23*). Most of these cases also occur sporadically, and they can be used as a sentinel phenotype for chromosome mutation. Table I gives some parameters estimated for the two tumors (*14*).

There are several centers in the world where consecutive data on the incidence of childhood malignancies, including the two tumors, are being collected from a large base population; hence the data already assembled can readily be utilized for surveillance, provided that an appropriate system for international collaboration, such as that for the ongoing Birth Defects Monitoring System (*4*) could be organized.

A difficulty of this approach lies in that whereas the diagnosis of a bilateral disease is definite, that of a unilateral case is only tentative because a tumor may develop later in the contralateral organ. However, in most bilateral cases, *i.e.*, about 80% of bilateral retinoblastomas and 70% of bilateral Wilms' tumors, the disease was already bilateral

TABLE I.   Some Estimated Parameters for Retinoblastoma and Wilms' Tumor

	Retinoblastoma	Wilms' tumor	Remarks
Approximate birth frequency in Japan	1: 16,000	1: 19,000	Based on data in Table V
Familial cases	3–5%	0.2% (0.1–1.5%)	Autosomal dominant inheritance with variable penetrance and expressivity
Cases with del(13q14) or del(11q13)	5%	1%	Mostly sporadic in origin
Of all sporadic cases Bilateral	30%	6% (2–12%)	Potential progenitor of familial cases
Unilateral	70%	94%	Mostly nonheritable
Fraction of sporadic unilateral cases that are heritable	10%	5–10%	

when the diagnosis in one eye or kidney was made, and in most sequentially bilateral cases, the ultimate diagnosis was made within 3 years after the first diagnosis; cases in which the interval exceeds 3 years are exceptional (1, 2, 6, 7, 22). Therefore, to confirm the diagnosis, unilateral cases should be followed up for at least 3 years, but extra efforts for this do not seem to pose a problem in countries where a childhood cancer registry has been established.

If a population is exposed to an environmental mutagen that induces germinal and/or somatic mutations, then after a latency period of a few years, there will be a rise in the incidence of sporadic cases of retinoblastoma and Wilms' tumor above the baseline level. Analyses of data from familial cases of retinoblastoma or Wilms' tumor suggested that patients with early onset are inherently more susceptible to the induction of either tumor than are those with late onset (13, 14). Probably the same applies to patients with a nonhereditary tumor that constitutes 90% or more of the sporadic unilateral cases. Therefore, to make early detection of an increase in mutation rates possible, attention should be paid to the change in the incidence of sporadic cases with early onset (say, under 1 year of age). However, the age of patients at diagnosis can be influenced considerably by socioeconomic factors such as availability of medical care services and medical awareness by the public. In Japan, for example, the mean age at diagnosis of patients with unilateral retinoblastoma has been lowered from 31.5 months to 23.6 months, and that of bilateral cases from 17.1 months to 10.4 months during the last 30 years (13). If a change in the pattern of age-specific incidence occurs (21), the data should be examined cautiously.

It is well known that both retinoblastoma and Wilms' tumor show, among all childhood cancers, least geographic and ethnic variation in frequency, although their incidence is never constant worldwide (3). The recurrent mutations responsible for most of these tumors may be caused by some intrinsic biological mechanisms common to all individuals, and not by mutagens found in our daily environment that varies from place to place and from time to time. However, if a significant rise in the incidence could be detected under constant surveillance, then the *excess* could be attributed to the introduction of environmental mutagens. In bilateral cases either paternal or maternal exposure prior to the conception of the index child should be suspected, whereas in unilateral cases the child's exposure before or after birth should be suspected. In the past most case-control studies failed to identify a causal agent. However, a recent report by Shiono *et al.* (20) is encouraging. By studying 40 children with malignant neoplasms (including 3 with retinoblastoma and 7 with Wilms' tumor) and 80 matched controls, these authors demonstrated that mothers of the case children had been exposed to X-rays significantly more often before and during pregnancy.

Childhood Cancer Registry in Japan

In Japan, a nationwide registration of childhood cancers has been conducted continuously since 1969 by joint effort of the Pediatric Association and the Pediatric Surgeon's Society of Japan, with the support of the Children's Cancer Association. Its primary aim is stated as being to register all malignant neoplasms observed in all children under 15 years of age country-wide when they first visit a hospital (8). Japan is divided into 7 districts from north to south, and each district has its own registration center. Data for newly registered cases in each center are sent annually to the National Cancer

Center, Tokyo, and the results of registration are reported periodically in a tabulated form. The total number of childhood malignancies registered during the 10 year period from 1969 to 1978 was 11,595, including 819 cases of retinoblastoma and 533 cases of Wilms' tumor (8, 12). No information is available concerning laterality and sporadic or familial occurrence of the disease. It is not known to what extent the data represents the actual number of new cases in the whole country, although Hanawa (8) guessed the rate of registration for all childhood cancers to be about 50%. Thus, the current data are not satisfactory for population surveillance because of incomplete ascertainment.

As a subset of this activity, registration of all retinoblastoma cases was initiated in 1975 by an *ad hoc* committee of the Ophthalmologists Society of Japan. A standard formula for recording family history, clinical observations and pathologic findings, the method of treatment, and the follow-up of the patients is sent each year to about 150 major hospitals in various parts of Japan, asking that physicians fill out the form and return to Minoda at the Teikyo University Ichihara Hospital in Ichihara (17).

Table II gives the number of registered cases from 1975 to 1980, as reported annually by Minoda. "Revisiting cases" refer to those patients who visited a hospital in the respective year but in whom the diagnosis had been made previously. For example, among the 37 revisiting cases registered in 1976 there may be some who were new cases in 1975 but were overlooked in registration as such. Correcting for such delayed reporting, Table III shows data on annual incidence of retinoblastoma. While the size of the base population remained almost the same during the 6 years, the number of new cases has been declining gradually, most probably as a result of the declining rate of registration. Regarding the data for the first 2 years, the registration appears to have ascertained nearly all cases, as suggested by the estimated incidence of 1 per about

TABLE II.   Data from National Registration of Retinoblastoma in Japan,
as Reported Annually by Midoda

Year	No. of:		Total
	New cases	Revisiting cases	
1975	121	342	463
1976	107	37	144
1977	77	7	84
1978	79	16	95
1979	78	44	122
1980	70	2	72
Total	532	448	980

TABLE III.   Annual Incidence of Retinoblastoma in Japan (1975–1980)

Year	Population under 15 years	No. of new cases			Birth frequency
		Sporadic	Familial	Total	
1975	27,035,000	119	8	127	1: 14,200
1976	27,267,000	114	6	120	1: 15,150
1977	27,462,000	103	3	106	1: 17,270
1978	27,522,000	84	2	86	1: 21,330
1979	27,479,000	82	3	85	1: 21,550
1980	27,353,300	75	4	79	1: 23,080

TABLE IV. Annual Incidence of Sporadic Retinoblastoma by Laterality in Japan (1975–1980)

Year	No. of new sporadic cases			Birth frequency
	Bilateral (%)	Unilateral	Total	
1975	31 (26.1)	88	119	1: 15,100
1976	34 (29.8)	80	114	1: 15,950
1977	30 (29.1)	73	103	1: 17,770
1978	29 (34.5)	55	84	1: 21,800
1979	25 (30.5)	57	82	1: 22,340
1980	27 (36.0)	48	75	1: 24,300
Total	176 (30.5)	401	577	

TABLE V. Number of New Cases of Childhood Malignancies Occurring in
Kanagawa Prefecture (1975–1982)

Year	Retinoblastoma	Wilms' tumor	All childhood malignancies	Population under 15 years
1975	11	7	177	1,632,000
1976	7	9	178	1,675,000
1977	4	3	168	1,706,000
1978	4	3	181	1,729,000
1979	9	9	198	1,740,000
1980	8	2	171	1,703,000
1981	7	5	189	1,702,000
1982	7	10	196	1,676,000
Total	57	48	1,458	13,563,000
Incidence per newborn	6.3×10^{-5} (1: 15,900)	5.3×10^{-5} (1: 18,840)	1.6×10^{-3} (1: 620)	

15,000 live-births, which is much higher than that (1 per 22,000) previously obtained in Hokkaido (15). Table IV gives data on sporadic bilateral and unilateral cases separately. The proportion of bilateral cases fluctuates around an average of about 30%, and no secular trend is seen.

On the other hand, there are a few local centers that are making efforts to register childhood cancers at the prefectural level. Since 1971 childhood cancers have been among a number of "designated diseases" for which the cost of medical treatment is defrayed, upon application, by central and local governments. By reviewing the application forms submitted by patients to each local government, it is feasible to achieve a nearly complete ascertainment of new cases of childhood neoplasms within the prefecture. Table V shows results of such a survey carried out at the Kanagawa Children's Medical Center since 1975 (9, 19). No clear trend can be seen in the incidence of the two tumors during the 8 years from 1975 to 1982. Because the average incidence of retinoblastoma is close to that for the whole country in 1975 and 1976 (Table III), it is reasonable to assume that the ascertainment was also nearly complete for other malignancies. It is interesting to note that Wilms' tumor is less common than retinoblastoma in Japan while it is more common for US white and black children (24). This finding supports the notion of Breslow and Langholz (3) who, by international comparison of data on cancer incidence, pointed out that Wilms' tumor rate among Japanese is approximately 60% of the rates in North America and Britain. It is impor-

TABLE VI. Statistical Power of Detecting a Significant Rise in the Combined Incidence
of Sporadic Cases of Retinoblastoma and Wilms' Tumor in Japan

| | Base-line incidence/year | | Total |
	Bilateral	Unilateral	
Retinoblastoma	26	62	88
Wilms' tumor	4	70	74
Total	30	132	162
S.D.	5.5	11.5	12.7
Critical incidence ($p<0.01$)	45	162	195
Increase	50%	23%	20%

tant that the central government encourage such population surveys to be carried out in other prefectures also to obtain comparable data.

Finally, a word should be said about the statistical power of detecting a significant rise in the incidence of these tumors throughout the country. With approximately 1.4 million births a year and the incidence of retinoblastoma and Wilms' tumor being 1 per 16,000 and 1 per 19,000 newborns respectively, the annual number of new cases of the two tumors combined would be about 162, of which about 30 may be affected bilaterally and 132 unilaterally. If this is taken as a standard, then the borderline above which a rise in the incidence would be statistically significant at the 1% level would be 45 for the bilateral and 162 for the unilateral cases (Table VI). Thus the minimal increase in the rates of germinal and somatic mutations that can be detected by this approach is 50% and 23%, respectively.

In conclusion, the proposed system of using retinoblastoma and Wilms' tumor as sentinel phenotypes for population surveillance seems to be workable if the childhood cancer registry is supported strongly by the central government and if the need for surveillance is well recognized by physicians.

Acknowledgment

This paper, contribution no. 1726 from the National Institute of Genetics, was supported by a grant-in-aid from the Ministry of Education, Science and Culture, Japan.

REFERENCES

1. Bishop, H. C. and Hope, J. W. Bilateral Wilms' tumors. *J. Pediat. Surg.*, **1**, 476–487 (1966).
2. Bond, J. V. Bilateral Wilms' tumor: Age at diagnosis, associated congenital anomalies, and possible pattern of inheritance. *Lancet*, **ii**, 482–484 (1975).
3. Breslow, N. E. and Langholz, B. Childhood cancer incidence: Geographic and temporal variation. *Int. J. Cancer*, **32**, 703–716 (1983).
4. Flynt, J. W. and Hay, S. International clearinghouse for birth-defects monitoring systems. *Contr. Epidemiol. Biostat.*, **1**, 44–52 (1979).
5. Francke, U., Holmes, L. B., Atkins, L., and Riccardi, V. M. Aniridia-Wilms' tumor association: Evidence for specific deletion of 11p13. *Cytogenet. Cell Genet.*, **24**, 185–192 (1979).
6. Garrett, R. A. and Donohue, J. P. Bilateral Wilms' tumors. *J. Urol.*, **120**, 586–588 (1978).
7. Gordon, H. Family studies in retinoblastoma. *Birth Defects* **X** (10), 185–190 (1974).

8. Hanawa, Y. All Japan Children's Cancer Registration, 1969–1973. Children's Cancer Association of Japan, Tokyo (1975).

9. Hanawa, Y. Childhood malignant neoplasms in Kanagawa prefecture. *Kanagawa Children's Medical Center J.*, **5**, 241–245 (1976).

10. ICPEMC Committee 5 final report. Mutation epidemiology: Review and recommendations. *Mutat. Res.*, **123**, 1–11 (1983).

11. Knudson, A. G., Jr. and Strong, L. C. Mutation and cancer: A model for Wilms' tumor of the kidney. *J. Natl. Cancer Inst.*, **48**, 313–324 (1972).

12. Kobayashi, N. All Japan Children's Cancer Registration, 1974–1978. Children's Cancer Association of Japan, Tokyo (1982).

13. Matsunaga, E. Hereditary retinoblastoma: Host resistance and age at onset. *J. Natl. Cancer Inst.*, **63**, 933–939 (1979).

14. Matsunaga, E. Genetics of Wilms' tumor. *Hum. Genet.*, **57**, 231–246 (1981).

15. Matsunaga, E. and Ogyu, H. Genetic study of retinoblastoma in a Japanese population. *Jpn. J. Hum. Genet.*, **4**, 156 (1959).

16. McKusick, V. A. Mendelian inheritance in man. "Catalogs of Autosomal Dominant, Autosomal Recessive, and X-linked Phenotypes," 7th ed. (1986). The Johns Hopkins Univ. Press, Baltimore and London.

17. Minoda, K. National registration of retinoblastoma children in 1975. *Acta Soc. Ophthalmol. Jpn.*, **80**, 1648–1657 (1976).

18. Mulvihill, J. J. and Czeizel, A. Perspectives in mutation epidemiology: 6. A 1983 view of sentinel phenotypes. *Mutat. Res.*, **114**, 425–447 (1983).

19. Nishihira, K. Childhood malignant neoplasms in Kanagawa prefecture. *Kanagawa Children's Medical Cancer J.*, **6**, 286–289 (1977); **7**, 406–409 (1978); **8**, 274–276 (1979); **9**, 355–357 (1980); **11**, 55–56 (1982); **12**, 62–63 (1983); **13**, 49–50 (1984).

20. Shiono, P. H., Chung, C. S., and Myrianthopoulos, N. C. Preconception radiation, intrauterine diagnostic radiation, and childhood neoplasia. *J. Natl. Cancer Inst.*, **65**, 681–686 (1980).

21. Sugahara, T. A possible population monitoring system on environmental mutagens: Statistical studies on retinoblastoma in Japan. *Mutat. Res.*, **30**, 137–142 (1975).

22. Tsunoda, A., Taguchi, H., and Akiyama, H. Bilateral Wilms' tumor (Second report). *Geka*, **33**, 83–90 (1971).

23. Vogel, F. Genetics of retinoblastoma. *Hum. Genet.*, **52**, 1–54 (1979).

24. Young, J. L., Jr. and Miller, R. W. Incidence of malignant tumors in U.S. children. *J. Pediat.*, **86**, 254–258 (1975).

FAMILY CLUSTERING OF CANCER: ANALYSIS OF CANCER REGISTRY DATA

Hiroshi Ogawa, Suketami Tominaga, and Ikuko Kato

*Division of Epidemiology, Aichi Cancer Center Research Institute**

Family cancer history was examined for 9,131 cancer patients who were reported to the Aichi Cancer Registry. A significant site concordance between patients and their family members with cancer was observed for cancer of the stomach, colon and rectum, and breast. The percentage of patients who had a family history of each of the above cancers was significantly higher for patients with cancer of the same site than for patients with cancer of a different site. When the patients were limited to highly familial cases, incidence rate of the above cancer among family members was higher for the families of patients with cancer of the same site than for the families of patients with cancer of a different site. These results suggest that cancer of the stomach, colon and rectum, and breast tends to cluster in a family. By case-control analysis, family clustering of these cancers was observed independently from life style factors such as smoking, consumption of alcohol, marital status and occupation. A bimodal age distribution was observed for colon and rectum cancer patients who had family history of this cancer. Bimodal age distribution was also obseved for patients with multiple primary cancer involving colon and rectum cancer. The cancer registry is useful for the study of family cancer.

One important aim in the study of family cancer is to gather evidence on environmental risk factors, genetic background, and the interaction of these conditions in human carcinogenesis. Cancer incidence and death rate largely changes with time, place, person, and even migration. Much epidemiologic research has pointed to the more important role of "nurture" than "nature" in human carcinogenesis. It is estimated that about 70% of the cancer deaths in the United States of America are attributable to tobacco, diet, and alcohol (3). This evidence suggests the possibility that family clustering of cancer may be explained in some part by common family exposure to such life style factors. However, cancer of a specific histopathologic type, multifocal or bilateral lesions, and early age at onset, tends to aggregate in a family through inherited susceptibility (18). It is also known that cancer-prone diseases such as polyposis coli, retinoblastoma, xeroderma pigmentosum, and others are heritable (12).

Another aim of the study of family cancer is cancer control. Identification of families with multiple cancer patients, and intervention with these high risk families are very important in public health practice. For example, oral supplementation of calcium to persons at high risk of non-polyposis familial colonic cancer seems a promising preventive measure (7). Regulation of exposure to sunlight for patients with xeroderma

---

* 1-1, Kanokoden, Chikusa-ku, Nagoya 464, Japan (小川　浩, 富永祐民, 加藤育子).

pigmentosum and prophylactic colectomy by the age of 20 years to those with multiple polyposis are recommended (12).

There are three kinds of family study: 1) genealogy, 2) case-control study, and 3) population-based study. The last one has a methodological advantage, because it minimizes sampling variation and bias which is always present in the first and second types of study (18). A community cancer registry gives us an opportunity to conduct a population-based family study, if information on family history is compiled. This article is to examine the family clustering of cancer among patients using such data from the Aichi Cancer Registry. Some of the results have already been reported elsewhere (14).

Cancer Registry Data

The Aichi Cancer Registry covers inhabitants in Aichi Prefecture (population 6,455,000 in 1985). It was started in 1962 and the number of reported cases had reached 133,015 in 1984, with 7,771 cases reported that year from 194 medical facilities in Aichi Prefecture. This registry is unique because it has compiled information on family history of cancer, smoking, consumption of alcohol, marital status, and occupation, in addition to medical items (2). Data processing by computer began in 1979.

The initial study population consisted of 13,539 cancer patients reported between 1979 and 1981. Patients of unknown sex or age, and patients under 20 years old at diagnosis were excluded. Among the remaining 13,162 patients, the percentage of those on which complete information was available was 69.4% for family history of cancer in parents and siblings, 76.4% for smoking, 75.1% for drinking, 94.4% for marital status, and 90.7% for occupation. No difference was observed in age and sex distribution between patients with and without complete information on each item. Data analysis was limited for the 9,131 cancer patients (4,653 males and 4,478 females) for whom complete information was obtained on family cancer history. Ages ranged from 20 to 98 years and was 58.5 years in average.

Family History of Cancer in Cancer Patients

The rate of cancer patients who had a history of cancer in their first degree families, except children, was 24.4% in males, 24.6% in females, or 24.5% for all patients. The rate by cancer sites for study patients ranged between 21.9% and 28.6%, and no sizeable difference was observed. The rate by the family relationship was 9.2% for father, 8.4% for mother, 6.0% for brothers, and 5.2% for sisters.

The rate of family history of cancer of all sites and specific sites is shown in Table I. Overall, the rate of family history by site was 12.2% for stomach cancer, 2.1% for colon and rectum cancer, 2.0% for liver cancer, 1.5% for lung cancer, 1.2% for breast cancer, 2.9% for uterus cancer, and 4.5% for other cancers. In viewing the figures in Table I it is noticed that there is a phenomenon of site concordance between study patients and families with cancer. In family history of stomach cancer, the rate ranged from 6.4% to 16.5%, and the highest rate was observed among stomach cancer patients. In family history of liver and breast cancers, the highest rates, 3.4% and 3.1% for each, were observed among patients with cancer of the same sites. In colon and rectum cancer a high rate of family history of this cancer was observed among patients with cancer of this site.

TABLE I. Rates of Cancer Patients with Family History of Cancer of Specific Sites[a,b]

Family history	Study patients							
	Stomach $n=2,848$	Colon and rectum $n=1,071$	Liver $n=252$	Lung $n=884$	Breast $n=870$	Uterus $n=646$	Others $n=2,560$	All sites $n=9,131$
Stomach	16.5	11.5	6.4	10.3	11.1	9.8	9.6	12.2
Colon and rectum	1.9	4.2	7.0	1.5	2.5	1.5	1.8	2.1
Liver	2.2	1.7	3.4	1.1	2.1	2.7	1.9	2.0
Lung	2.2	1.3	0.3	1.4	1.6	0.8	1.1	1.5
Breast	0.9	1.0	0.2	0.8	3.1	0.9	1.1	1.2
Uterus	2.3	2.5	3.9	3.7	4.0	3.7	3.2	2.9
Others	4.6	4.4	5.5	4.6	3.3	4.4	5.0	4.5
All sites	28.6	23.3	23.7	21.9	25.4	23.1	21.6	24.5

[a] Age- and sex-adjusted percentages.
[b] Breast cancer only in females.

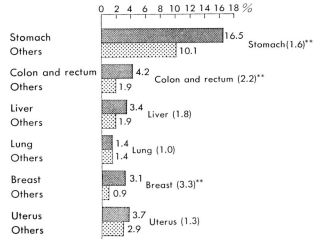

FIG. 1. Rates of cancer patients with family cancer history: comparison between patients with cancer of specific sites and other sites[a-c]

[a] Age- and sex-adjusted percentages. [b] Breast cancer only in females. [c] Ratio in parenthesis. ** $p<0.01$. From Ogawa et al. (14).

Figure 1 illustrates comparison of the rates of family history for a specific site and other sites. Significant site concordance was observed for cancer of the stomach, colon and rectum, and breast. The rate of family history of stomach cancer was 16.5%, and this is 1.6 times higher than the corresponding rate of 10.1% in other cancer patients ($p<0.01$). Similarly, the rate ratio was 2.2 for colon and rectum cancer ($p<0.01$), and 3.3 for breast cancer ($p<0.01$). The site concordance for these cancers was consistently observed for every family relationship. The rate ratios for stomach cancer were 1.6 for father, 1.5 for mother, 1.8 for brothers, and 2.2 for sisters. The ratios for colon and rectum cancer were 2.1 for father, 2.2 for mother, 2.8 for brothers, and 3.1 for sisters. The ratios for breast cancer were 3.5 for mother and 3.6 for sisters. These results suggest that cancer of the stomach, colon and rectum, and breast tend to cluster in a family.

Case-control Analysis

Information on smoking, drinking, marital status, and occupation have been compiled in the Aichi Cancer Registry. This information is useful to discern whether the observed family clustering of cancer of the stomach, colon and rectum, and breast is or is not modified by such life style factors, and if so, how it is modified. Case-control analysis was applied to estimate relative risk of these cancers for family history in combination with life style factors. In this analysis, patients with cancer of sites other than the stomach, colon and rectum, liver, lung, breast, and uterus were used as control patients. The Mantel-Haenszel estimate of relative risk adjusted for sex and age was calculated (*11*).

The results of case-control analysis for family history and smoking are shown in Table II. Study and control patients were divided into four groups: 1) those who had no family history of cancer of the same site, and had never smoked [− −], 2) those who had family history and had never smoked [+ −], 3) those who had no family history and had been in the past or were now a smoker (ex-smoker or smoker) [− +], and 4) those who had a family history and had smoked [+ +].

Relative risk of stomach cancer was 1.67 ($p<0.01$) in [+ −], 0.99 in [− +], 1.83 ($p<0.01$) in [+ +]. The risk was consistently high whenever patients had a family history of stomach cancer. A similar pattern of risk was observed in breast cancer: 3.21

TABLE II. Case-control Analysis of Major Cancer Sites in
Relation to Family History and Smoking[a–d]

Case-control analysis	Family history and smoking			
	[− −]	[+ −]	[− +]	[+ +]
Stomach cancer patients	937	164	859	192
Control	967	101	765	89
RR	1.00	1.67**	0.99	1.83**
Colon and rectum cancer patients	477	19	334	10
Control	1,055	13	839	15
RR	1.00	3.21**	0.73**	1.21
Liver cancer patients	65	2	103	6
Control	1,049	19	840	14
RR	1.00	1.79	1.42**	4.16**
Lung cancer patients	225	4	494	12
Control	1,057	11	841	13
RR	1.00	1.69	2.23**	3.64**
Breast cancer patients	537	16	89	6
Control	744	7	108	3
RR	1.00	3.21**	1.13	2.94
Uterus cancer patients	405	18	75	4
Control	727	24	105	6
RR	1.00	1.31	1.27*	1.20

[a] Family history of cancer of the same site: + presence; − absence.
[b] Smoking: + smoker and ex-smoker; − never smoked.
[c] Control: patients with cancer of sites other than stomach, colon and rectum, liver, lung, breast, and uterus.
[d] Mantel-Haenszel estimate of relative risk (RR) adjusted for sex and age.
* $p<0.05$, ** $p<0.01$.

($p<0.01$) in [+ −], 1.13 in [− +], and 2.94 in [+ +]. In cancer of the colon and rectum, the risk was 3.21 ($p<0.01$), 0.73 ($p<0.01$), and 1.21 in each corresponding combination pattern. The high risk for family history and low risk for smoking were counterbalanced in this cancer when both factors were combined. These results suggest that in cancer of the stomach, colon and rectum, and breast, family history is a risk factor which is independent from smoking.

Case-control analysis of family history was also conducted in combination with consumption of alcohol, marital status, and occupation. The results do not differ from those observed in combination with smoking. The risk of cancer of the stomach, colon and rectum, and breast was always significantly high where patients had family history of these cancers. These results enable us to conclude that family clustering of these cancers is not explained by life style factors such as smoking, consumption of alcohol marital status, or occupation.

It may be interesting to see the result for lung cancer, which is well known to be causally associated with smoking. As shown in Table II, the risk of lung cancer was 1.69 for family history alone [+ −], 2.23 ($p<0.01$) for smoking alone [− +], and 3.64 ($p<0.01$) where family history and smoking were combined [+ +]. The evidence that the risk of lung cancer for smokers increases in combination of family history of lung cancer has been reported in other studies (15, 21). The excess risk for combination of family history and smoking was also observed in liver cancer.

Age Distribution

Some studies have reported that familial cancer patients were younger than non-familial cancer patients, especially in cancer of the large bowel and the breast (1, 8, 13, 22). The distribution of age at diagnosis was examined for patients with cancer of the stomach, colon and rectum, and breast. The patients were divided into three groups: 1) those with a family history of cancer of the same site, 2) those with a family history of cancer of different sites, and 3) those with no family history of cancer of any site. Table III shows mean and standard deviation of the age at diagnosis for patients in each group. Significant age difference was observed among the three groups only in colon and rectum cancer patients. Those with a family history of the same site were significantly younger than the other two groups of patients ($p<0.01$ and $p<0.05$). The age distribution curve for each of the three groups with colon and rectum cancer is illustrated in Fig. 2. The curve of patients with a family history of this cancer is quite different than the other two groups. It was shifted in a younger direction, and was bimodal

TABLE III. Mean and Standard Deviation of Patients with Cancer of the Stomach, Colon and Rectum, and Breast by Pattern of Family History of Cancer

Site of patient cancer	Patients								
	With family history of same cancer			With family history of different cancer			Without family history of cancer		
	N	$\bar{X}$	S.D.	N	$\bar{X}$	S.D.	N	$\bar{X}$	S.D.
Stomach cancer	476	59.0	12.1	312	57.6	11.8	2,060	58.7	13.5
Colon and rectum cancer	40	55.8	13.9	203	61.2	11.0	828	60.1	13.1
Breast cancer	29	51.9	10.1	187	53.2	11.0	654	51.1	12.3

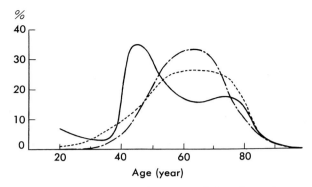

Fɪɢ. 2.   Age distribution of patients with cancer of the colon and rectum by family history of cancer
——— patients with family history of colon and rectum cancer ($n=40$); —·— patients with family history of other cancers ($n=203$); and - - - patients without family history of cancer ($n=828$). From Ogawa *et al.* *(14)*.

Tᴀʙʟᴇ IV.   Cancer Sites, Age, Sex, and Family History of Cancer for Patients with Multiple Primary Cancers Involving Colon and Rectum Cancer

Sex		Site and age				Family history
Male						
No.	1	Colon	35	Stomach	42	—
	2	Colon	44	Liver	45	—
	3	Colon	46	Stomach	46	+ (Mo-stomach)
	4	Colon	47	Lung	50	—
	5	Stomach	46	Colon	47	—
	6	Colon	49	Rectum	49	—
	7	Stomach	45	Colon	50	?
	8	Stomach	44	Colon	50	—
	9	Colon	51	Rectum	51	—
	10	Colon	52	Rectum	54	—
	11	Colon	67	Stomach	68	—
	12	Colon	68	Brain	69	—
	13	Colon	71	Rectum	71	?
	14	Stomach	71	Rectum	72	—
	15	Colon	73	Stomach	73	—
	16	Colon	73	Liver	73	?
	17	Rectum	73	Liver	73	+ (Mo-uterus)
	18	Colon	75	Stomach	75	+ (Fa-stomach)
	19	Colon	76	Stomach	76	—
	20	Colon	78	Rectum	78	—
	21	Rectum	81	Stomach	81	—
Female						
No.	1	Uter. corp.	45	Colon	47	+ (Bro-colo. rect., Sis-other)
	2	Colon	53	Breast	54	+ (Mo-stomach)
	3	Colon	55	Thyroid	55	+ (Fa-stomach)
	4	Colon	61	Stomach	61	+ (Fa-liver)
	5	Rectum	63	Stomach	63	—
	6	Rectum	71	Stomach	71	—
	7	Rectum	85	Liver	85	—

+ case with family history; — case without family history; ? family history is unknown; Fa, father; Mo, mother; Bro, brothers; Sis, sisters.

with a larger peak in the 40s and a smaller peak in the 70s. This result suggests the existence of two different etiological backgrounds for cancer of the colon and rectum. The younger peak may be related to inherited host conditions, and the older peak to environmental risk factors such as food habits.

As some studies reported that patients with multiple primary cancer involving colon and rectum cancer tended to be young and to have a family cancer history (*13, 22*), analysis of age was extended for these individuals. Twenty eight cases with multiple primary cancers were identified from among the 1,642 colon and rectum cancer patients in this study. A profile of these cases is shown in Table IV. It is noteworthy that the distribution of age at diagnosis for the initial cancer was rather bimodal: 9 cases (32.1%) age 49 years or less, 8 cases (28.6%) age 50s and 60s, and 11 cases (39.3%) age 70 years or more. Special attention should be given to females No. 1, No. 2, and No. 3 in Table IV, because they are rather young, involve cancer of the corpus uterus, breast, or thyroid, and have a family history of cancer. These characteristics partially satisfy the criteria for the cancer family syndrome (*9*).

Familial Cancer Patients

The word, "familial" refers here to the occurrence of cancer in two or more categories of father, mother, brothers, and sisters. From the 9,131 total study patients, 348 cases (3.8%) were identified as familial. Among them, 104 (29.9%) were reported from the Aichi Cancer Center Hospital. Sex ratio was 54/50 (m/f) and average age was 59.7 years. Medical records of these familial cases were reviewed to examine family clustering of specific cancers.

The number of family members in the familial cases was 104 fathers, 104 mothers, 245 brothers, and 289 sisters for a total of 742. Incidence rate of cancer of all sites was 32.7% (243/742). The families were divided into seven groups by the cancer site for the proband, and incidence rate of cancer of each specific site was calculated for each

TABLE V. Cancer Incidence (%) in Families with Multiple Cancer History[a,b]

Family member cancer	Cancer of probands							
	Stomach cancer	Colon and rectum cancer	Lung cancer	Breast cancer	Uterus cervix cancer	Uterus corpus, endometrium cancer	Other cancers	All cancers
	$N=30$ $n=214$	$N=11$ $n=67$	$N=11$ $n=70$	$N=13$ $n=100$	$N=12$ $n=96$	$N=7$ $n=50$	$N=20$ $n=145$	$N=104$ $n=742$
Stomach cancer	15.9	16.4	14.3	7.0	7.3	12.0	12.4	12.5
Colon and rectum cancer	0.9	10.4	2.9	1.0	4.2	4.0	2.8	3.0
Lung cancer	3.3	1.5	1.4	1.0	0.0	0.0	0.0	1.5
Breast cancer	1.0	5.4	2.6	8.9	1.8	0.0	1.2	2.8
Uterus cancer	6.9	8.1	10.5	8.9	7.1	10.0	3.7	8.1
Liver cancer	3.7	1.5	4.3	7.0	3.1	4.0	2.1	4.0
Other cancers	5.1	4.5	5.7	4.0	7.3	6.0	6.2	5.9
All cancers	32.7	41.8	35.7	30.0	27.1	36.0	31.7	32.7

N, number of families; *n*, number of total family members (parents and siblings).

[a] Probands were excluded in calculation.

[b] Breast cancer only in females.

family group. As shown in Table V, site concordance was again noticed for cancer of the stomach, colon and rectum, and breast. Incidence rate of stomach cancer was 15.9% in stomach cancer families and 16.4% in colon rectum cancer families. Both rates are high compared with the rates in other cancer families. Incidence rate of colon and rectum cancer was 10.4% in colon and rectum cancer families, which was 4.7 times higher than 2.2% in other cancer families ($p<0.01$). Incidence rate of breast cancer was 8.9% in breast cancer families, which is 5.4 times higher than the 0.9% in other cancer families ($p<0.01$). It should be noted that the rate of breast cancer was also high in colon and rectum cancer families (5.4%). These results are additional evidence of the family clustering of cancers of the stomach, colon and rectum, and breast.

DISCUSSION

In epidemiologic study on family clustering of cancer, a great effort is needed to identify familial cancer cases. The percentage of cancer patients who had a history of cancer of the same site in their parents or siblings was 3.1% to 4.2% for the major sites except stomach cancer (16.5%), as shown in Table I. The Aichi Cancer Registry, which has been compiling information on family cancer histories has enabled us to do a family study more efficiently. However, the reported cases in this registry, cover only 51% of the total estimated incidences in Aichi Prefecture in 1982 (2). Furthermore, information on family history was not obtained for 30.6% of all reported cases; therefore, a sampling bias must be assumed in this study.

Another problem is that the results on family clustering were obtained by internal comparison among only cancer patients. The rate of family history of a specific cancer was compared between patients with this cancer and patients with other cancers. In case-control analysis, patients with cancer of a site other than major sites were used as a control group. Therefore, it is possible that the present results of family clustering may be an underestimation. Comparison with the general population is preferable, but this is impossible because the Registry does not cover information on family size or age of members. Even if such information were available, there is no data on family cancer history in a comparable general population. These limitations on the present data must be kept in mind.

The significant site concordance observed between patients and family members for cancer of the stomach, colon and rectum, and breast cancer means that these cancers tended to aggregate in a family. The rate of family history of stomach cancer for stomach cancer patients was 1.7 times higher than the corresponding rate for other cancer patients. Similarly, the ratio was 2.2 in cancer of the colon and rectum, and 3.3 in breast cancer. Further, the incidence of stomach cancer for families of stomach cancer patients with multiple family history of cancer was 1.4 times higher than that for families of other cancer patients with multiple history of cancer. The ratio was 4.7 for colon and rectum cancer, and 5.4 for breast cancer. These results are in line with those in previous studies. The risk of stomach cancer has been reported to be 1.5 to 3.4 times higher for families of the proband with this cancer, compared with families of control or general population (6, 10, 19, 20). The ratio was 2.2 (22) and 3.1 (10) for colon and rectum cancer, and 1.8 to 5.9 for breast cancer (1, 4, 16, 17).

Many risk factors, both host and environmental, have been suggested for these cancers (5) and are candidates to explain family clustering. In stomach cancer, intake of salty and smoked food, cereals and starch, low intake of green-yellow vegetables and dairy foods, smoking, and blood type A are suspected. Cancer of the colon and rectum may be associated with familial polyposis, animal fat, beer drinking, low intake of dietary fiber, and inflammatory bowel disease. Breast cancer is suspected to be related to early menarche, later menopause, late first pregnancy, lower parity, unmarried state, and large body constitution. The present study revealed that in cancer of the stomach, colon and rectum, and breast, family history was a risk factor independent from smoking, consumption of alcohol, marital status, or occupation.

It is advocated that these risk and familial factors should be examined in combination in a single study. Environmental risk factors have been apt to be excluded from data intake or data analysis in previous family studies on cancer. In contrast, many case-control or cohort studies seemed to have ignored family cancer history. It is also recommended that environmental risk factors, host factors, and family cancer history should be examined in relation to age at onset, histologic type, and locality of lesion of cancer, as well as precancerous conditions. Biological assay such as inducibility of aryl-hydrocarbon hydroxylase (AHH) and sister chromatid exchange (SES) seems promising for the study of highly familial cases.

Cancer registries offer a great potential for future studies on the family clustering of cancer. If information on family cancer history is compiled in the registry, detection of familial cases, search for specific causes of family clustering, and control of cancer in high risk familes may be more effectively pursued.

REFERENCES

1. Anderson, D. E. Breast cancer in families. *Cancer*, **40**, 1855–1860 (1977).
2. Department of Public Health, Aichi Prefectural Government. Cancer registry of Aichi Prefecture, 1982, Nagoya (1986).
3. Doll, R. and Peto, R. The causes of cancer: Quantitative estimates of avoidable risks of cancer in the United States today. *J. Natl. Cancer Inst.*, **66**, 1191–1308 (1981).
4. Fukushima, I. A study on the familial aggregation of cancer. Part I. Observations on the cases of breast cancer. *Tohoku Med. J.*, **53**, 239–252 (1956).
5. Hirayama, T., Waterhouse, J.A.H., and Fraumeni, J. F., Jr. (eds.) "Cancer Risks by Site," (1980). UICC Tech. Rep. Ser., Vol. 41, Geneva.
6. Lehtola, J. Family study of gastric carcinoma; with special reference to histological types. *Scand. J. Gastroenterol.*, **13** (Suppl.), 1–54 (1978).
7. Lipkin, M. and Newmark, H. Effect of added dietary calcium on colonic epithelial-cell proliferation in subjects at high risk for familial colonic cancer. *N. Engl. J. Med.*, **313**, 1381–1384 (1985).
8. Lipkin, M., Scherf, S., Schechter, L., and Braun, D., Jr. Memorial Hospital Registry of population groups at high risk for cancer of the large intestine: Age of onset of neoplasms. *Prev. Med.*, **9**, 335–345 (1980).
9. Lynch, H. T., Krush, A. J., Thomas, R. J., and Lynch, J. Cancer family syndrome. *In* "Cancer Genetics," ed. H. T. Lynch, pp. 355–388 (1976). Charles C Thomas, Springfield.
10. Macklin, M. T. Inheritance of cancer of the stomach and large intestine in man. *J. Natl. Cancer Inst.*, **24**, 551–571 (1960).
11. Mantel, N. and Haenszel, W. Statistical aspects of the analysis of data from retrospective studies of disease. *J. Natl. Cancer Inst.*, **22**, 719–748 (1959).
12. Mulvihill, J. J. Clinical genetics of human cancer. *In* "Host Factors in Human Carcinogenesis," ed. H. Bartsch and B. Armstrong, pp. 107–117 (1982). IARC Scientific Pub-

lications No. 39, Lyon.

13. Murata, M. and Takahashi, T. An epidemiological study on familial predisposition to large bowel cancer. *Jpn. J. Cancer Cin.*, **30**, 243–250 (1984).

14. Ogawa, H., Kato, I., and Tominaga, S. Family history of cancer among cancer patients. *Jpn. J. Cancer Res. (Gann)*, **76**, 113–118 (1985).

15. Ooi, W. L., Elston, R. C., Chen, V. W., Bailey-Wilson, J. E., and Rothschild, H. Increased familial risk for lung cancer. *J. Natl. Cancer Inst.*, **76**, 217–222 (1986).

16. Richardson, S., Gerber, M., and Pujol, H. Familial risk in a case-control study on breast carcinoma. *In* "Familial Cancer," ed. H. J. Müller and W. Weber, pp. 31–33 (1985). Karger, Basel.

17. Sattin, R. W., Rubin, G. L., Webster, L. A., Huezo, C. M., Wingo, P. A., Ory, H. W., and Lyde, P. M. Family history and the risk of breast cancer. *JAMA*, **253**, 1908–1913 (1985).

18. Schull, W. J. and Weiss, K. M. Genetic and familial factors in cancer: A population perspective. *In* "Host Factors in Human Carcinogenesis," ed. H. Bartsch and B. Armstrong, pp. 87–106 (1982). IARC Scientific Publications No. 39, Lyon.

19. Sugiuchi, H. A statistical study on the familial aggregation of stomach cancer. *Tohoku Med. J.*, **62**, 39–53 (1960).

20. Takei, K. Statistical investigations on genetic aspects of gastric carcinoma. *Jpn. J. Hum. Genet.*, **13**, 67–80 (1968).

21. Tokuhata, G. K. Cancer of the lung: Host and environmental interaction. *In* "Cancer Genetics," ed. H. T. Lynch, pp. 213–232 (1976). Charles C Thomas, Springfield.

22. Utsunomiya, J., Iwama, T., Matsumura, K., Ichikawa, T., and Tanimura, M. A study of non-polyposis familial large bowel cancer. *Surgery*, **43**, 881–889 (1981).

FAMILIAL ASPECTS OF BREAST CANCER

Motoi Murata,[*1] Goi Sakamoto,[*2] and Fujio Kasumi[*3]

Division of Epidemiology, Chiba Cancer Center[*1] *and Department of Pathology*[*2] *and Department of Surgery,*[*3] *Cancer Institute Hospital*

Epidemiologic studies on the familial clustering of human breast cancer and its relation to certain physical and endocrinological traits were reviewed with special reference to the characteristics of the disease in Japanese as a low-risk population. The author's earlier published and current studies were also included. Relative familial risk of breast cancer in siblings of patients with the same disease is 2- to 3-fold that of the controls, independent of whether the study is conducted in high- or low-risk countries. From the generally hormone dependent nature of this disease and also from its stronger familial predisposition to premenopausal onset, one can suspect that the relevant genetic trait involves some endocrine factors, especially ovarian hormone. Our data indicate that early age at menarche is associated with a positive family history of breast cancer. Although this is but indirect evidence, it suggests that early puberty may create later favorable condition for the development of mammary tumor.

Among human cancers of various organs, breast cancer has been the most extensively documented for its familial nature by numerous investigators in the world; even if confined to those case-control studies primarily concerned with the familial risk of breast cancer, the number of reports would be more than twenty. Interestingly, the risk of breast cancer in close relatives of patients of this disease is always 2- to 3-fold higher than that of the control population (36), independent of whether the respective studies are originated in low-risk or high-risk countries. Thus there is presently no doubt of the familiality of this disease from the statistical point of view. However, despite recent studies exploring a genetic linkage relationship between various marker traits and liability for this disease, none revealed any definitely attributable evidence (21).

Environmental factors, such as nutritional intake, reproductive life-style and socio-economic status, are also known to be significantly influential in breast cancer (18). In Japan the annual age-standardized incidence rate of this cancer has steadily increased during the last decade, which is probably due to the changing pattern of dietary habits from traditional Japanese to a westernized one. Nevertheless, the incidence rate is still far below that of most western countries. Familial aggregation of the disease also corresponds to its prevalence in the general population. In our own data on the family history of breast cancer observed among 39,500 mid-aged normal women (details will be referred to later on), 0.6% had a mother with this disease, whereas the corresponding rate is usually more than 4% in the majority of family studies conducted in the United States. This suggests that a major part of the familial aggregation of the disease may be ascribable either to the effects of certain environmental factors or of genetic-environ-

---

[*1] 666-2, Nitona-cho, Chiba 280, Japan (村田　紀).

[*2], [*3] 1-37-1, Kami-Ikebukuro, Tokyo 170, Japan (坂元吾偉, 霞　富士雄).

mental interactions. It would be very worthwhile to analyze the familial predisposition for this disease in Japan as a low-risk country and compare the result with the findings obtained in other high-risk countries.

Breast Cancer in Japan

In Fig. 1 is shown changes in the incidence rate of breast cancer in Japan from 1965 to 1980 for different age groups (10), in comparison with that in the United States (40). As often pointed out, variations of incidence between high- and low-risk countries is more notable in the post- than in the premenopausal age ranges. Accordingly, it had been expected that breast cancer in Japan would increase as a result of the westernization of dietary habits more promptly in older than in younger age groups. However, this is not obviously recognized in Fig. 1. At least up until 1980, the rate of increased incidence is more or less the same throughout all age groups, and it remains far below that of the United States.

Distribution of the histological types of breast cancer is also quite different between the two countries. Sakamoto et al. (33) carried out a comparative study on this problem by examining all the specimens from breast cancer cases surgically treated at Cancer Institute Hospital (CIH) in Japan and at Vanderbilt University Hospital in the United States. The proportion of papillotubular carcinoma is larger and that of scirrhous and lobular carcinomas is smaller in Japanese than in American breast cancers. He also examined the time trend of those histological types in Japan and found that their frequency was moving very slowly toward the pattern of the United States (32). Thus observations on both incidence rate and histological types indicate that breast cancer in Japan remains in quite a different state than that of western countries.

Since Carrol (8) showed the clear correlation of breast cancer mortality in different

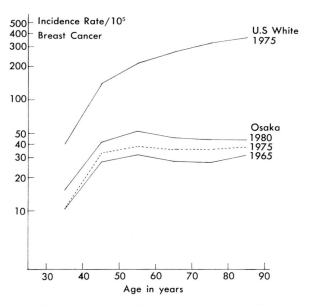

FIG. 1.   Age-specific incidence rates of breast cancer in Japan (Osaka prefecture) in different years and that of the United States

countries to the per capita consumption of dietary (especially animal) fat and protein, dietary habit has been regarded as the most important factor responsible for the international difference in incidence of this disease. In Japan a cohort study done by Hirayama (16), which followed a population of 140,000 unselected women for many years, revealed that the risk of breast cancer was 2.4 times higher in those eating meat daily than those eating it only rarely. On the other hand, Hirohata et al. (17) found no significant association of a high-fat diet to breast cancer risk in a case-control study.

Together with the dietary habit, obesity is also an important risk factor for breast cancer, especially in the postmenopausal age period. Sakamoto (32) compared the average degree of obesity between breast cancer cases and controls in the Cancer Institute Hospital by adopting Broca's index (weight (kg)/(height (cm)$\times 0.9-90$)). In comparison to the group with an index value of 1.0 or less, a significant elevation of relative risk was observed in those with a value of 1.1 or more and it was even more remarkable in older age women. A similar result was obtained in a preliminary study done in Chiba Cancer Center (CCC) in Japan, as will be described in a later section.

A number of studies have already demonstrated that various kinds of female reproductive history are etiologically relevant to breast cancer. Particularly, late age at first full-term pregnancy or no child-bearing is regarded as a factor of definite influence. Hirayama (16) and Hirohata et al. (17) both confirmed that this situation is observable in Japan.

The positive association of both obesity and female reproductive history to breast cancer is suggestive of some endogenous hormonal conditions being an underlying etiological factor. In a series of studies on various endocrine profiles of normal Japanese and British women (7, and others), a significantly lower adrenal androgen level was revealed in the former group, whereas no convincing difference in pituitary and ovarian hormone levels was found. A comparative epidemiologic study of breast cancer in high- and low-risk countries with special reference to female endocrinological status would be useful. Fifty-seven percent of premenopausal breast cancer in Japan is of the estrogen receptor positive type, and this rate is more or less the same in the United States: for postmenopausal breast cancers, however, there is a significant difference; 50% in the former and 79% in the latter country (20). Furthermore, in Japanese cases, the proportion was larger in obese than in non-obese patients of postmenopausal ages. These findings again suggest that breast cancer in Japan, even postmenopausal, may have different characteristics from those of the western countries, at least at the time of these studies.

Family Study

Multiple occurrences of breast cancer in certain families was reported in European countries even in the last century. A method of statistical analysis on family history of cancer patients was later developed. Mohri and Futagami (23) first reported this type of study in Japan on various cancers. They detected a history of breast cancer in one sister among siblings of 27 patients with the same disease, while none of 53 female stomach cancer patients had siblings affected with breast cancer. The method of statistical analysis of family history has been further improved to one which can now compare observed and expected incidence rates of the disease in family members. Fukushima (13) was the first author who reported this type of family study on breast cancer in Japan.

He studied families of 897 patients and found 4 mothers and 9 sisters with the same disease in contrast to the expected numbers of 2.2 and 2.0, respectively. Relative risk was estimated at 3.0 as a whole. Nakano (26) investigated 603 families and observed 19 mothers and 17 sisters with breast cancer as compared with the expected numbers of 1.2 and 4.4, respectively. This observed number in the mothers seems rather super- fluous, because the estimated relative risk was unusually higher than those obtained by other authors (36): the average value calculated from those of most published papers is 2.3 in the mothers and 2.5 in the sisters of probands.

One of the present authors (MM) conducted a case-control study of 642 breast cancer patients who were surgically treated at CCC from 1973 to 1986, and the same number of hospital controls selected by matching birth year and residence. The control group comprised patients who were admitted to the same hospital for treatment of various kinds of alimentary and gynecologic cancers or benign diseases. Comparative features of the case and control groups with respect to certain physical traits are shown in Table I. Breast cancer patients were significantly more obese and more hypertensive than controls. When patients were divided into two groups by age at diagnosis, i.e., those of less than 50 years and 50 years and over, the obese and hypertensive characteristics were more remarkable in the older group. Values for the patients with positive family history in Table I will be discussed later.

TABLE I.   Physical Traits of Breast Cancer Patients in CCC, Patients with Positive Family History and Controls (mean±S.E.)

Subjects	Body height	Body weight	Obesity	Systolic B. P.	Diastolic B. P.	Age at menarche
All ages						
Controls	151.8±0.2	51.4±0.3	1.11±0.01	125.8±0.9	74.5±0.5	14.4±0.1
Patients	152.0±0.2	52.5±0.3*	1.13±0.01*	128.6±0.9*	77.7±0.6**	14.4±0.1
F.H. (+)	151.8±1.2	53.5±1.2	1.16±0.04	126.2±3.3	78.3±2.6	13.5±0.4†
<50 years						
Controls	153.3±0.3	52.8±0.4	1.10±0.91	122.5±0.9	73.1±0.7	14.2±0.1
Patients	153.8±0.3	52.6±0.4	1.09±0.01	122.3±1.0	75.3±0.71	14.0±0.1
F.H. (+)	153.1±1.3	52.6±1.2	1.14±0.04	125.3±3.2	79.3±2.04	13.6±0.4
≥50 years						
Controls	149.8±0.4	49.6±0.5	1.11±0.01	130.1±1.7	76.2±0.8	14.9±0.2
Patients	149.6±0.4	52.4±0.6**	1.18±0.01**	136.6±1.5**	80.7±0.8**	15.1±0.2
F.H. (+)	148.6±2.0	56.0±3.1	1.29±0.10	135.6±8.6	83.2±8.6	13.2±0.9†

Significantly different from controls at 5% level (*) and at 1% level (**).
Significantly different from nonfamilial patients at 5% level (†).

TABLE II.   Number of Cases with Positive Family History of Cancer in First Degree Relatives among Breast Cancer Patients and Controls in CCC

Subjects	Total number	Family history of:						
		Stomach cancer	Colorect. cancer	Liver cancer	Lung cancer	Breast cancer	Uterine cancer	Brain tumor
Patients	642	60	14	12	23	19[a]	18	1
Controls	642	84	20	15	13	7	29	9

[a] Difference between patients and controls is significant at 5% level.

We could not adopt the method of comparing observed and expected incidences among the family members, because their detailed age structure was not known. Accordingly we compared the proportion with positive family history, not distinguishing either single or multiple occurrences within a family, between the case and control groups (Table II). If confined to the first degree relatives, family history of breast cancer was positive in 19 (3.0%) of the cases and 7 (1.1%) of the controls, which gave an odds ratio of 2.8 (confidence interval was 1.2–6.6). In the patient group, 8 cases were mothers and 12 were sisters, while in the control group 2 were mothers and 5 were sisters. It appeared that the relative risk was slightly larger in mothers than in sisters. Lung cancer was also more frequently observed in families of breast cancer patients than in controls, which conceivably reflected a more westernized life style of the former group. Further observed was a peculiar feature in the family history of brain tumor. Contrary to the other family histories, however, its positive rate was larger in the control than in the case groups. Out of 9 controls with a positive family history of brain tumor, 5 were patients of myoma uteri; we are presently not sure whether or not there is any biological relationship.

No other type of epidemiologic study on the familial predisposition to breast cancer, such as determination of the incidence rate of the disease in a cohort population or investigation of the concordance rate in twins, has yet been done in Japan. One of the present authors (MM) is now conducting a prospective study on a population of participants in a cervical cancer screening program. The population was started in 1978 and was followed by checking with the computer file of a population-based cancer registry. This study is continuing and a preliminary result will be presented here. The fundamental source of information on family and other history of the participants was a questionnaire completed at their clinics. Thus information was based entirely upon personal documentation and was not verified by medical doctors. By the end of 1985, 474 cancers were detected among around 39,500 cohorts. By matching the birth year and residence, 474 women were chosen within the same cohort population who were so far unaffected with any cancer, and who were not listed in the population-based cancer registry. Then the family history of various cancers was compared between the affected and unaffected womens (Table III).

TABLE III. Number of Cases with Positive Family History of Cancer among Cancer Patients (P) and Controls (C) in a Cohort Population in Urban/Rural Residences

Site of cancer in patients	Residence	Total number	Stomach cancer		Colorect. cancer		Breast cancer		Uterine cancer	
			P	C	P	C	P	C	P	C
Stomach	Urban	46	13	11	3	1	1	1	2	5
	Rural	60	13	13	0	4	3	0	9	8
Colorect.	Urban	26	3	5	3	0	0	1	2	2
	Rural	17	4	4	0	0	0	0	0	2
Breast	Urban	62	7	12	1	0	3	1	1	8[a]
	Rural	53	10	10	0	0	1	0	3	2
Uterus	Urban	29	4	8	2	2	0	2	1	4
	Rural	36	8	4	0	0	0	1	4	2

[a] Difference between patients and controls is significant at 5% level.

Among 115 women affected with breast cancer, four had a family history of the same disease, whereas among unaffected women the number was one. Although the numbers were not large enough to reflect a statistical significance, at face value the relative risk of 4.0 seems to conform to the result of many case-control studies. Furthermore, there seemed a slight urban-rural difference in the family history of cancer. For instance, the history of cancers of the colo-rectum and breast was more prominent in the urban than rural areas, which may reflect the involvement of urbanized life styles in the familial predisposition to cancer. Family history of uterine cancer was quite different between those affected and unaffected with breast cancer, especially in the urban area. We have no adequate explanation for this finding.

Anderson (1) demonstrated that a stronger familial risk was observed in the premenopausal and/or bilateral breast cancer than in the postmenopausal and/or unilateral. Several other authors have confirmed this relationship (3, 4, 9, 39). In Japan, Sakamoto et al. (34) also provided supportive evidence for the stronger familial predisposition in the bilateral breast cancer in CIH: proportion with a positive family history in first degree relatives was 6/92 (6.5%) in bilateral patients and 11/490 (2.2%) in unilateral patients. On the other hand, the differential familial risks in either pre- or postmenopausal onset of the disease probably depend on how this disease has achieved a notable elevation of incidence in the general population in postmenopausal age ranges. In Japan it was not achieved until very recent years. According to Murata et al. (25), who studied about 3,900 breast cancer patients admitted to CIH during the period 1946–1977, the mean age at diagnosis was 47.2±0.7 years in familial patients as compared with 48.5± 0.2 years in total cases, the difference not being significant. In the above mentioned case-control study performed in CCC, the proportion with a positive family history among total cases was 14/362 (3.9%) in those diagnosed before age 50 and 5/280 (1.8%) for those diagnosed at or over age 50. In the control group, the corresponding numbers were 3/362 and 4/280. Comparison between the cases and controls shows a significant difference only in the younger age group ($X^2=6.0$, $d.f.=1$, $p<0.05$). Thus a familially

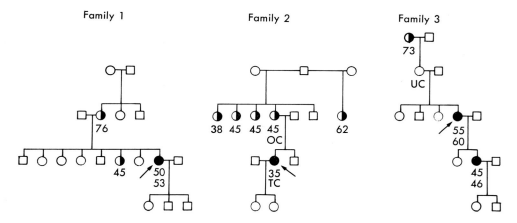

FIG. 2.   Families of patients with bilateral breast cancer detected in CIH
    Arrows indicate the proband. Shaded and half-shaded circles respectively indicate unilateral and bilateral breast cancer. Numbers presented for each patient indicate age at diagnosis or death. OC, oesophagus cancer; TC, thyroid cancer; UC, uterine cancer.

predisposed woman is more likely to be affected with premenopausal breast cancer. We occasionally experience a familial clustering of this disease in which patients are affected at successively younger ages as the generations advance (Fig. 2).

Genetic Factors

As discussed in the previous section, results of most of the published epidemiologic studies dealing with the familial risk of breast cancer indicate that certain predisposing conditions apparently run in a patient's family. The subsequent question is whether these conditions are caused by any hereditary or nonhereditary factors, and if hereditary, what the mode of inheritance is. First, we shall consider environmental factors. As mentioned, the rate of familial aggregation depends on the general prevailing incidence of the disease. For breast cancer, a positive family history in mothers in the United States is over 4-fold that in Japan, which obviously indicates that family members share a similar life style such as dietary habits (1). Nevertheless, according to the results of many family studies, the relative risk thus estimated for the familial predisposition is quite comparable between the two countries. Moreover, several published epidemiologic studies (11, 37) which dealt simultaneously with family history and other nonhereditary factors, elucidated that the effect of a positive family history of breast cancer was independent of other confounding factors such as reproductive histories, obesity and oral contraceptive use; dietary factors, however, were not included among them. Hence it seems very probable that a familial predisposition to breast cancer is ascribable to some hereditary factors.

Before exploring any genetic trait which might be involved in the etiology of this disease, we should inspect its mode of inheritance. Since we rarely encounter typical instances of either dominantly or recessively inherited families, a multifactorial or polygenic control has been generally accepted. However, since Lynch et al. (22) proposed the concept of the cancer family syndrome, families of a dominantly inherited cancer have been reported by many authors. In Japan, too, several examples of breast cancer families have been reported (e.g., 27). In consequence, monogenic and polygenic causes should both be hypothesized in investigating genetic factors of this cancer.

From the hormone-dependent nature of this disease, one might also conceive that the possible relevant genetic trait is associated with some endocrine systems. One bit of circumstantial evidence comes from the relationship between the age at onset of the disease and its familiality. As stated above, a larger risk of positive family history is usually observed in younger than in older patients, in other words, there is more pre- than postmenopausal onset of disease. Furthermore, Sattin et al. (35) found that the risk in the familially predisposed was elevated in both pre- and postmenopausally diagnosed diseases, but not in the perimenopausal one. A similar finding was made by Vorherr and Messer (38), who cited the data of Anderson (2) in a modified manner. According to them, the cumulative percentage of blood relatives affected by the disease is successively increased with advancing age except at the age of about 50 years, which means that the excess risk ascribable to the familial predisposition was not observed in this age range. Thus the following conclusion may be made. Familial predisposition certainly plays a part in at least premenopausal breast cancer and is less effective in peri- or postmenopausal cancer. The suspected genetic trait is most likely relevant to a hormonal factor whose activity is reduced in the peri- or postmenopausal ages.

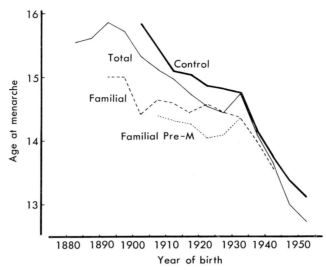

FIG. 3.   Mean age at menarche in Japanese women by their birth years
Control, healthy women; total, breast cancer patients admitted in CIH, 1946–
1977; familial, familial breast cancer patients; familial Pre-M, familial premenopausal patients.

Murata *et al.* (*25*) demonstrated that a patient of familial breast cancer was characterized by having been of earlier age at menarche and taller in stature than nonfamilial
patients; this was particularly remarkable in premenopausal patients (Fig. 3). Age at
menarche and body height are generally recognized as being highly correlated traits and
both are, to some extents, genetically controlled. This may be interpreted as both of
these traits being influenced by an underlying common hormonal factor which acts on
the pubertal condition of a woman and thus plays a role in the later onset of breast cancer.

    One of the present authors (MM) recently attempted to confirm this finding in
the case-control and cohort studies whose materials and methods were referred to above.
In the cohort study using participants in a cervical cancer screening program, 115 patients affected with breast cancer showed mean age at menarche of 14.3 ± 0.1 years
which was not different from 14.3 ± 0.2 years of the non-affecteds. Mean age at menarche
of those four patients with positive family history was 13.3 ± 0.2 years, which was slightly
but not significantly younger than that of the other patients. Results of the case-control
study using data on patients at CCC are presented in Table I. Among various physical
traits examined, only the age at menarche was significantly different between the family
history positive and negative patients ($t=2.1$, $p<0.05$), while the mean body height
was comparable. Thus our former finding on the positive association of the earlier age
at menarche and taller stature with the familial predisposition to breast cancer is yet
to be confirmed.

    In Japan studies exploring the biological factors associated with familial predisposi-
tion to breast cancer are very few. Nomura *et al.* (*28*) observed a slightly higher proportion of estrogen receptor positive breast cancer in those with than without a positive
family history (63.2% *vs.* 56.2%). The proportion was also slightly higher in those
with taller than shorter stature if confined to premenopausal breast cancer. On the other

hand, in postmenopausal breast cancer, the proportion was elevated in those with any one of the non-genetic risk factors, *i.e.*, obesity, unmarried state, older age at first child delivery and fewer instances of child bearing. These findings suggest that the suspected endocrine condition favoring the disease development is differently influenced by other endogenous and exogenous risk factors in either pre- or postmenopausal stages, and that at least in the former stage some component of the ovarian estrogen profiles might be genetically controlled. A number of hypotheses have been postulated which interpret the familial risk for breast cancer using various endocrinological entities, but none yet appears overwhelmingly plausible (*5, 6, 12, 15, 24, 30*).

Apart from the endocrinological traits, other kinds of studies have also been conducted exploring either a cytogenetic abnormality or biochemical marker traits possibly linked or correlated with the disease liability (*19, 29, 31*). So far, however, reports on these aspects are rather sporadic and have not been confirmed by other authors.

Concluding Remarks

Familial risk of breast cancer has been fully ascertained by numerous epidemiologic studies and we are now convinced of the influence of genetic susceptibility on this disease. However, as is obvious from the variable pedigree patterns of its familial occurrence, there are at least two types of hereditary breast cancer, *i.e.*, dominantly inherited and multifactorial. This may have contributed to the conflict in past investigations of possible genetic defects responsible for familial risk. We need still more advanced pedigree analysis on the genetic linkage of various marker traits with the disease liability. As one marker trait, DNA polymorphisms may become more and more important in investigating any genetic disease, including cancer susceptibility. In this connection, a recent finding that human estrogen receptor gene has extensive homology with v-*erb*-A gene in their DNA sequences as well as their biological functions is quite interesting (*14*). Although the chromosomal localization of human estrogen receptor gene (No. 6) and c-*erb*-A (the counterpart of v-*erb*-A) gene (No. 17) is known to be different, there may be some common underlying mechanism with respect to the role of estrogen in the function of both genes. Thus this oncogene might be one of the clues for study subjects of DNA markers.

Acknowledgment

This work was supported in part by a Grant-in-Aid for Cancer Research from the Ministry of Health and Welfare in Japan.

REFERENCES

1. Anderson, D. E. A genetic study of human breast cancer. *J. Natl. Cancer Inst.*, **48**, 1029–1034 (1972).
2. Anderson, D. E. A high risk group for breast cancer. *Cancer Bull.*, **25**, 23–25 (1973).
3. Bain, C., Speizer, F. E., Rosner, B., Belanger, C., and Hennekens, C. Family history of breast cancer as a risk indicator for the disease. *Am. J Epidemiol.*, **111**, 301–308 (1980).
4. Bodian, C. and Haagensen, C. D. Family history of breast carcinoma predisposing to the disease. *In* "Disease of the Breast," ed. C. D. Haagensen, pp. 408–423 (1986). Saunders Co., Philadelphia.

5. Boffard, K., Clark, G.M.G., Irvine, J.B.D., Knyba, R. E., Bulbrook, R. D., Wang, D. Y., and Kwa, H. G. Serum prolactin, androgens, oestradiol and progesterone in adolescent girls with or without a family history of breast cancer. *Eur. J Cancer Clin Oncol.*, **17**, 1071–1077 (1981).

6. Bruning, P. F., Bonfrer, J.M.G., and Hart, A.A.M. Non-protein bound estradiol, sex hormone binding globulin, breast cancer and breast cancer risk. *Br. J Cancer*, **51**, 479–484 (1985).

7. Bulbrook, R. D., Swain, M. C., Wang, D. Y., Hayward, J. L., Kumaoka, S., Takatani, O., Abe, O., and Utsunomiya, J. Breast cancer in Britain and Japan: plasma oestradiol-17, oestrone and progesterone and their urinary metabolites in normal British and Japanese women. *Eur. J Cancer*, **12**, 725–735 (1976).

8. Carrol, K. K. Experimental evidence of dietary factors in hormone-dependent cancers. *Cancer Res.*, **35**, 3374–3383 (1975).

9. Craig, T. J., Comstock, G. W., and Geiser, P. B. Epidemiologic comparison of breast cancer patients with early and late onset of malignancy and general population controls. *J. Natl. Cancer Inst.*, **53**, 1577–1581 (1974).

10. Department of Health and Welfare of Osaka Prefecture. Cancer Registry in Osaka Prefecture, No. 17–39 (1971 to 1985).

11. Farewell, V. T. The combined effect of breast cancer risk factors. *Cancer*, **40**, 931–936 (1977).

12. Fishman, J., Fukushima, D. K., O'Connor, J., and Lynch, H. T. Low urinary estrogen glucuronides in women at risk for familial breast cancer. *Science*, **204**, 1089–1091 (1979).

13. Fukushima, I. A study on the familial aggregation of cancer. Part 1. Observations of cases of breast cancer. *Tohoku Med. J.*, **53**, 239–252 (1956).

14. Green, S., Walter, P., Kumar, V., Krust, A., Bornert, J. M., Argos, P., and Chambon, P. Human oestrogen receptor cDNA: sequence, expression and homology to v-*erb*-A. *Nature*, **320**, 134–139 (1986).

15. Henderson, B. E., Gerkins, V., Rosario, I., Casagrande, J., and Pike, M. S. Elevated serum levels of estrogen and prolactin in daughters of patients with breast cancer. *N. Engl. J. Med.*, **293**, 790–795 (1975).

16. Hirayama, T. Epidemiology of breast cancer with special reference to the role of diet. *Prevent. Med.*, **7**, 173–195 (1978).

17. Hirohata, T., Shigematsu, T., Nomura, A.M.Y., Nomura, Y., Horie, A., and Hirohata, I. Occurrence of breast cancer in relation to diet and reproductive history: A case-control study in Fukuoka, Japan. *Natl. Cancer Inst. Monogr.*, **69**, 187–190 (1985).

18. Kelsey, J. L. A review of the epidemiology of human breast cancer. *Epidemiol. Rev.*, **1**, 74–109 (1979).

19. King, M. C., Go, R.C.P., Elston, R. C., Lynch, H. T., and Petrakis, N. L. Allele increasing susceptibility to human breast cancer may be linked to the glutamate-pyruvate transaminase locus. *Science*, **208**, 406–408 (1980).

20. Kuno, K., Fukami, A., Hori, M., and Kasumi, F. Hormone receptors and obesity in Japanese women with breast cancer. *Breast Cancer Res. Treat.*, **1**, 135–139 (1981).

21. Lynch, H. T. (eds.) "Genetics and Breast Cancer," pp. 1–253 (1981). Van Nostrand Reinhold Company, New York.

22. Lynch, H. T., Krush, A. J., Thomas, R. J., and Lynch, J. Cancer family syndrome. *In* "Cancer Genetics," ed. H. T. Lynch, pp. 355–388 (1976). Thomas, Springfield.

23. Mohri, S. and Futagami, S. Studies of heredity in man. 1. Heredity of tumor. *Juzenkai J.*, **48**, 158–186 (1942).

24. Morgan, R. W., Vakil, D. V., Brown, J. B., and Elinson, L. Estrogen profiles in young women: effect of maternal history of breast cancer. *J. Natl. Cancer Inst.*, **60**, 965–967 (1978).

25. Murata, M., Kuno, K., Fukami, A., and Sakamoto, G. Epidemiology of familial predisposition for breast cancer in Japan. *J. Natl. Cancer Inst.*, **69**, 1229–1234 (1982).

26. Nakano, K. Genetical studies of malignant tumor. I. Genetical studies of breast cancer. *Kumamoto Med. J.*, **20**, 1040–1050 (1967).

27. Nomizu, T. and Watanabe, I. Clinical investigation of familial clustering of cancer. *Jpn. J. Cancer Clin.*, **32**, 485–492 (1986).

28. Nomura, Y., Tashiro, H., Hamada, Y., Saeki, K., and Shigematsu, T. Estrogen receptors in breast cancer in relation to risk factors in Japanese pre- and postmenopausal patients. *Jpn. J. Cancer Clin.*, **28**, 1701–1708 (1982).

29. Olsson, H., Berger, R., Bernheim, A. Kristoffersson, U., and Mitelman, F. C-band heteromorphism in breast cancer patients. *In* "Familial Cancer," ed. H. J. Müller and W. Weber, pp. 44–45 (1985). Karger, Basel.

30. Ottman, R., Hoffman, P. G., and Siiteri, P. K. Estrogen receptor assays in familial and nonfamilial breast cancer. Banbury Report 8. *In* "Hormones and Breast Cancer," ed. M. C. Pike, P. K. Siiteri, and C. W. Welsch, pp. 197–211 (1981). Cold Spring Harbor Laboratory, New York.

31. Petrakis, N. L., Emster, V. L., Sacks, S. T., King, E. B., Schweitzer, R. J., Hunt, T. K., and King, M. C. Epidemiology of breast fluid secretion: association with breast cancer risk factors and cerumen type. *J. Natl. Cancer Inst.*, **67**, 277–284 (1981).

32. Sakamoto, G. Breast cancer in Japan—past trends and future prospects. *Jpn. J. Cancer Chemother.*, **11**, 703–708 (1984).

33. Sakamoto, G., Sugano, H., and Hartmann, W. H. Comparative pathological study of breast carcinoma among American and Japanese women. *In* "Breast Cancer," ed. W. L. McGuire, Vol. 4, pp. 211–231 (1981). Plenum Medical Book Company, New York.

34. Sakamoto, G., Sugano, H., and Kasumi, F. Bilateral breast cancer and familial aggregation. *Prevent. Med.*, **7**, 225–229 (1978).

35. Sattin, R. W., Rubin, G. L., Webster, L. A., Huezo, C. M., Wingo, P. A., Ory, H. W., and Layde, P. M. Cancer and Steroid Hormone Study. Family history and the risk of breast cancer. *JAMA*, **253**, 1908–1913 (1985).

36. Thomas, D. B. Epidemiologic and related studies of breast cancer etiology. *In* "Review in Cancer Epidemiology," ed. A. M. Lilienfeld *et al.*, pp. 153–217 (1980). Elsevier, New York.

37. Tulinius, H., Day, N. E., Bjarnason, O., Geirsson, G., Yohannesson, G., de Gonzalez, M.A.L., Sigvaldason, H., Bjarnadottier, G., and Grimsdottier, K. Familial breast cancer in Iceland. *Int. J. Cancer*, **29**, 365–371 (1982).

38. Vorherr, H. and Messer, R. H. Breast cancer: Potentially predisposing and protecting factors. Role of pregnancy, lactation and endocrine status. *Am. J Obstet. Gynecol.*, **130**, 335–358 (1978).

39. Wynder, E. L., MacCornack, F. A., and Stellman, S. D. The epidemiology of breast cancer in 785 United States caucasian women. *Cancer*, **41**, 2341–2354 (1978).

40. Young, J. L., Jr., Percy, C. L., and Asire, A. J. Surveillance, epidemiology, and end result: incidence and mortality data, 1973–77. *Natl. Cancer Inst. Monogr.*, **57**, 1–1082 (1981).

CHROMOSOMES AND
GENE MUTATIONS

Gann Monograph on Cancer Research 35, 1988

CHROMOSOME ABERRATIONS IN LEUKEMIA AND LYMPHOMA IN JAPAN

Masaharu SAKURAI

Department of Cancer Chemotherapy, Saitama Cancer Center Hospital*

Chromosome aberrations reported in Japanese patients with leukemia and lymphoma were reviewed from the literature. Although there were no significant differences in the positivity of the Ph[1] translocation in chronic myelogenous leukemia (CML), and in the incidence of various additional abnormalities between Japan and the United States or Europe, significant differences existed in the distribution of the various chromosome abnormalities seen in acute nonlymphocytic leukemia (ANLL) between Japan and Western countries. In Japan, translocations such as t(8; 21) and t(15; 17) were overrepresented while abnormalities of chromosomes 5 and/ or 7 seemed to be underrepresented. The latter abnormalities, however, were frequently observed in atomic bomb-related hematologic diseases. No features specific to acute lymphocytic leukemia (ALL) in Japan were noted, probably because of the paucity of the relevant reports. Distribution of chromosome abnormalities in non-Hodgkin's malignant lymphoma may be different in Japan from that in the United States or European countries. The difference may not be entirely due to the endemic occurrence of adult T-cell leukemia/lymphoma (ATL) in southwestern Japan. While there were a considerable number of cases with Burkitt's lymphoma also in Japan, the incidence of t(14; 18) appeared to be lower than in other countries. In respect to ATL and other T-cell neoplasms, some of the problems to be solved are: the presence or absence of differences in the distributions of various types of chromosome abnormalities between ATL and non-ATL lymphomas in Japan, between ATL cases in different areas within Japan, and between non-ATL lymphomas in Japan and in other countries. Still more thorough chromosome studies will be necessary to fully understand the nature of leukemia and lymphoma in Japan.

It has long been recognized that there are differences in the incidence of certain types of leukemia or lymphoma between Japan and the United States or Europe. A well-known example is chronic lymphocytic leukemia (CLL) (77); Japan and some other Asian countries are known for lower incidences of the disease as compared with the United States or Europe. Japan is also known by the rarity of Hodgkin's disease (21).

In more recent years, some specific chromosome abnormalities have been considered to be unevenly distributed among various countries. Thus, t(8; 21)(q22; q22), a reciprocal translocation between chromosomes 8 and 21 at their q22 bands seen in acute myeloblastic leukemia (AML), has been found more commonly among leukemia patients in Japan than among those in the United States or Europe (6, 57, 62). On the

---

* 818 Komuro, Ina, Saitama 362, Japan (桜井雅温).

contrary, +12, trisomy of chromosome 12, which is an abnormality commonly seen among patients with chronic lymphocytic leukemia in the United States or Europe (12, 60), is rare in Japan; the finding coincides with the rarity of this type of leukemia in this country.

Adult T-cell leukemia-lymphoma (ATL) is a disease endemic in southwestern Japan (73), and arises mainly in association with the adult T-cell leukemia virus or human T-lymphotropic virus type I (ATLV/HTLV-I) (16, 50). A number of reports on chromosome studies in this disease have been published since the turn of the decade (8, 38, 39, 52, 58, 74). Certain discrepancies seem to exist among the findings in these reports, however. A current concern in the study of chromosomes in ATL is the incidence of the abnormality in the proximal portion of the long arm of chromosome 14. The abnormalities with a break in 14q11–13 are commonly seen in T-cell leukemia or lymphoma (15), but whether or not the incidence is higher in ATL than in other T-cell diseases awaits elucidation.

In Hiroshima and Nagasaki, it has been noted that the incidence of leukemia and other malignant diseases is higher among the atomic bomb survivors than among the general population (17). Whether or not the chromosome abnormalities found in atomic bomb (A-bomb)-related leukemia are different from those in *de novo* leukemia is also a point of interest.

In this article, I will survey the literature in the field of cytogenetics in leukemia and lymphoma in Japan, and try to shed light on the problems the Japanese cytogeneticists studying leukemia and lymphoma are now facing.

Chronic Myelogenous Leukemia (CML)

There seems to be no significant difference in the incidence of Philadelphia (Ph[1]) chromosome-positive cases among the reports published in Japan. Thus, most papers report the presence of the Ph[1] translocation in more than 90% of patients with CML (19, 37, 44, 46, 72) (Table I). The report by Ishihara et al. (19) was a summary of studies carried out in 10 institutions throughout Japan, from Kochi in Shikoku in the south, to Sapporo in Hokkaido in the north, and the Ph[1]-positivity rate of 96% is considered to be the representative figure for CML of Japan. According to the report, 143 (27.8%) of the 514 Ph[1]-positive patients had additional abnormalities. Of 424 patients in the

TABLE I.   Chromosome Findings in CML Patients Reported in Japan

Total no. of patients	Ph[1]-positive cases				Ph[1]-negative cases (%)	Reference
	Total Ph[1]-positive cases (%)	Cases with a standard transloca-tion[a]	Cases with a variant transloca-tion[b]	Cases with a complex transloca-tion[c]		
50	48 (96)	48			2 (4)	37
534[d]	514 (96)	497	2	15	20 (4)	19
42	39 (93)	37		2	3[e](7)	46

[a] Cases with t(9; 22)(q34; q11).
[b] Cases with a translocation between band 22q11 and a band other than 9q34.
[c] Cases with a translocation involving one or more band in addition to bands 9q34 and 22q11.
[d] Data collected from 10 institutions in Japan.   The data include most cases reported in refs. 44 and 72.
[e] One patient showed a standard Ph[1] translocation and other abnormalities at relapse.

tween the incidences of these conditions in Japan and the United States or Europe.

It is to be noted that Yamada and Furusawa (76) reported a high incidence of trisomy 8, and that of trisomy or monosomy of chromosome 21 in leukemia or preleukemia. These abnormalities were rather rare in other reports (Table II).

Myelodysplastic Syndromes (MDS)

Only several cases have been reported on chromosomes in MDS in Japan. Okada et al. (48) reported on 4 cases with MDS; one case with refractory anemia with excess of blasts (RAEB) had diploidy, one case with sideroblastic anemia showed a hypodiploid complex karyotype with an interstitial deletion of 5q, and two cases with RAEB had a marker chromosome and a karyotype with a 17p+ chromosome, respectively. Miura (36) reported chromosome abnormalities in 4 of 5 patients with MDS; one patient with RAEB had only cells with a diploid karyotype, another patient with RAEB had a karyotype showing deletion of 20q, and the other patient with RAEB had a hyperdiploid complex karyotype with karyotypic instability. Two patients with RAEB in transformation (RAEB in T) had elongation of 2q (2q+) and loss of a Y chromosome, respectively. The paucity of reports on MDS may at least partly be related to the putative rarer occurrence of MDS cases in Japan than in the United States or Europe although no reliable statistics are available concerning the precise incidence of MDS in various countries. Cases with primary MDS in the United States or Europe frequently had 5q−, −7, +8, or 20q− (20, 64).

Atomic Bomb (A-bomb)-related Hematologic Diseases

The high incidence of the development of leukemia has been well established among the A-bomb survivors (17). Thus, the incidence of all types of leukemia except for CLL increased, and the increased risk for leukemia development still persists among them. Sadamori et al. (53) studied chromosomes of 9 A-bomb survivors and 9 non-exposed patients with MDS. While they found structural chromosome abnormalities in 7 exposed patients, including 5q− in 3, 5q translocation in one, and 7q− in two, only two of the 9 non-exposed patients had such abnormalities; one had 5q translocation, and the other had 5q− (p=0.025). Monosomy 7 and trisomy 8 were found in both groups. Although a significant correlation between the exposure to the A-bomb and the presence of structural abnormalities existed, no abnormalities were preferentially involved in MDS that developed in A-bomb survivors. They also studied chromosomes in both exposed and non-exposed patients with ANLL, CML, acute lymphocytic leukemia (ALL), and multiple myeloma, but did not see any appreciable difference between the exposed and the non-exposed groups in any of these conditions.

Kamada et al. (22) studied chromosomes in 167 patients with A-bomb-related hematologic diseases, i.e., 70 with ANLL, 61 with CML, 36 in the blastic phase of CML, and 7 with RAEB, and compared the findings with those obtained from 307 patients with such diseases unrelated to radiation. Among the ANLL patients, all the 10 who had received more than 200 rads of radiation exhibited 3.0 chromosome abnormalities on the average in their main leukemic clones. In contrast, only 53.3% and 55.6% of 15 and 18 patients who had received between 1 and 200 rads or less than 1 rad, respectively, exhibited average 1.07 and 0.89 chromosome abnormalities in the main clones. There was no increase in the number of chromosome abnormalities in ANLL which developed in people having entered the hypocenter area immediately after the bombing, or in children one or both of whose parents had been within 2 km of the hypocenter at the bomb explosion. The same authors presented the karyotypes of the 10 ANLL patients who had received more than 200 rads; 3 patients had a hypodiploid mode, 5 a pseudo-diploid mode, and 2 a hyperdiploid mode. Five patients had 3 or more abnormalities in the main clone. Thus, the more radiation a patient had received, the more chromosome abnormalities he or she possessed in the leukemic cells. Three patients had a 5q— (or Bq—), and one patient had a —5. Four of the 10 patients had a diagnosis of erythroleukemia, 3 of AML, 2 of AMOL, and one of APL. The hypo- or pseudodiploid complex karyotype is commonly seen not only in radiation- or drug-induced leukemia, but also in *de novo* ANLL in elderly people particularly in the United States or Europe (*6, 13, 32, 35, 51, 56, 59, 60*). Exposure to the A-bomb explosion seems to have increased the development of leukemia with this MAKA-type abnormality which is otherwise rare in this country. The same authors also compared the numbers of chromosome abnormalities in the blastic phase of CML among the patients who had received 1 rad or more, those who had received less than 1 rad or entered the hypocenter area after the bombing, and those who were not exposed to the A-bomb. They found that the number was significantly greater in the first group of patients than in the other 2 groups; the patients in the first group had 6.46 abnormalities in their main clones on the average, while those in the second group and the last-mentioned (unexposed) group had only average 3.57 and 3.75 abnormalities, respectively. They compared karyotypes of exposed and non-exposed RAEB patients, but, different from Sadamori *et al.*'s report (*53*), found no difference between the 2 groups; both groups of patients had structural abnormalities, often including 5q—, and sometimes had complex abnormalities.

Acute Lymphocytic Leukemia (ALL)

Acute lymphocytic leukemia is frequently seen in children, and is seen commonly though less frequently in adults as well. The Third International Workshop on Chromosomes in Leukemia held in 1980 reported that t(9; 22) or the Ph[1] translocation was the abnormality most frequently found in patients with ALL (*71*). Among 40 serially studied ALL patients in Japan (*24, 36, 45, 69*) (Table V), t(9; 22) was also the most frequently observed abnormality, and was seen in 5 patients (13%), all with L2 of the FAB morphology. Other structural abnormalities observed included 6q— or 6q+, t(13q14q), i(17q), and rearrangements of 1p, 1q, 2p, 2q, 4q, 7p, 8q, 9p, 9q, 11p, 11q, 12p, 13q,

TABLE V.   Chromosome Findings in Patients with ALL Reported in Japan

Total no. of patients	Number of cases with:					Reference
	t(9; 22)	Near-haploidy	≥50 chromosomes	Other changes	Normal diploidy	
5 (adults)	1			2	2	69
17 (9 children, 8 adults)		1	6	9	1	24
12 (adults)	2			2	8	45
6 (3 children, 3 adults)	2		1	1	2	36
40	5	1	7	14	13	

17q, 18p, and 18q. Seven patients had a hyperdiploid karyotype with 50 or more chromosomes. Usually these patients were 15 years old or younger, and achieved and maintained remission. The Third Workshop also reported an excellent prognosis for childhood patients with this type of hyperdiploidy (71).

As many as 34% of the cases with ALL submitted to the Third International Workshop had no chromosome abnormalities (71). Many of these patients may possibly have possessed abnormalities since leukemic cells of ALL tend to grow poorly *in vitro*, and abnormal metaphases could be easily missed or ignored because of the fuzziness or poor delineation of the chromosomes (59). In fact, some studies report the presence of chromosome abnormalities in virtually all patients with ALL (24, 78). Since there have been no studies on a sizeable group of ALL patients in Japan, thorough, and preferably prospective studies may be necessary to obtain good estimates of the true incidences of various abnormalities found in ALL in Japan. Also, a majority of cases with an 11q23 abnormality were classified in ALL (26). A patient with the 11q23 translocation can have a myeloid nature, a lymphoid nature, or both (14, 26, 43). Leukemia with this type of translocation in the very same patient can sometimes be classified as myeloid or lymphoid according to the features of the cells considered for the classification. Whichever category it may be classified in, the cellular and other clinical characteristics should be meticulously examined, and the correlation between these characteristics and the different transolcation partners should also be carefully studied in cases with a break in 11q23. The 1; 19 translocation, which has been known in other countries, was reported also in 6 Japanese children (65).

Non-Hodgkin's Lymphoma (NHL)

Although a geographic difference in the distribution of various histologic types of non-Hodgkin's lymphoma exists necessitating modification of the internationally utilized classification system (70) for use in Japan (68), and chromosome findings are expected to be different in Japan from those in the United States or Europe, we find only one study on chromosomes of serial patients with non-Hodgkin's lymphoma in Japan. In the 22 cases of NHL included in Kaneko *et al.*'s studies (23), there were no cases with t(8; 14), and only one case with t(14; 18). Some cases with t(8; 14) have also been reported in Japan as will be discussed later. On the other hand, t(14; 18) has been rare in Japan, and this fact coincides with the putative paucity of follicular lymphoma in this country (21). Kaneko *et al.* gave precise breakpoints in each case, and revealed that the arms frequently involved in the translocations or deletions were 1q, 2q, 6q, 8q, 11q, 14q, 18q, and 19q. The arm 14q was involved in 9 of the 22 cases; 14q32 in 7, 14q11 and 14q22 in one each. Band 14q32 was the most frequently involved of all chromosome bands. The immunoglobulin H-chain gene was mapped later in 14q32, and the T-cell receptor α-chain gene in 14q11. The arm 6q is special in that it was involved almost exclusively in the deletion. Thus, deletion 6q was found in 5 cases. The deletion was reported terminal, and the breakpoint was in band q21 in 4, and in q23 in one. The long arm of chromosome 11 was also involved in 6 patients, with an unidentified chromosome segment attached at 11q23 or 25 in 4 patients, and terminal or interstitial deletion with a break in 11q23 in one each. Although no patient had a break at 8q24, there were 4 patients with an 8q abnormality; 3 with a break in 8q22, and one with that in 8q11. Four patients had an 18q abnormality; 3 had an unknown chromosome segment attached to chromosome 18 at q23, and one had a t(14; 18)(q32; q21). Four patients had a 19q abnormality, 3 with an unknown chromosome segment and one with part of 4p attached to band q13. These studies had been done before the current gene map became available. However, some breaks were occurring in bands where oncogenes, immunoglobulin genes, or T-cell receptor genes were mapped later. There were two patients with a deletion distal to 7p15 and 7p22, respectively. Also, two patients had a terminal deletion with a break in 7q32. The breakpoints in these patients coincide with the locations of the genes for T-cell receptor γ- and β-chains, respectively. Despite the frequent occurrence of breaks in the locations of T cell-related genes, no surface marker studies were done on these patients. Thus, large-scale histologic, immunologic and cytogenetic studies will still be necessary to know correlation of the karyotype with the various morphologic and immunologic parameters in malignant lymphoma in Japan.

Chromosome findings in Burkitt's lymphoma and ATL will be discussed separately in the following sections.

1) Burkitt's lymphoma

Among 16 Japanese patients with Burkitt's lymphoma reported from Saitama, Kochi, and Kyoto, 11 had t(8; 14), 2 had t(2; 8), one had t(8; 22), and 2 had a 14q+ chromosome (10, 40, 54) (Table VI). These findings indicate that chromosome findings of Burkitt's lymphoma in Japan are not different from those in the United States, Europe or Africa. Fukuhara et al. also reported t(8; 14) in 6 patients with lymphomas other than Burkitt's or with ALL, i.e., 3 with large non-cleaved cell lymphoma, one with unspecified small non-cleaved cell lymphoma, and 2 with ALL of the FAB-L3 classification (10). All these conditions are considered to be related to Burkitt's lymphoma.

2) Adult T-cell leukemia-lymphoma (ATL)

Adult T-cell leukemia-lymphoma is a disease endemic in southwestern Japan (73), and especially common among the carriers of ATLV/HTLV-I (16, 50). Numerous reports on chromosomes in ATL patients have been published thus far in this country (8, 38, 39, 52, 58, 67, 74) (Table VII). The data reported from different institutions have often contradicted one another; there have been studies reporting high incidences of abnormalities of 14q11 (52), 14q32 (52, 67), trisomy 3 (39, 58), deletion of 6q (39), or trisomy 7 or 7q abnormality (39, 58, 74). Also, 7 of the 8 with trisomy 18 were reported from a single laboratory (39). When the results of these contradicting reports are combined, no abnormalities seem to emerge that have a high incidence characteristically in ATL. Among the 90 patients collected for Table VII, 10 (11%) had a break in 14q11–13, and 23 (26%) had a 14q32 abnormality. Thus, some cases with ATL certainly had an abnormality in 14q11–13, but whether or not its incidence is higher in

TABLE VI.   Chromosome Abnormalities in Japanese Patients with Burkitt's Lymphoma

Total no. of patients	Number of cases with:				Reference
	t(8; 14)	t(2; 8)	t(8; 22)	14q+	
5	3	1		1	54
8	5	1	1	1	40
3	3				10
16	11	2	1	2	

TABLE VII.   Chromosome Abnormalities in Japanese Patients with ATL

| Total no. of patients | Number of cases with: | | | | | | | | Reference |
	14q11–13	14q32	+3	6q−	+7	7q abnormality	+18	Normal diploidy	
15		2[a]	1		3	1		1	74
30	1	8[b]	10	16	1	7	7		39
8		4[e]	1	1					67
18		1[a]	5	1	5	1	1	4	58
8	6	6[c]	2	1	1				52
11	2[d]	2[b]	2	2	1	3			8
90	9	23	21	21	11	12	8	5	

[a] Breakpoints were not described.
[b] One case with an involvement of 14q32 in inv(14)(q11q32) is included.
[c] Two cases and one case with an involvement of 14q32 in inv(14)(q11q32) and t(14;14)(q11;q32), respectively, are included.
[d] Four other patients had a 14p12 abnormality.
[e] Breakpoint was not described in one patient.

ATL than in other types of T-cell diseases, or in ATL in some geographical areas than in others, remains open to question. Similar problems also exist regarding the incidence of trisomy 3, deletion of 6q, trisomy 7, 7q abnormality, *etc.* Although not mentioned specifically, abnormalities of 1p, 10p, and 10q were described in 13, 14, and 11 patients of the 90, respectively. Abnormalities of 5q and 6p were also common, and were found in 9 and 6 patients, respectively. Abnormalities of 7p and 9p were reported in 4 patients each.

Sanada *et al.* (58) observed that while 8 of 9 patients with acute ATL had chromosome abnormalities including trisomy 3 and/or trisomy 7, none of 6 patients with chronic ATL exhibited such aberrations although 5 of them had other chromosome abnormalities. They also noted that all 3 patients with smoldering ATL exhibited only diploid karyotypes. Miyamoto *et al.* reported earlier that 3 ATL patients with a normal karyotype were alive 12, 14, and 21 months after diagnosis while the average survival time of 12 ATL patients with an abnormal karyotype was less than 5 months (38). They noted rather similar clinical pictures in both groups of patients. Other studies indicated the presence of chromosome abnormalities in 9 of 42 patients with pre-ATL, including a 14q11–13 abnormality in 4 (18), or in 3 of 5 ATL-associated antigen (ATLA) antibody-positive healthy individuals, including 14q11–13 abnormality in one (9). These studies, if confirmed, would seem to indicate that the chromosome abnormalities emerge, and the karyotype evolves nonrandomly in the course of development and progression of ATL, a phenomenon similar to that seen in the relation between MDS and ANLL. A study on HTLV-positive leukemia-lymphoma in the United States reported the high frequency of deletion of 6q with various breakpoints (75).

It has been established that ATLV/HTLV-I is causally related to the development of ATL. It is known, however, that there are ATL cases in which ATLA antibody and ATLV/HTLV-I genomes are not detected, and which are thought to have developed without the involvement of ATLV/HTLV-I (66). Whether or not there are differences in the karyotype between these two categories of ATL, and also between ATL and other types of T-cell lymphomas or leukemias is also a matter of interest.

To solve these problems, karyotypes should be determined as precisely as possible for each patient. Thus, an *ad hoc* karyotype review committee was established in Japan, and reviewed karyotypes of ATL and other T-cell lymphomas submitted from various institutions throughout the country to improve them. The committee will publish results of its activities.

CONCLUSION

The involvement of chromosome abnormalities in the carcinogenesis or leukemogenesis is being implicated at the molecular level (*3, 4*). Thus, translocations, such as t(9; 22) in CML or ALL, and t(8; 14) in Burkitt's lymphoma, and deletion of 13q or 11p in retinoblastoma or Wilms' tumor, are now believed to play a fundamental role in the development of the diseases from the findings in molecular studies. To clarify the significance of each chromosome abnormality in leukemogenesis or lymphomagenesis, more thorough and precise studies on chromosomes in leukemia and lymphoma will be necessary in Japan, particularly since these diseases seem to have aspects in this country different from those in the United States or Europe.

Acknowledgments

I am grateful to Drs. Y. Kaneko and N. Maseki for helpful discussions and comments. This work was supported in part by a Grant-in-Aid from the Ministry of Health and Welfare for a Comprehensive 10-year Strategy for Cancer Control, Japan, and by Grants-in-Aid for Cancer Research from the Ministry of Education, Science and Culture of Japan.

REFERENCES

1. Bennett, J. M., Catovsky, D., Daniel, M. T., Flandrin, G., Galton, D.A.G., Gralnick, H. R., and Sultan, C. Proposals for the classification of the acute leukaemias. *Br. J. Haematol.*, **33**, 451–458 (1976).
2. Berger, R., Bernheim, A., and Flandrin, G. Absence d'anomalie chromosomique et leucémie aiguë: relations avec les cellules médullaires normales. *C. R. Acad. Sci. Paris*, **290**, 1557–1559 (1980).
3. Bishop, J. M. The molecular genetics of cancer. *Science*, **235**, 305–311 (1987).
4. Croce, C. M. Chromosome translocations and human cancer. *Cancer Res.*, **46**, 6019–6023 (1986).
5. First International Workshop on Chromosomes in Leukaemia. Chromosomes in Ph¹-positive chronic granulocytic leukaemia. *Br. J. Haematol.*, **39**, 305–309 (1978).
6. Fourth International Workshop on Chromosomes in Leukemia, 1982. Overview of association between chromosome pattern and cell morphology, age, sex, and race. *Cancer Genet. Cytogenet.*, **11**, 265–274 (1984).
7. Fourth International Workshop on Chromosomes in Leukemia, 1982. *Translocation* (8; 21)(q22; q22) in acute nonlymphocytic leukemia. *Cancer Genet. Cytogenet.*, **11**, 284–287 (1984).
8. Fujita, K., Fukuhara, S., Nasu, K., Yamabe, H., Tomono, N., Inamoto, Y., Shimazaki, C., Ohno, H., Doi, S., Kamesaki, H., Ueshima, Y., and Uchino, H. Recurrent chromosome abnormalities in adult T-cell lymphomas of peripheral T-cell origin. *Int. J. Cancer*, **37**, 517–524 (1986).
9. Fukuhara, S., Hinuma, Y., Gotoh, Y., and Uchino, H. Chromosome aberrations in T

lymphocytes carrying adult T-cell leukemia-associated antigens (ATLA) from healthy adults. *Blood*, **61**, 205–207 (1983).

10. Fukuhara, S., Kita, K., Nasu, K., Kannagi, M., Kamezaki, T., Ohno, H., Yamazowa, M., Nishigori, M., Uchino, H., Yagita, M., Matsuo, N., Yamabe, H., and Tanaka, S. Karyotype evolution in B-cell lymphoid malignancy with an 8; 14 translocation. *Int. J. Cancer*, **32**, 555–562 (1983).

11. Fukushige, S., Matsubara, K., Yoshida, M. C., Sasaki, M., Suzuki, T., Semba, K., Toyoshima, K., and Yamamoto, T. Localization of a novel v-*erb*B-related gene, c-*erb*B-2, on human chromosome 17 and its amplification in a gastric cancer cell line. *Mol. Cell. Biol.*, **6**, 955–958 (1986).

12. Gahrton, G., Robert, K., Friberg, K., Zech, L., and Bird, A. G. Nonrandom chromosomal aberrations in chronic lymphocytic leukemia revealed by polyclonal B-cell-mitogen stimulation. *Blood*, **56**, 640–647 (1980).

13. Golomb, H. M., Alimena, G., Rowley, J. D., Vardiman, J. W., Testa, J. R., and Sovik, C. Correlation of occupation and karyotype in adults with acute nonlymphocytic leukemia. *Blood*, **60**, 404–411 (1982).

14. Hayashi, Y., Sakurai, M., Kaneko, Y., Abe, T., Mori, T., and Nakazawa, S. 11; 19 translocation in a congenital leukemia with two cell populations of lymphoblasts and monoblasts. *Leukemia Res.*, **9**, 1467–1473 (1985).

15. Hecht, F., Morgan, R., Kaiser-McCaw Hecht, B., and Smith, S. D. Common region on chromosome 14 in T-cell leukemia and lymphoma. *Science*, **226**, 1445–1447 (1984).

16. Hinuma, Y., Nagata, K., Hanaoka, M., Nakai, M., Matsumoto, T., Kinoshita, K., Shirakawa, S., and Miyoshi, I. Adult T-cell leukemia: Antigen in an ATL cell line and detection of antibodies to the antigen in human sera. *Proc. Natl. Acad. Sci. U.S.A.*, **78**, 6476–6480 (1981).

17. Ichimaru, M., Ohkita, T., and Ishimaru, T. Leukemia, multiple myeloma, and malignant lymphoma. *Gann Monogr. Cancer Res.*, **32**, 113–127 (1986).

18. Ikeda, S., Nishino, K., Momita., S., Amagasaki, T., Kamihira, S., Kinoshita, K., Ichimaru, M., Toriya, K., Kusano, M., Soda, H., Tomonaga, Y., and Tagawa, M. Pathophysiology of pre-ATL (preleukemic state of adult T cell leukemia). *Rinsho Ketsueki*, **27**, 677–685 (1986) (in Japanese).

19. Ishihara, T., Sasaki, M., Oshimura, M., Kamada, N., Yamada, K., Okada, M., Sakurai, M., Sugiyama, T., Shiraishi, Y., and Kohno, S. A summary of cytogenetic studies on 534 cases of chronic myelocytic leukemia in Japan. *Cancer Genet. Cytogenet.*, **9**, 81–92 (1983).

20. Jacobs, R. H., Cornbleet, M. A., Vardiman, J. W., Larson, R. A., Le Beau, M. M., and Rowley, J. D. Prognostic implications of morphology and karyotype in primary myelodysplastic syndromes. *Blood*, **67**, 1765–1772 (1986).

21. Kadin, M. E., Berard, C. W., Nanba, K., and Wakasa, H. Lymphoproliferative diseases in Japan and western countries: Proceedings of the United States-Japan Seminar, 1982, in Seattle, Washington. *Hum. Pathol.*, **14**, 745–772 (1983).

22. Kamada, N., Tanaka, K., Dohy, H., Takimoto, Y., Oguma, N., and Kuramoto, A. Cytogenetic studies on patients with leukemia and RAEB found in atomic bomb survivors. *Rinsho Ketsueki*, **25**, 156–163 (1984) (in Japanese).

23. Kaneko, Y., Abe, R., Sampi, K., and Sakurai, M. An analysis of chromosome findings in non-Hodgkin's lymphomas. *Cancer Genet. Cytogenet.*, **5**, 107–121 (1982).

24. Kaneko, Y., Hayashi, Y., and Sakurai, M. Chromosomal findings and their correlation to prognosis in acute lymphocytic leukemia. *Cancer Genet. Cytogenet.*, **4**, 227–235 (1981).

25. Kaneko, Y., Honma, C., Maseki, N., Sakurai, M., Toyoshima, K., and Yamamoto, T. Human c-*erb*B-2 remains on chromosome 17 in band q21 in the 15; 17 translocation associated with acute promyelocytic leukemia. *Jpn. J. Cancer Res.* (*Gann*), **78**, 16–19 (1987).

26. Kaneko, Y., Maseki, N., Takasaki, N., Sakurai, M., Hayashi, Y., Nakazawa, S., Mori, T.,

Sakurai, Mi., Takeda, T., Shikano, T., and Hiyoshi, Y. Clinical and hematologic characteristics in acute leukemia with 11q23 translocations. *Blood*, **67**, 484–491 (1986).

27. Kaneko, Y., Maseki, N., Takasaki, N., Sakurai, M., Kawai, K., and Sakurai, Mi. Possible association of a new translocation, t(7; 11)(p15; p15), with Ph[1] chromosome-negative chronic myelogenous leukemia. *Int. J. Cancer*, **36**, 657–659 (1985).

28. Knuutila, S., Vuopio, P., Borgström, G. H., and de la Chapelle, A. Higher frequency of 5q– clone in bone marrow mitoses after culture than by a direct method. *Scand. J. Haematol.*, **25**, 358–362 (1980).

29. Kondo, K. and Sasaki, M. Cytogenetic studies in four cases of acute promyelocytic leukemia (APL). *Cancer Genet. Cytogenet.*, **1**, 131–138 (1979).

30. Kondo, K. and Sasaki, M. Further cytogenetic studies on acute promyelocytic leukemia. *Cancer Genet. Cytogenet.*, **6**, 39–46 (1982).

31. Larson, R. A., Kondo, K., Vardiman, J. S., Butler, A. E., Golomb, H. M., and Rowley, J. D. Evidence for a 15; 17 translocation in every patient with acute promyelocytic leukemia. *Am. J. Med.*, **76**, 827–841 (1984).

32. Le Beau, M. M., Albain, K. S., Larson, R. A., Vardiman, J. W., Davis, E. M., Blough, R. R., Golomb, H. M., and Rowley, J. D. Clinical and cytogenetic correlations in 63 patients with therapy-related myelodysplastic syndromes and acute nonlymphocytic leukemia: Further evidence for characteristic abnormalities of chromosomes 5 and 7. *J. Clin. Oncol.*, **4**, 325–345 (1986).

33. Le Beau, M. M., Larson, R. A., Bitter, M. A., Vardiman, J. W., Golomb, H. M., and Rowley, J. D. Association of an inversion of chromosome 16 with abnormal marrow eosinophils in acute myelomonocytic leukemia. A unique cytogenetic-clinicopathological association. *N. Engl. J. Med.*, **309**, 630–636 (1983).

34. Maseki, N., Kaneko, Y., and Sakurai, M. Nonrandom additional chromosome changes in acute nonlymphocytic leukemia with inv(16)(p13q22). *Cancer Genet. Cytogenet.*, **26**, 309–317 (1987).

35. Mitelman, F., Brandt, L., and Nilsson, P. G. Relation among occupational exposure to potential mutagenic/carcinogenic agents, clinical findings, and bone marrow chromosomes in acute nonlymphocytic leukemia. *Blood*, **52**, 1229–1237 (1978).

36. Miura, I. Cytogenetic study of the significance of FAB classification. *Rinsho Ketsueki*, **27**, 1323–1331 (1986) (in Japanese).

37. Miyamoto, K. Chromosome abnormalities in patients with chronic myelocytic leukemia. *Acta Med. Okayama*, **34**, 367–382 (1980).

38. Miyamoto, K., Kitajima, K., Suemaru, S., and Tanaka, T. Karyotypic findings and prognosis of adult T-cell leukemia patients. *Gann*, **73**, 854–856 (1982).

39. Miyamoto, K., Tomita, N., Ishii, A., Nonaka, H., Kondo, T., Tanaka, T., and Kitajima, K. Chromosome abnormalities of leukemia cells in adult patients with T-cell leukemia. *J. Natl. Cancer Inst.*, **73**, 353–362 (1984).

40. Miyoshi, I. Japanese Burkitt's lymphoma: Clinicopathological review of 14 cases. *Jpn. J. Clin. Oncol.*, **13**, 489–496 (1983).

41. Mizutani, R., Shimizu, T., Yamada, O., Takahashi, M., Katahira, J., Totsuka, K., Motoji, T., Oshimi, K., and Mizoguchi, H. Studies of acute promyelocytic leukemia. Incidence and clinical features of the patients with t(15; 17). *Rinsho Ketsueki*, **23**, 1377–1382 (1982) (in Japanese).

42. Nagasaka, M., Maeda, S., Maeda, H., Chen, H., Kita, K., Mabuchi, O., Misu, H., Matsuo, T., and Sugiyama, T. Four cases of t(4; 11) acute leukemia and its myelomonocytic nature in infants. *Blood*, **61**, 1174–1181 (1983).

43. Nagasaka, M., Maeda, S., Sugiyama, T., Mabuchi, O., Misu, H., and Nakamura, S. Chromosomal analysis of childhood leukemia and lymphoma and relation to the clinical features. *Rinsho Ketsueki*, **25**, 1408–1416 (1984) (in Japanese).

44. Oguma, N. Cytogenetic study of 122 patients with chronic myelogenous leukemia. *Acta Haematol. Jpn.*, **43**, 536–549 (1980).

45. Ohyashiki, K. Nonrandom cytogenetic changes in human acute leukemia and their clinical implications. *Cancer Genet. Cytogenet.*, **11**, 453–471 (1984).

46. Ohyashiki, K. A chromosome survey of 42 cases of chronic myelogenous leukemia: Significance of the Philadelphia translocation. *Acta Haematol. Jpn.*, **47**, 972–981 (1984).

47. Ohyashiki, K., Oshimura, M., Uchida, H., Nomoto, S., Sakai, N., Tonomura, A., and Ito, H. Cytogenetic and ultrastructural studies on ten patients with acute promyelocytic leukemia, including one case with a complex translocation. *Cancer Genet. Cytogenet.*, **14**, 247–255 (1985).

48. Okada, M., Mizoguchi, H., Kubota, K., and Nomura, Y. Quantitative analysis of chromosomal G-bands in human hematopoietic disorders by methotrexate synchronization technique. *Cancer Genet. Cytogenet.*, **13**, 225–237 (1984).

49. Oshimura, M., Ohyashiki, K., Mori, M., Terada, H., and Takaku, F. Cytogenetic and hematologic findings in acute myelogenous leukemia, M2 according to the FAB classification. *Gann*, **73**, 212–216 (1982).

50. Poiesz, B. J., Ruscetti, F. W., Gazdar, A. F., Bunn, P. A., Minna, J. D., and Gallo, R. C. Detection and isolation of type C retrovirus particles from fresh and cultured lymphocytes of a patient with cutaneous T-cell lymphoma. *Proc. Natl. Acad. Sci. U.S.A.*, **77**, 7415–7419 (1980).

51. Rowley, J. D., Golomb, H. M., and Vardiman, J. W. Nonrandom chromosome abnormalities in acute leukemia and dysmyelopoietic syndromes in patients with previously treated malignant disease. *Blood*, **58**, 759–767 (1981).

52. Sadamori, N., Nishino, K., Kusano, M., Tomonaga, Y., Tagawa, M., Yao, E., Sasagawa, I., Nakamura, H., and Ichimaru, M. Significance of chromosome 14 anomaly at band 14q11 in Japanese patients with adult T-cell leukemia. *Cancer*, **58**, 2244–2250 (1986).

53. Sadamori, N., Tomonaga, Y., Tagawa, M., Kusano, M., Nishino, K., Yao, E., and Ichimaru, M. Cytogenetic studies on leukemia and preleukemic state in atomic bomb survivors. Structural abnormality of chromosomes as leukemia inducing factors (Preliminary report). *Hiroshima Igaku*, **33**, 417–424 (1980).

54. Sakurai, M., Hayashi, Y., Abe, R., and Nakazawa, S. Chromosome translocations, surface immunoglobulins, and Epstein-Barr virus in Japanese Burkitt's lymphoma. *Cancer Genet. Cytogenet.*, **8**, 275–276 (1983).

55. Sakurai, M., Kaneko, Y., and Abe, R. Further characterization of acute myelogenous leukemia with t(8; 21) chromosome translocation. *Cancer Genet. Cytogenet.*, **6**, 143–152 (1982).

56. Sakurai, M. and Sandberg, A. A. Chromosomes and causation of human cancer and leukemia. XIII. An evaluation of karyotypic findings in erythroleukemia. *Cancer*, **37**, 790–804 (1976).

57. Sakurai, M., Sasaki, M., Kamada, N., Okada, M., Oshimura, M., Ishihara, T., and Shiraishi, Y. A summary of cytogenetic, morphologic, and clinical data on t(8q−; 21q+) and t(15q+; 17q−) translocation leukemias in Japan. *Cancer Genet. Cytogenet.*, **7**, 59–65 (1982).

58. Sanada, I., Tanaka, R., Kumagai, E., Tsuda, H., Nishimura, H., Yamaguchi, K., Kawano, F., Fujiwara, H., and Takatsuki, K. Chromosomal aberrations in adult T cell leukemia: Relationship to the clinical severity. *Blood*, **65**, 649–654 (1985).

59. Sandberg, A. A. "The Chromosomes in Human Cancer and Leukemia" (1980). Elsevier North Holland, New York.

60. Sandberg, A. A. The chromosomes in human leukemia. *Semin. Hematol.*, **23**, 201–217 (1986).

61. Sasaki, M., Okada, M., Kondo, I., and Muramoto, J. Chromosome banding patterns in 27 cases of acute myeloblastic leukemia. *Proc. Jpn. Acad.*, **52**, 505–508 (1976).

62. Second International Workshop on Chromosomes in Leukemia (1979). Cytogenetic, morphologic, and clinical correlations in acute nonlymphocytic leukemia with t(8q−; 21q+). *Cancer Genet. Cytogenet.*, **2**, 99–102 (1980).

63. Second International Workshop on Chromosomes in Leukemia (1979). Chromosomes in acute promyelocytic leukemia. *Cancer Genet. Cytogenet.*, **2**, 103–107 (1980).

64. Second International Workshop on Chromosomes in Leukemia (1979). Chromosomes in preleukemia. *Cancer Genet. Cytogenet.*, **2**, 108–113 (1980).

65. Shikano, T., Kaneko, Y., Takazawa, M., Ueno, N., Ohkawa, M., and Fujimoto, T. Balanced and unbalanced 1; 19 translocation-associated acute lymphoblastic leukemias. *Cancer*, **58**, 2239–2243 (1986).

66. Shimoyama, M., Kagami, Y., Shimotohno, K., Miwa, M., Minato, K., Tobinai, K., Suemasu, K., and Sugimura, T. Adult T-cell leukemia/lymphoma not associated with human T-cell leukemia virus type I. *Proc. Natl. Acad. Sci. U.S.A.*, **83**, 4524–4528 (1986).

67. Shiraishi, Y., Taguchi, T., Kubonishi, I., Taguchi, H., and Miyoshi, I. Chromosome abnormalities, sister chromatid exchanges, and cell cycle analysis in phytohemagglutinin-stimulated adult T cell leukemia lymphocytes. *Cancer Genet. Cytogenet.*, **15**, 65–77 (1985).

68. Suchi, T., Tajima, K., Nanba, K., Wakasa, H., Mikata, A., Kikuchi, M., Mori, S., Watanabe, S., Mohri, N., Shamoto, M., Harigaya, K., Itagaki, T., Matsuda, M., Kirino, Y., Takagi, K., and Fukunaga, S. Some problems on the histopathological diagnosis of non-Hodgkin's malignant lymphoma. A proposal of a new type. *Acta Pathol. Jpn.*, **29**, 755–776 (1979).

69. Takeuchi, J., Ohshima, T., and Amaki, I. Cytogenetic studies in adult acute leukemias. *Cancer Genet. Cytogenet.*, **4**, 293–302 (1981).

70. The Non-Hodgkin's Lymphoma Pathologic Classification Project. National Cancer Institute sponsored study of classifications of non-Hodgkin's lymphomas. Summary and description of a working formulation for clinical usage. *Cancer*, **49**, 2112–2135 (1982).

71. Third International Workshop on Chromosomes in Leukemia (1980). Clinical significance of chromosomal abnormalities in acute lymphoblastic leukemia. *Cancer Genet. Cytogenet.*, **4**, 111–137 (1981).

72. Tomiyasu, T., Sasaki, M., Kondo, K., and Okada, M. Chromosome banding studies in 106 cases of chronic myelogenous leukemia. *Jpn. J. Hum. Genet.*, **27**, 243–258 (1982).

73. Uchiyama, T., Yodoi, J., Sagawa, K., Takatsuki, K., and Uchino, H. Adult T-cell leukemia: Clinical and hematologic features of 16 cases. *Blood*, **50**, 481–492 (1977).

74. Ueshima, Y., Fukuhara, S., Hattori, T., Uchiyama, T., Takatsuki, K., and Uchino, H. Chromosome studies in adult T-cell leukemia in Japan: Significance of trisomy 7. *Blood*, **58**, 420–425 (1981).

75. Whang-Peng, J., Bunn, P. A., Knutsen, T., Kao-Shan, C. S., Broder, S., Jaffe, E. S., Gelmann, E., Blattner, W., Lofters, W., Young, R. C., and Gallo, R. C. Cytogenetic studies in human T-cell lymphoma virus (HTLV)-positive leukemia-lymphoma in the United States. *J. Natl. Cancer Inst.*, **74**, 357–369 (1985).

76. Yamada, K. and Furusawa, S. Preferential involvement of chromosomes No. 8 and No. 21 in acute leukemia and preleukemia. *Blood*, **47**, 679–686 (1976).

77. Wakisaka, G., Uchino, H., Yasunaga, K., Nakamura, T., Sakurai, M., Miyamoto, K., Yoshino, T., and Moriga, M. Statistical investigations of leukemia in Japan from 1956 to 1961. *Path. Microbiol.*, **27**, 671–683 (1964).

78. Williams, D. L., Harber, J., Murphy, S. B., Look, A. T., Kalwinsky, D. K., Rivera, G., Melvin, S. L., Stass, S., and Dahl, G. V. Chromosomal translocations play a unique role in influencing prognosis in childhood acute lymphoblastic leukemia. *Blood*, **68**, 205–212 (1986).

Gann Monograph on Cancer Research 35, 1988

CHROMOSOMAL ABERRATIONS IN ATOMIC BOMB SURVIVORS

Akio A. Awa

*Department of Genetics, Radiation Effects Research Foundation**

Radiation-induced chromosomal aberrations have persisted for many years in the somatic cells of atomic bomb survivors in Hiroshima and Nagasaki. Based on the T65DR dose estimates, a statistically significant dose-response relationship for chromosomal aberration frequencies exists in both cities, but the coefficient of linear regression for aberration frequencies is higher in Hiroshima than in Nagasaki by a factor of 2. A preliminary analysis of cytogenetic data at ABCC-RERF** indicates that the inter-city difference observed with the T65DR doses becomes less pronounced with the new dosimetry system (DS86), although the regression coefficient is still higher in Hiroshima than in Nagasaki.

The majority of chromosomal aberrations detectable to date are of the stable type, such as reciprocal translocations and inversions, and they are major components contributing to the dose-response relationship.

In 1960, a simple and reliable culture technique was developed for obtaining preparations of mitotic cells from peripheral blood lymphocytes using mitogens (*35*). The technique has enabled us not only to analyze accurately somatic chromosomes in the normal and diseased states but also to determine the effect of various clastogens, including ionizing radiation, on the induction of structural chromosomal aberrations in the somatic cells of man. Since the work of Tough *et al.* (*50*), who first observed gross chromosome damage in cells from blood cultures of two patients after X-ray therapy for ankylosing spondylitis, evidence has accumulated that there is a positive relationship between the frequency of cells with induced chromosomal aberrations and increasing radiation dose which persists over many years following *in vivo* exposure (*9, 10, 16, 17, 24–26, 31*, for details see *41*).

The atomic bomb (A-bomb) survivors of Hiroshima and Nagasaki constitute a unique human population, since they received acute whole-body exposure to a large dose of ionizing radiation with a high dose rate. It was thus anticipated that radiation-induced structural rearrangements of chromosomes would be observed in both somatic and germ cells of A-bomb survivors.

The present paper will describe the current status of knowledge on the chromosomal aberrations in the somatic cells of A-bomb survivors in Hiroshima and Nagasaki,

* 5-2, Hijiyama Park, Minami-ku, Hiroshima 732, Japan (阿波章夫).

** ABCC (Atomic Bomb Casualty Commission) was established in Hiroshima and Nagasaki by the United States government in 1947 to initiate long-term follow-up surveys on the late health effects of atomic bomb radiation. ABCC was soon joined in its research activities by a branch laboratory of the Japanese National Institute of Health.

In 1975, responsibility for these studies was assumed by the Radiation Effects Research Foundation (RERF), an independent binational institution equally funded by the two governments.

with special emphasis on the relationship between chromosomal aberration frequencies and the estimated radiation doses assigned to individual survivors. As will be mentioned later in this chapter, it was impossible until recently to determine the effect of A-bomb radiation on human germ cell chromosomes due to technical limitations. In this context, this article will deal exclusively with the somatic chromosome data on the survivors.

Cytogenetic Studies of Atomic Bomb Survivors

1) A historical review

Cytogenetic investigations of the survivors of the atomic bombing of Hiroshima and Nagasaki were initiated by Masuo Kodani as early as the late 1940s, using a classic paraffin-section technique. The limitations of this technique were so many that his findings are of historical interest only.

The presence of radiation-induced chromosomal aberrations in cultured peripheral leukocytes was demonstrated independently, but almost simultaneously, by Doida *et al.* (*18*), and by Kumatori and Ishihara (*24*).

Doida *et al.* (*18*) performed detailed karyotype analysis on 7 A-bomb survivors, 2 in Hiroshima and 5 in Nagasaki. They reported that 18 out of the 40 metaphases analyzed had structural anomalies derived presumably from either translocations or inversions, although they failed to observe any dicentric, ring, or acentric fragment among the 705 cells examined. They further suggested the possible presence of clonal cells with an identical abnormal karyotype.

Ishihara and Kumatori (*24*) examined cytogenetically 6 survivors, 2 in Hiroshima and 4 in Nagasaki, and demonstrated an increase in the frequency of induced chromosomal aberrations characterized by the presence of dicentrics, rings, acentrics, and abnormal monocentric chromosomes.

Iseki (*23*) studied 25 survivors (4 in Hiroshima and 21 in Nagasaki) and 10 non-exposed controls. Since acute radiation symptoms are sensitive biological indicators reflecting the radiation doses absorbed by the survivors, the exposed group was further divided by their symptoms, mainly epilation and bleeding, into two groups: 12 cases with symptoms and 13 cases without. The frequencies of induced chromosome-type aberrations (such as acentric fragments, dicentrics, rings, and abnormal monocentrics) were higher in the exposed than in the controls. Among the exposed, the aberration frequency was greater in survivors with acute radiation symptoms than in those without symptoms, suggesting a possible association between aberration frequencies and radiation dose.

Using blood samples cultured for three days, Bloom and his colleagues (*11, 12*) studied a large number of young (less than 30 years of age at the time of bombing) and old (30 years of age or more at that time) A-bomb survivors in Hiroshima and Nagasaki. They found an increase in the frequency of cells with induced chromosomal aberrations in the exposed individuals, and the frequency of survivors bearing chromosomally aberrant cells was significantly higher in the proximally exposed than in the distally exposed in both cities. When the young and old groups were compared, a predominance of cells with stable chromosomal exchanges was observed among older survivors. Bloom *et al.* (*12*) and Honda *et al.* (*20*) reported the presence of cells of clonal origin in the heavily exposed survivors. Clones were characterized by cells with identical stable aberrations occurring in more than 3 cells per individual.

Time in culture for blood lymphocytes is considered an important factor in the determination of the frequency of chromosomal aberrations induced *in vivo* in irradiated persons. At around 48 hr, after incubation of phytohemagglutinin (PHA)-stimulated cultures, the majority of the dividing cells are in their first mitosis *in vitro*. However, a small proportion will already be in their second *in vitro* mitosis due in part to the asynchrony of cell proliferation in culture. It is known that asymmetrical chromosomal aberrations (dicentrics, rings, and acentrics) are unstable at mitosis, and may result in cell death (8, 16, 36, 45). Thus the proportion of chromosomally aberrant cells, relative to normal ones, seen in the second or later cell divisions may be considerably reduced as compared with the proportion seen in the first mitosis in culture. The relative decrease of aberrant cells over cytogenetically normal ones will be more makred as culture time increases. In order to obtain the best estimates of aberration frequency, it is essential to examine cells at their first mitosis in culture. For this reason, a 2-day (or 48 hr) culture time has been widely used for obtaining estimates of maximum aberration frequency in lymphocytes from persons irradiated *in vivo* (*cf. 41*).

With the above view in mind, Sasaki and Miyata (*44*) examined 51 Hiroshima survivors and 11 controls more than 20 years after A-bomb exposure. Their observations on 2-day-culture preparations indicated an increased frequency of induced chromosomal aberrations of both stable and unstable types among survivors, and the frequencies of both types were proportional to the distance from the hypocenter for each individual. They further attempted to correlate the chromosome aberration frequency, as an indicator of biological dose, with the physical dose estimate, by proposing an approach termed the Q_{dr} method, a quality value measured by dicentrics and rings. Basically this method considers the yield of dicentrics and rings from those cells which contain unstable aberrations, termed X_1Cu cells, and assumes that these cells were formed at the time of exposure and were present without any mitosis. Q_{dr} is given by

$$Q_{dr} = \frac{X}{(X_1Cu)} = \frac{Y_{dr}}{1 - \exp(-Y_{del} - Y_{dr})}$$

where (X_1Cu) is the number of X_1Cu cells, X is the number of dicentrics and rings in X_1Cu cells, and Y_{dr} and Y_{del} are the dose-relationships for dicentrics plus rings, and terminal plus interstitial deletions, respectively.

Both Y_{dr} and Y_{del} can be obtained from *in vitro* dose-response curves for X-rays. By this method, they were able to obtain reasonable dose estimates for individual A-bomb survivors when transmission factors from shielding were taken into account for each of the survivors, *i.e.*, those who were exposed either in reinforced concrete buildings, in Japanese type houses, or without any shielding (*43*). They further reported the presence of cells with an identical abnormal karyotype, providing unequivocal evidence of clonal proliferation of lymphocytes *in vivo*.

2) *Cytogenetic studies at ABCC-RERF*

Since the early work of Bloom and his colleagues, cytogenetic studies of A-bomb survivors have continued and they are now one of the major investigative efforts at ABCC-RERF designed to evaluate the biological effects of A-bomb radiation (*1–6*).

The objectives of this expanded program are (a) to determine the type and frequency of radiation-induced chromosomal aberrations in the somatic cells of A-bomb survivors in Hiroshima and Nagasaki, (b) to correlate the observed aberration frequencies from individual survivors with their physical dose estimates, and (c) to provide information for use in evaluating radiation risk to human health.

Subjects of the study were drawn from participants in the RERF Adult Health Study cohort, who visit the RERF clinic biennially for periodical health examinations. The study samples consist of two groups of survivors selected on the basis of the estimated radiation dose (T65DR) assigned to each individual survivor (34): (a) proximally exposed survivors (within 2,000 m from the hypocenter) with an estimated dose of 0.01 Gy or more, and (b) distally exposed survivors with an estimated dose of less than 0.01 Gy, the latter serving as controls for the proximally exposed. Excluded from this study were those survivors who had received radiotherapy or radioisotope exposure at any time in the past, as well as those whose doses were estimated to have exceeded 1,000

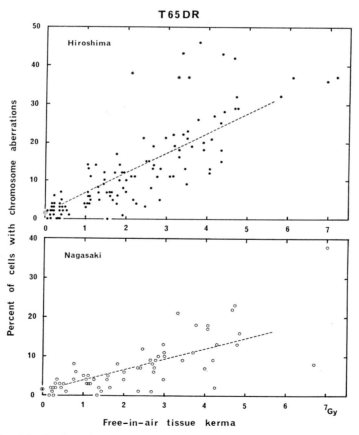

Fig. 1.   Distribution of aberrant cell frequencies for individual A-bomb survivors plotted against the T65DR tissue kerma

Top: Hiroshima, 116 cases (closed circles). Bottom: Nagasaki, 62 cases (open circles). Double circles indicate mean values from distally exposed controls. Linear regressions for the dose-aberration relationship are indicated by dashed lines.

rad. Microscopic slides were coded and examined without knowledge of the survivor's exposure status.

Blood samples drawn from each donor were cultured for 52 hr, and chromosome slides were prepared according to the routine procedure using conventional Giemsa stain. Cultures were judged successful when a minimum of 30 metaphases were analyzable karyotypically, but no more than 100 metaphases were scored for each case with non-banded preparations.

a) Dose-response relationship

Figure 1 gives the chromosomal aberration frequencies plotted against free-in-air tissue kerma (kinetic energy released in material) from individual survivors by city. There is an increase in the frequency of cells with chromosomal aberrations as the dose increases; however, the variability in aberration frequency at a given dose is large. Nevertheless, as a first approximation, linear regression coefficients can be obtained for Hiroshima and Nagasaki, with the following equation

$$Y = k + aD$$

where Y is the frequency of aberrant cells in percent, k is a constant, a is the regression coefficient, and D is the T65DR tissue kerma in gray. Based on the data shown in Fig. 1, the values of a are 5.2 for Hiroshima and 2.6 for Nagasaki, respectively, and k is 1.5 in both cities. Thus, regression coefficients differ between Hiroshima and Nagasaki by a factor of 2.

b) Types of chromosomal aberrations

Among the cells with chromosomal abnormalities, stable aberrations, such as reciprocal translocations and inversions, predominated strikingly in all dose ranges, and

TABLE I. Type and Frequency of Chromosomal Aberrations in Hiroshima A-bomb Survivors (6)

Exposure status	Proximally exposed		Distally exposed (control)	
	No.	(%)	No.	(%)
No. of cases examined	386		263	
Mean T65DR dose (Gy)	2.70		0	
No. of cells examined	35,564		24,409	
No. of aberrations				
Unstable				
dic[a]	191	(0.54)	58	(0.24)
r	51	(0.14)	5	(0.02)
f[b]	155	(0.44)	59	(0.24)
Total unstable	397	(1.12)	117	(0.48)
Stable				
t	2,369	(6.66)	137	(0.56)
inv	348	(0.98)	18	(0.07)
del[c]	389	(1.09)	35	(0.14)
Total stable	3,106	(8.73)	190	(0.78)
Total aberrations	3,503	(9.85)	307	(1.26)

Abbreviations for chromosomal aberrations are used according to ISCN (*21, 22*). dic, dicentrics; r, rings; f, fragments; t, translocations; inv, inversions; del, deletions.

[a] Including tricentrics scored as two dicentrics.

[b] Including both terminal and interstitial types.

[c] Defined as deletions without fragments.

these aberrations constituted the major contributors to the dose-response relationship (Fig. 1, Table I). Cells with unstable aberrations, *i.e.*, dicentrics, rings, and acentrics, were less frequent, being less than 10% of the total aberrant cells in the exposed group. However, there was still an increase in unstable aberrations with increasing dose.

The predominance of cells with stable aberrations over unstable ones in the A-bomb survivor data strongly suggests that cells with dicentrics and rings would have been eliminated after radiation exposure from the *in vivo* lymphocyte population through mitosis (*8, 17, 36*), provided the assumptions that (a) the proportion of peripheral blood lymphocytes with stable aberrations has remained unchanged (*8, 17*), and (b) the incidence of unstable and stable aberrations was equal at the time of aberration induction are true (*15, 16, 45*).

The number of aberrations per aberrant cell increased with increasing dose. This implies that the higher the dose absorbed, the greater the number and the complexity of the chromosomal aberrations induced in an aberrant cell.

Radiation-induced chromosome breaks and subsequent rejoining between breaks to form exchanges seem to occur in a random fashion. Therefore, it is assumed that the probability of a given chromosome being involved in an exchange is proportional to its relative length. On the basis of this assumption, all of the identifiable chromosomes involved in the aberrations were classified according to the chromosome groups from A to G. Expected values were derived from the relative lengths of metaphase chromosomes described in the ISCN (*21, 22*), while the observed values in each chromosome group were determined by the number of chromosomes involved in the exchanges. The observed frequency of dicentrics was not statistically different from the expected. This suggests that cells with dicentrics have been eliminated randomly with time following exposure from the *in vivo* lymphocyte population. For reciprocal translocations, the counterpart of dicentrics, there was a statistical difference between the observed and expected values. Although it is conceivable that this effect is real, it is more likely to be attributable to the difficulty in identifying aberrations formed by the C group chromosomes, all of which are alike both in shape and length.

The frequency of aberrant cells does not increase indefinitely with increasing dose but plateaus. The highest frequency of cells with induced aberrations among the heavily exposed survivors in Hiroshima examined so far has never exceeded 60%. This phenomenon is explicable if there is a saturation in the capacity of aberration production at the high dose range, or preferential loss of cells with unstable chromosomal aberrations with postexposure time lapse or both. Although stable chromosomal rearrangements are considered not to give rise to mechanical disturbances at mitosis, they may result in genetic imbalance in daughter cells, and thus may result in somewhat lowered proliferative potential eventually leading to cell death.

Littlefield and Joiner (*32*) conducted detailed cytogenetic examinations on six men accidentally exposed to fission neutron and gamma radiation in 1958. Their findings are very similar to those on the A-bomb data, *i.e.*, most aberrations observed 16–17 years postexposure were of the stable type (translocations and inversions), and the frequency of lymphocytes with residual aberrations were roughly correlated with dose.

From non-banded conventional and G-banded preparations, Kamada and his associates (*28, 48*) undertook an extensive cytogenetic study of Hiroshima A-bomb survivors. They reported strikingly similar findings to those of the RERF study group; in the PHA-stimulated T lymphocytes from the survivors, they found (a) a dose-depen-

to be no specific cytogenetic patterns in these leukemic cases ascribable to A-bomb radiation exposure. The same was true for 20 Hiroshima cases diagnosed as having chronic granulocytic leukemia among the directly exposed, where no specific abnormalities other than the presence of the Ph[1] chromosome were observed. It is interesting to note that a smaller G chromosome, resembling the Ph[1] in morphology, was noted persistently in the bone marrow cells of an apparently healthy, but heavily exposed male survivor for more than 12 years through serial examinations. He later developed Ph[1]-positive chronic granulocytic leukemia. This suggests the possible association between the persistence of a small G chromosome during the healthy period and the presence of a Ph[1] in the diseased state (28).

The incidence of hematologic disorders other than leukemia is known to be high in heavily exposed survivors. Chromosome analysis of patients with refractory anemia (RA) showed the absence of any structural aberrations of chromosomes, while patients having refractory anemia with an excess of blasts (RAEB) showed abnormal karyotypes, mostly due to deletions of certain chromosomes. Here again, it was impossible to correlate the cytogenetic abnormalities with the nature of the hematological disorder (28).

Cytogenetic Data for A-bomb Dosimetry Reassessment

Serious doubts concerning the validity of the T65DR system of dosimetry began to emerge in 1976 (for details, see 30). Since then, extensive efforts have been made by a US-Japan team of experts (39, 40) to develop a more appropriate system for specifying individual exposures. The work now is complete and the data for individual survivors will be available shortly.

The major change known to date in the new dosimetry system (DS86) as compared with the old one (T65DR) is that the free-in-air tissue kerma in Hiroshima was mostly contributed by gamma rays, and the neutron component was significantly less than previously estimated. There is also a considerable change in the transmission factors for gamma rays associated with Japanese-type houses by which the majority of survivors were shielded at the time of bombing. In this context, the proportion of neutrons to the total kerma is greatly reduced, especially in Hiroshima, from an average of about 25% for the T65DR to about 5% for the DS86, while no such drastic changes are observed in Nagasaki.

Preliminary analysis of the existing chromosomal aberration data indicates that the difference in the dose-response relationship between Hiroshima and Nagasaki seen with T65DR data is less pronounced when the DS86 system is used (7, 19). The regression coefficient in Hiroshima is still approximately 30% higher than in Nagasaki, when the RBE of neutrons is assumed to be 1. Detailed analysis of the cytogenetic data on the A-bomb survivors in Hiroshima and Nagasaki is now in progress, and the results will appear elsewhere in the near future.

Concluding Remarks

It is now well established that the frequency of chromosomal aberrations in the peripheral blood lymphocytes can be used for the purpose of dose assessment, since the frequency of induction of chromosomal aberrations, both *in vivo* and *in vitro*, responds very sensitively to exposure to ionizing radiation. In this context, it is not surprising that one can see a dose-dependent increase in the frequency of cells with induced chromosomal aberrations with increasing radiation dose among the survivors of the atomic bombings of Hiroshima and Nagasaki. Cytogenetic data on the A-bomb survivors are being utilized as reliable biological endpoints for the A-bomb dosimetry reassessment, though there still exist some technical limitations to be resolved.

As repeatedly mentioned in the preceding sections, A-bomb survivors received acute whole-body exposure, so that the increased frequency of chromosomal aberrations observable in T lymphocytes was induced at the time of the bombings not only in the mature lymphocytes in the circulating blood but also in other lymphocyte-producing organs, such as bone marrow, spleen, thymus, and lymph nodes. All of the cytogenetic reports have pointed to a common feature among the survivors; namely, the persisting presence of cells carrying a dicentric and its accompanying acentric fragment strongly suggests that the affected lymphocytes have existed for many decades in the circulating blood. Thus, a small fraction of mature T lymphocytes have an unusually long life-span in a dormant state without mitosis. The presence of clones formed by cells with identical karyotypic abnormalities among the heavily exposed survivors indicates that whole-body exposure to ionizing radiation can cause cytogenetic damage in the lymphopoietic stem cells without any impaired proliferative potential.

The biological and clinical significance of cells with radiation-induced chromosomal aberrations has remained unresolved. It is probable, however, that chromosomal aberrations have persisted in somatic cells other than those of the blood-forming tissues. The kind and frequency of these aberrations should follow, more or less, a pattern similar to that of T lymphocytes. This may imply an association between the specific sites of chromosome breaks in the exchanges and the activation of oncogenes situated at or nearby the break sites. King et al. (31), however, indicated no positive correlation of increased aberration frequency with any findings on the past clinical examinations. In addition, the majority of the survivors were, in fact, healthy at the time of examination. It may thus be that the chromosomal aberrations are not associated with any specific clinical manifestations in the heavily irradiated survivors. As the survivors have become older, the incidence of morbidity as well as mortality from cancer is increasing in relation to aging. It is crucial at this moment to conduct a correlated cytogenetic, clinical, and epidemiological study in order to evaluate the relationship between the observed cytogenetic abnormalities and radiation risk to human health, especially to radiation carcinogenesis.

A new cytogenetic technique for obtaining preparations of human sperm chromosomes using hamster ova as recipients has been developed in the last few years, and is available for the evaluation of acquired chromosomal damage in male germ cells (see 14, 29, 33, 42). Although this technique has not yet been applied to A-bomb survivors, for various reasons, such technological developments will undoubtedly facilitate an expansion of research possibilities in the field of human radiation cytogenetics.

REFERENCES

1. Awa, A. A. Cytogenetic and oncogenic effects of the ionizing radiations of the atomic bombs. In "Chromosomes and Cancer," ed. J. German, pp. 637–674 (1974). John Wiley & Sons, New York.
2. Awa, A. A. Review of thirty years study of Hiroshima and Nagasaki atomic bomb sur-

vivors. II. Biological effects. G. Chromosome aberrations in somatic cells. *J. Radiat. Res.* (Suppl.), 122–131 (1975).

3. Awa, A. A. Chromosome damage in atomic bomb survivors and their offspring—Hiroshima and Nagasaki. *In* "Radiation-induced Chromosome Damage in Man," ed. T. Ishihara and M. S. Sasaki, pp. 433–453 (1983). Alan R. Liss, Inc., New York.

4. Awa, A. A. Radiation-induced chromosome aberrations in A-bomb survivors—a key to biological dosimetry. *In* "Atomic Bomb Survivor Data: Utilization and Analysis," ed. R. L. Prentice and D. J. Thompson, pp. 99–111 (1984). SIAM, Philadelphia.

5. Awa, A. A., Neriishi, S., Honda, T., Yoshida, M. C., Sofuni, T., and Matsui, T. Chromosome-aberration frequency in cultured blood-cells in relation to radiation dose of A-bomb survivors. *Lancet*, **ii**, 903–905 (1971).

6. Awa, A. A., Sofuni T., Honda, T., Itoh, M., Neriishi, S., and Otake, M. Relationship between the radiation dose and chromosome aberrations in atomic bomb survivors of Hiroshima and Nagasaki. *J. Radiat. Res.*, **19**, 126–140 (1978).

7. Awa, A. A., Sofuni, T., Honda, T., Hamilton, H. B., and Fujita, S. Preliminary reanalysis of radiation-induced chromosome aberrations in relation to past and newly revised dose estimates for Hiroshima and Nagasaki A-bomb survivors. *In* "Biological Dosimetry," ed. W. G. Eisert and M. L. Mendelsohn, pp. 77–82 (1984). Springer-Verlag, Berlin.

8. Bauchinger, M. Chromosomenaberrationen und ihre zeitliche Veranderung nach Radium-Roentgentherapie gynaekologischer Tumoren. *Strahlen-therapie*, **135**, 553–564 (1968).

9. Bender, M. A. and Gooch, P. C. Persistent chromosome aberrations in irradiated human subjects. *Radiat. Res.*, **16**, 44–53 (1962).

10. Bender, M. A. and Gooch, P. C. Persistent chromosome aberrations in irradiated human subjects. II. Three and one-half year investigation. *Radiat. Res.*, **18**, 389–396 (1963).

11. Bloom, A. D., Neriishi, S., Kamada, N., Iseki, T., and Keehn, R. Cytogenetic investigation of survivors of the atomic bombings of Hiroshima and Nagasaki. *Lancet*, **ii**, 672–674 (1966).

12. Bloom, A. D., Neriishi, S., Awa, A. A., Honda, T., and Archer, P. G. Chromosome aberrations in leukocytes of older survivors of the atomic bombings of Hiroshima and Nagasaki. *Lancet*, **ii**, 10–12 (1967).

13. Bloom, A. D., Neriishi, S., and Archer, P. G. Cytogenetics of the *in-utero* exposed of Hiroshima and Nagasaki. *Lancet*, **ii**, 10–12 (1968).

14. Brandriff, B., Gordon, L., Ashworth, L., Watchmaker, G., Carrano, A., and Wyrobek, A. Chromosomal abnormalities in human sperm: comparisons among four healthy men. *Hum. Genet.*, **66**, 193–201 (1984).

15. Buckton, K. E. Identification with G and R banding of the position of breakage points induced in human chromosomes by *in vitro* X-irradiation. *Int. J. Radiat. Biol.*, **29**, 475–488 (1976).

16. Buckton, K. E. Chromosome aberrations in patients treated with X-irradiation for ankylosing spondylitis. *In* "Radiation-induced Chromosome Damage in Man," ed. T. Ishihara and M. S. Sasaki, pp. 491–511 (1983). Alan R. Liss, Inc., New York.

17. Buckton, K. E., Hamilton, G. E., Paton, L., and Langland, A. O. Chromosome aberrations in irradiated ankylosing spondylitis patients. *In* "Mutagen-induced Chromosome Damage in Man," ed. H. J. Evans and D. C. Lloyd, pp. 142–150 (1978). Edinburgh University Press, Edinburgh.

18. Doida, Y., Sugahara, T., and Horikawa, M. Studies on some radiation-induced chromosome aberrations in man. *Radiat. Res.*, **26**, 69–83 (1965).

19. Fujita, S., Awa, A. A., Pierce, D. A., Kato, H., and Shimizu, Y. Re-evaluation of biological effects of atomic bomb radiation by changes of estimated dose. Proc. IAEA Symp. "Biological Effects of Low-level Radiation," pp. 55–60 (1983). IAEA, Vienna.

20. Honda, T., Kamada, N., and Bloom, A. D. Chromosome aberrations and culture time.

Cytogenetics, **8**, 117–124 (1969).

21. ISCN. An International System for Human Cytogenetic Nomenclature. *In* "Birth Defects: Original Article Series," ed. D. G. Harnden and H. P. Klinger, Vol. 14, No. 8, (1978). The National Foundation, New York.

22. ISCN. An International System for Human Cytogenetic Nomenclature. *In* "Birth Defects: Original Article Series," ed. D. G. Harnden and H. P. Klinger, Vol. 21, No. 1 (1985). March of Dimes Birth Defects Foundation, New York.

23. Iseki, T. Cytogenetic studies in atomic bomb survivors. *J. Jpn. Soc. Int. Med.*, **55**, 76–83 (1966).

24. Ishihara, T. and Kumatori, T. Chromosome aberrations in human leukocytes irradiated *in vivo* and *in vitro*. *Acta Haematol. Jpn.*, **28**, 291–307 (1965).

25. Ishihara, T. and Kumatori, T. Cytogenetic studies on fishermen exposed to fallout radiation in 1954. *Jpn. J. Genet.*, **44**, 242–251 (1969).

26. Ishihara, T. and Kumatori, T. Cytogenetic follow-up studies in Japanese fishermen exposed to fallout radiation. *In* "Radiation-induced Chromosome Damage in Man," ed. T. Ishihara and M. S. Sasaki, pp. 475–490 (1983). Alan R. Liss, Inc., New York.

27. Kamada, N., Kuramoto, A., Katsuki, T., and Hinuma, Y. Chromosome aberrations in B lymphocytes of atomic bomb survivors. *Blood*, **53**, 1140–1147 (1979).

28. Kamada, N. and Tanaka, K. Cytogenetic studies of hematological disorders in atomic bomb survivors. *In* "Radiation-induced Chromosome Damage in Man," ed. T. Ishihara and M. S. Sasaki, pp. 455–474 (1983). Alan R. Liss, Inc., New York.

29. Kamiguchi, Y. and Mikamo, K. An improved, efficient method for analyzing human sperm chromosomes using zona-free hamster ova. *Am. J. Hum. Genet.*, **38**, 724–740 (1986).

30. Kerr, G. D., Tajima, E., Edington, C. W., and Roesch, W. C. Foreword. *In* "Reassessment of Atomic Bomb Radiation Dosimetry in Hiroshima and Nagasaki." Final Report on the Proceedings of the Third and Fourth U.S.-Japan Joint Workshops, RERF, Hiroshima, in press.

31. King, R. A., Belsky, J. L., Otake, M., Awa, A. A., and Matsui, T. Chromosome abnormalities: Correlation with findings on examination. *ABCC Tech. Rep.*, 15–72 (1972).

32. Littlefield, L. G. and Joiner, E. E. Cytogenetic follow-up studies in six radiation accident victims (16 and 17 years post-exposure). *In* "Late Biological Effects of Ionizing Radiation," Vol. 1, pp. 297–308 (1978). IAEA, Vienna.

33. Martin, R. H. A detailed method for obtaining preparations of human sperm chromosomes. *Cytogenet. Cell Genet.*, **35**, 252–256 (1983).

34. Milton, R. C. and Shohoji, T. Tentative 1965 radiation dose (T65D) estimation for atomic bomb survivors, Hiroshima and Nagasaki. *ABCC Tech. Rep.* 1–68 (1968).

35. Moorhead, P. S., Nowell, P. C., Mellman, W. J., Battips, D. M., and Hungerford, D. A. Chromosome preparations of leukocytes cultured from human peripheral blood. *Exp. Cell Res.*, **20**, 613–616 (1960).

36. Norman, A., Sasaki, M. S., Ottoman, R. E., and Fingerhut, A. G. Elimination of chromosome aberrations from human lymphocytes. *Blood*, **27**, 706–714 (1966).

37. Ohtaki, K., Shimba, H., Awa, A. A., and Sofuni, T. Comparison of type and frequency of chromosome aberrations by conventional and G-staining methods in Hiroshima atomic bomb survivors. *J. Radiat. Res*, **23**, 441–449 (1982).

38. Ohtaki, K., Shimba, H., and Awa, A. A. Comparison of chromosome aberrations by ordinary staining and G-staining methods in Hiroshima A-bomb survivors. *Jpn. J. Hum. Genet.*, **31**, 220–221 (1980).

39. Proc. US-Japan Joint Workshop for Reassessment of Atomic Bomb Radiation Dosimetry in Hiroshima and Nagasaki. RERF, Hiroshima (1983).

40. Proc. Second US-Japan Workshop for Reassessment of Atomic Bomb Radiation Dosimetry in Hiroshima and Nagasaki. RERF, Hiroshima (1983).

41. Report of the United Nations Scientific Committee on the Effects of Atomic Radiation. Annex C, Radiation-induced chromosome aberrations in human cells. General Assembly Official Records: Twenty-fourth Session, Suppl. 13 (A/7613), United Nations, New York (1969).

42. Rudak, E., Jacobs, P. A., and Yanagimachi, R. Direct analysis of the chromosome constitution of human spermatozoa. *Nature*, **274**, 911–913 (1978).

43. Sasaki, M. S. Use of lymphocyte chromosome aberrations in biological dosimetry. *In* "Radiation-induced Chromosome Damage in Man," ed. T. Ishihara, M. S. Sasaki, pp. 585–604 (1983). Alan R. Liss, Inc., New York.

44. Sasaki, M. S. and Miyata, H. Biological dosimetry in atomic bomb survivors. *Nature*, **220**, 1189–1193 (1968).

45. Savage, J.R.K. and Papworth, D. G. Frequency and distribution studies of asymmetrical *versus* symmetrical chromosome aberrations. *Mutat. Res.*, **95**, 7–18 (1982).

46. Seabright, M. A rapid banding technique for human chromosomes. *Lancet*, **ii**, 971–972 (1971).

47. Sofuni, T., Shimba, H., Ohtaki, K., and Awa, A. A. A cytogenetic study of Hiroshima atomic bomb survivors. *In* "Mutagen-induced Chromosome Damage in Man," ed. H. J. Evans and D. C. Lloyd, pp. 108–114 (1978). Edinburgh University Press, Edinburgh.

48. Tanaka, K., Kamada, N., Ohkita, T., and Kuramoto, A. Nonrandom distribution of chromosome breaks in lymphocytes of atomic bomb survivors. *J. Radiat. Res.*, **24**, 291–304 (1983).

49. Tonomura, A., Kishi, K., and Saito, F. Types and frequencies of chromosome aberrations in peripheral lymphocytes of general populations. *In* "Radiation-induced Chromosome Damage in Man," ed. T. Ishihara and M. S. Sasaki, pp. 605–616 (1983). Alan R. Liss, Inc., New York.

50. Tough, I. M., Buckton, K. E., Baikie, A. G., and Court-Brown, W. M. X-ray induced chromosome damage in man. *Lancet*, **ii**, 849–851 (1960).

BIOCHEMICAL MUTATIONS IN THE CHILDREN
OF ATOMIC BOMB SURVIVORS[*1]

Chiyoko SATOH[*2] and James V. NEEL[*3]

*Department of Genetics, Radiation Effects Research Foundation[*2]
and Department of Human Genetics, University of
Michigan Medical School[*3]*

Genetic effects of atomic bombs in the children of survivors in Hiroshima and Nagasaki were studied employing two biochemical indicators. The participating children were composed of two groups. The first group of children were born to "proximally exposed" parents, that is, one or both of whom were within 2,000 meters of the hypocenter at the time of the bomb (ATB). The second group of children were born to "distally exposed" parents, *i.e.*, who were either more than 2,500 meters from the hypocenter ATB or were not in the city.

A total of 13,052 children of the proximally exposed parents and 10,609 children of the distally exposed were examined with respect to rare variants of 30 blood proteins by one-dimensional gel electrophoresis. In the children of the proximally exposed, 3 mutations altering electrophoretic mobility of proteins were identified among 667,404 locus tests. This corresponds to a mutation rate of 0.45×10^{-5} per locus per generation with a 95% confidence interval of 0.1×10^{-5} and 1.3×10^{-5}. In the children of the distally exposed, 3 mutations among 466,881 locus tests were seen, yielding a mutation rate for electromorphs of 0.64×10^{-5} per locus per generation with a 95% confidence interval of 0.1×10^{-5} and 1.9×10^{-5}. The average gonad doses in rad received by the proximally exposed parents have been estimated under the dose schedule developed in 1965 (T65 DR) as follows: Hiroshima fathers, 16.9 for gamma and 3.4 for neutron; Hiroshima mothers, 14.0 and 1.3; Nagasaki fathers, 26.2 and 0.3; Nagasaki mothers 19.7 and 0.1. These estimates are now being revised downwards, principally with respect to the neutron exposures, but the magnitude of the reduction is currently unclear. The distally exposed parents received either negligible amounts (<1 rad) or no radiation.

A subset of the children was screened for variants in 9 erythrocyte enzymes with activity $\leq 66\%$ of normal value. There was one mutation

---

[*1] After the manuscript was sent to the publisher in March 1987, Dosimetry System 1986 (DS86) doses became available for a large part of the proximally exposed parents of children under study, although for others they are still unavailable. Parental gonad doses were calculated using DS86 procedure for the former group of parents and a hybrid procedure for the latter that calculates organ radiation dose on the basis of the DS86 Kerma in air, tissue transmission factors and T65 DR physical shielding factors. Combining the doses from both procedures, estimated doses in Gy for the proximally exposed parents are as follows: Hiroshima fathers, 0.204 for gamma and 0.002 for neutron; Hiroshima mothers, 0.231 and 0.001; Nagasaki fathers, 0.216 and 0.001; Nagasaki mothers, 0.223 and 0.0001 (J. V. Neel, C. Satoh *et al.*, *Am. J. Hum. Genet.*, **42**, 663–676, 1988)

[*2] 5-2, Hijiyama Park, Minami-ku, Hiroshima 732, Japan (佐藤千代子).

[*3] Ann Arbor, MI 48109, U.S.A.

resulting in the loss of enzyme activity in 60,529 tests conducted on the children of the proximally exposed parents but no mutations in 61,741 tests on the distally exposed. When the results of these two approaches are combined, the mutation rates are 0.60 and 0.64×10^{-5} per locus per generation in the former and the latter, respectively.

Studies of the genetic effects of the atomic bombs were at first, of necessity, primarily morphological (21) but in 1968, as the techniques for the study of human cytogenetics matured, a search for chromosomal abnormalities in the children of proximally and distally exposed parents was initiated (4) and in 1972, as human biochemical genetics became an active field of study, an effort was begun to use protein variants as indicators of mutation. The first technique to be employed in this context was electrophoresis (23) but later studies of enzyme activity were also undertaken (32). In this paper we will summarize the present status of these biochemical studies, which have been completed, with particular reference to some of the biochemical issues which arise in the course of such a study. The findings with respect to the children of the distally exposed have already been presented (26) and brief reports on the findings in the children of the proximally exposed have also been presented (35, 36) and a detailed report will be submitted as soon as the new gonad doses are available. Thus what we present here constitutes an interim report.

The General Plan of the Study

There has in the past been considerable conjecture concerning the possibility that a substantial proportion of the genetic damage induced by the atomic bombs was recessive in nature, finding expression in the later generations of the descendants of exposed persons. Earlier studies on the genetic effects of the bombs, dealing with congenital defect, survival, and the sex-ratio, and later cytogenetic studies on sex-chromosome aneuploids and reciprocal translocations all deal predominantly with what technically are dominant effects. The present study, by contrast, deals with what must be termed recessive effects, since the electrophoretic variants and the losses of enzyme activity towards which this study was directed would not in the heterozygous condition be expected to influence the child's gross phenotype.

Classical experimental studies on the genetic effects of radiation were conducted in the era before it was convenient to screen for biochemical variants of proteins. At the time this study was initiated, there were therefore no experimental studies to set even an approximate expectation for the frequency of spontaneous and induced mutations for electromorphs. There still are only very limited studies using radiation as the mutagenic agent, but several of the more recent, extensive studies on the mutagenic effects of a variety of chemicals have employed some of the techniques used in the present study; there is considerable evidence concerning the efficacy of chemicals in producing the types of mutations towards which the present techniques are directed (18). We suggest that in view of the need to put in perspective the relative mutagenic risks of ionizing radiation and various chemical exposures, this fact alone would justify the design of the present study.

Primarily because most radiation-induced mutations are lethal when homozygous, and because of the well-demonstrated ability of radiation to produce easily visualized damage to chromosomes, it has been assumed that most radiation-induced mutations are small deletions or rearrangements in the DNA. This may be so, but in fact the techniques most commonly employed in experimental genetics to study "point" mutations, such as the murine 7-locus test of Russell (*30*), probably would not detect the majority of the kinds of variants revealed by electrophoresis. It is our hope, now that this study has been completed, that a parallel study will be conducted on an experimental animal.

The present investigation was undertaken as one aspect of the Genetic Program of the Radiation Effects Research Foundation (RERF, the former Atomic Bomb Casualty Commission). An early feature of this program was the establishment of two matched cohorts of liveborn children for a study of the effects of parental exposure to the atomic bombs on the survival of their children. One cohort was born to parents residing in Hiroshima or Nagasaki, one or both of whom were within 2,000 meters of the hypocenter at the time of the bomb (ATB), the so-called proximally exposed. The other cohort is comprised of an age-sex matched set of children born to parents also residing in these two cities, who were either more than 2,500 meters from the hypocenter ATB (the so-called distally exposed) or were not in the city at that time (*22, 38*). These latter parents are presumed to have received either very negligible amounts (<1 rad) or no radiation ATB. The first cohort now includes virtually all of the children born in these cities to proximally exposed parents between 1946 and 1980. The children from whom blood samples were obtained for the present study were drawn from these two cohorts when they were 13 years of age or older.

These blood samples were examined for variants of a series of proteins carefully selected for their suitability for such a study (see "Biochemical Indicators and Procedures"). Most of the effort was directed towards electrophoretic studies, but a subset of the proteins functioning as enzymes was examined for variants resulting in approximately half-normal levels of enzyme activity. Whenever such a variant was encountered, family studies were undertaken to determine if it had been inherited or was the result of a fresh mutation.

The significance of this study for an understanding of the genetic effects of radiation on a human population depends in the final analysis upon the amount of radiation absorbed by the gonadal tissues of the survivors. Unfortunately, at this writing no reliable estimate is available. For some years the RERF (and its predecessor, the Atomic Bomb Casualty Commission) employed a system of estimating organ doses designated T65 DR (*3, 19*). Serious doubts concerning the validity of this system began to surface in 1976 and several scientific groups tried to reevaluate the atomic bomb doses (*17*); these have prompted a whole-scale reevaluation of the "dosage question," a reevaluation now nearing completion (*28*). However, organ doses under the new schedule are not yet available, and we must still be guided by the T65 DR estimates. The principal departure of the new dosage estimates from the T65 DR estimates will be to reduce substantially the neutron component in the Hiroshima spectrum of radiation but to somewhat increase the gamma. There will also be changes in the estimate of the shielding conferred by presence in a Japanese house ATB, and in the penetration of body tissue by gamma rays. Because the radiation spectrum is mixed gamma and neutron, the biological dose must be expressed in *rem*. Since the relative biological effectiveness (RBE) of neutrons increases, as dose decreases, the loss in the neutron exposure will be partially compensated by the higher RBE of the remaining neutron component in the exposure. Thus, whereas an RBE of 5 was employed in our earlier analysis (*23*) and in the present study, we now feel that in the future, with the lower neutron exposures, a figure of 20 is more appropriate for genetic end-points (*10, 12, 13*). Though the magnitude of the reduction is currently unclear, as a *very rough* guide, we expect that the new estimates of gonad doses, in *rem*, will be roughly 70–80% of the T65 DR estimates employing an RBE of 5.

Biochemical Indicators and Procedures

1) Definition of biochemical indicators

Rare electrophoretic variants with allele frequencies <0.01 were employed as candidate indicators for mutations altering electrophoretic mobility of proteins. In this series of 30 blood proteins examined by electrophoresis, they were encountered about once in each 500 examinations of any particular protein of the serum or erythrocyte. Common variants encountered as genetic polymorphisms, observed in 9 protein systems of this series, are not studied as candidates for mutation because of a relatively low probability of being the result of a mutation. We also excluded two relatively high frequency "rare" variants of transferrin (TF) and ceruloplasmin (CP), TF D_{CHI} and CP C_{NG1} with allele frequencies of 0.006 and 0.009 in our population, respectively, as candidate indicators of mutation for the same reason.

In enzyme activity measurements, variants with activity ≤66% of normal value in any of 9 erythrocyte enzymes examined were chosen as indicators of mutation resulting in the loss of enzyme activity. The rationale for this definition has been described (*32*). On the assumptions that (a) the activity measured is due to the gene products of alleles of a single locus and (b) there is no biochemical compensation, an individual heterozygous for a variant devoid of activity should exhibit 50% of the normal activity for the enzyme in question. The most favorable opportunity for detecting such variants is provided by enzymes with a coefficient of variation (CV) <11% (*20, 32*). Six of 9 enzymes under study meet the criterion of CV <11% and one is close to it (*32*). On the assumption that the same CV of 11% should apply to the heterozygotes, heterozygotes for a normal allele and a variant allele which codes either no protein at all or a protein with no activity, should exhibit values ≤66% of normal. However, we anticipate some contamination of these presumed null heterozygotes by a class of alleles characterized by reduced activity or marked instability of associated gene products. No genetic polymorphisms of enzyme activity variants were encountered in this study, so that all such variants were employed as indicators of mutation.

2) Electrophoretic studies

Children of proximally and distally exposed parents living in Hiroshima and Nagasaki were examined with respect to rare electrophoretic variants of 30 proteins. Haptoglobin (HP), TF, CP, and albumin (ALB) are plasma proteins. The following 26 systems are erythrocyte proteins: hemoglobin A1 and A2 (HB A1 and HB A2), adenosine deaminase (ADA), 6-phosphogluconate dehydrogenase (PGD), adenylate kinase-1 (AK1), phosphoglucomutase-1, -2, and -3 (PGM1, PGM2, and PGM3), acid phosphatase-1 (ACP1), triosephosphate isomerase (TPI), nucleoside phosphorylase (NP), esterase A1, B, and D (ESA1, ESB and ESD), peptidase A and B (PEPA and PEPB), glucosephosphate isomerase (GPI), isocitrate dehydrogenase-1 (IDH1), lactate dehydrogenase (LDH), malate dehydrogenase-1 (MDH1), carbonic anhydrase-1 and -2

(CA1 and CA2), glucose-6-phosphate dehydrogenase (G6PD), glutamate-oxaloacetate transaminase-1 (GOT1), glutamate-pyruvate transaminase-1 (GPT1), and phosphoglycerate kinase-1 (PGK1). Twenty nine proteins were examined with starch gel electrophoresis and one (G6PD) was examined with polyacrylamide gel electrophoresis. Blood samples were mixed with formula A, acid-dextrose (ACD) solution (6) as an anticoagulant and separated into plasma and erythrocytes as previously described (9). Depending on the laboratory schedule, they were immediately used for examination or preserved at $-70°C$ or in liquid nitrogen. Samples preserved at $-70°C$ were used in 2 or 3 days and no difference in either mobility or intensity of unstable variants was observed. When samples were preserved in liquid nitrogen, even the very faint bands characteristic of certain variants could be detected after 10 years. The methods for preparation of hemolysates of a 1:1 dilution from erythrocytes as well as those of electrophoresis and staining of protein bands are those previously described (9, 31, 41, 42). For the classification of rare variants, differences in mobility and isoelectric point were precisely compared using polyacrylamide gel electrophoresis and polyacrylamide gel isoelectric focusing. Biochemical characteristics such as thermostability, stability against denaturing reagents, values for K_m and K_i and optimal pH of erythrocyte enzymes were also examined. Procedures recommended by WHO (5) were employed for the classification of G6PD variants.

3) Enzyme activity measurements

A subset of children examined for electrophoretic variants was also screened for variants with activity $\leq 66\%$ of normal value in the following 9 erythrocyte enzymes: PGD, AK1, TPI, GPI, LDH, GOT1, PGK1, glyceraldehyde phosphate dehydrogenase (GAPD), and hexokinase (HK). Our procedures in general followed the recommendations of the International Committee for Standardization in Haematology (7). A portion of the erythrocyte fraction separated for electrophoretic examination was freed from contaminating leukocytes and the resulting erythrocyte samples were immediately used for preparation of hemolysates or preserved in liquid nitrogen when analyses were planned for later. A 1:20 dilution of hemolysates was used in the examinations for hemoglobin concentration and activity of 7 enzymes. For TPI and GAPD, a 1:800 and a 1:200 dilution were employed, respectively. Enzyme activities determined at 30°C using a centrifugal fast analyzer, Aminco Rotochem IIa/36, were converted to International Units (IU) per gram of hemoglobin. Precise procedures and conditions for the preparation of samples and activity measurements and efforts employed to minimize the contribution of technical or biological factors were previously described (32).

4) Family studies for putative mutations

All the parents of children having variants suitable for indicators of mutation (see above) were asked to donate their blood to determine whether the variants had been inherited or were the results of mutation. Their blood samples were examined for all of the protein systems included in the test batteries for electrophoretic studies and enzyme activity measurements. On the relatively few occasions when neither parent exhibited the variant, and there was no other evidence that the child was not the biological offspring of these parents, genetic typings appropriate to detecting discrepancies between legal and biological parentage were performed. These included A1 and B of the ABO system; M, N, S, and s of the MNSs system; C, D, E, c, and e of the Rh system,

Fy^a of the Duffy system; and the α_1-anti-trypsin types. Among the 30 proteins studied for the occurrence of mutation, polymorphisms useful for the detection of parentage discrepancies occur in the following: HP, ADA, PGD, PGM1, PGM3, ACP1, ESD, GOT1, and GPT1. In addition, major histocompatibility complex typings were obtained, involving 12 antigens of the A complex, 32 of the B complex, and 4 of the C complex. If the putative mutation involved one of the proteins included in the test battery, the findings with reference to that protein were excluded from the calculation of exclusion probabilities.

Findings in the Electrophoretic Studies

Among a total of 16,702 children born to proximally exposed parents and contacted for study, 13,052 children (78%) could be examined by electrophoresis. For the children of distally exposed, the corresponding numbers were 13,993 and 10,609 (76%). There are many families in which multiple siblings participated in the study. Thus, in the proximally exposed, 38% of children are siblings to some member of the remaining 62% while 30% of children are siblings in the distally exposed.

On the basis of T65 DR and attenuation tables prepared by Kerr (16), we have estimated the average gonad doses (rad) received by the proximally exposed parents of the examined children as follows: Hiroshima fathers, 16.9 for gamma and 3.4 for neutron; Hiroshima mothers, 14.0 and 1.3; Nagasaki fathers, 26.2 and 0.3; Nagasaki mothers 19.7 and 0.1. Employing an RBE for neutron of 5, the conjoint parental exposure, expressed in *rem*, in Hiroshima is 54.4, and in Nagasaki is 47.8, and for the two cities averaged 51.2.

Results obtained in the electrophoretic studies are shown in Tables I and II. The entry "total loci screened" corresponds to the number of locus tests. For an autosomal trait and a sex-linked trait in females, it is twice the number of electrophoretic tests but for sex-linked trait in males, it is the actual number of electrophoretic tests. HB A1 and HB A2 are tetramers that share a common polypeptide of α-globin. HB A1 has the composition of $\alpha_2\beta_2$ and HB A2 has $\alpha_2\delta_2$ composition. There are two loci encoding for the α-globin. In the examination of HB A1, 8 α-globin variants were encountered in 7 children of proximally exposed parents and one child of distally exposed and 4 β-globin variants were detected in 4 children of proximally exposed. However, the existence of these 8 α-globin variants could not be recognized in the examination of HB A2. Thus, the number of electrophoretic tests of HB A1 is used for calculating numbers of α and β locus tests while that of HB A2 is used for calculating the number of δ locus tests. Accordingly, the number of α locus tests is 4 times the number of electrophoretic tests of HB A1 and the numbers of β and δ locus tests are each twice the number of electrophoretic tests of HB A1 and HB A2, respectively. LDH is a tetramer composed of two A-subunits and two B-subunits. These 2 types of polypeptides are products of two independent loci, *LDHA* and *LDHB*. Therefore, the numbers of locus tests for *LDHA* and *LDHB* are each twice the number of electrophoretic tests of LDH. In earlier publications, we treated the three esterase A1 isozymes as dimers of a shared polypeptide with three independently coded gene products. However, since all of the 34 variants of this isozyme encountered in this study appear to involve all three isozyme bands (11), we now feel it more appropriate to consider these isozymes as products of a single locus. Thus the total number of different gene products examined becomes 33.

TABLE I.   Results of Examinations for the Occurrence of Mutations Altering Electrophoretic
Mobility: Data from Children of Proximally Exposed Parents

| Protein | EC no. | Locus symbol | Total loci screened | Rare variants | | Variants, both parents ex- amined | Equiv- alent locus tests | Excep- tional children |
				No. of types	Total			
Haptoglobin		*HP*	25,734	9	29	25	22,184	1[a]
Transferrin		*TF*	26,096	12	132	108	21,351	
Ceruloplasmin		*CP*	26,068	5	17	13	19,934	
Albumin		*ALB*	26,102	4	34	27	20,728	
Hemoglobin A1		*HBA1 +HBA2*	52,168	2	7	7	52,168	
		HBB	26,084	3	4	2	13,042	
Hemoglobin A2		*HBD*	26,088	0	0	0	26,088	
Adenosine deaminase	3.5.4.4	*ADA*	26,092	2	7	3	11,182	
6-Phosphogluconate dehydrogenase	1.1.1.44	*PGD*	26,054	7	11	10	23,685	
Adenylate kinase-1	2.7.4.3	*AK1*	25,164	0	0	0	25,164	
Phosphoglucomutase-1	2.7.5.1	*PGM1*	25,046	13	78	61	19,587	
Phosphoglucomutase-2	2.7.5.1	*PGM2*	25,064	4	9	8	22,279	1
Phosphoglucomutase-3	2.7.5.1	*PGM3*	5,962	0	0	0	5,962	
Acid phosphatase-1	3.1.3.2	*ACP1*	25,014	1	1	1	25,014	
Triosephosphate isomerase	5.3.1.1	*TPI*	21,916	2	2	2	21,916	
Nucleoside phosphorylase	2.4.2.1	*NP*	24,160	4	24	20	20,133	1
Esterase A1	3.1.1.1	*ESA1*	23,776	5	14	14	23,776	
Esterase B	3.1.1.1	*ESB*	22,878	0	0	0	22,878	
Esterase D	3.1.1.1	*ESD*	24,126	1	1	1	24,126	
Peptidase A	3.4.11.-	*PEPA*	26,002	1	18	15	21,668	
Peptidase B	3.4.11.-	*PEPB*	26,104	2	14	12	22,375	
Glucosephosphate isomerase	5.3.1.9	*GPI*	26,100	7	132	105	20,761	1[a]
Isocitrate dehydrogenase-1	1.1.1.42	*IDH1*	26,050	4	25	20	20,840	
Lactate dehydrogenase	1.1.1.27	*LDHA*	26,068	1	1	1	26,068	
		LDHB	26,068	3	4	3	19,551	
Malate dehydrogenase-1	1.1.1.37	*MDH1*	26,098	2	3	3	26,098	
Carbonic anhydrase-1	4.2.1.1	*CA1*	25,958	3	17	15	22,904	
Carbonic anhydrase-2	4.2.1.1	*CA2*	26,060	0	0	0	26,060	
Glucose-6-phosphate dehydrogenase	1.1.1.49	*G6PD* Male	2,488	3	5	3	1,493	
		Female	5,774	3	9	6	3,849	
Glutamate-oxaloacetate transaminase-1	2.6.1.1	*GOT1*	17,292	3	53	42	13,703	
Glutamate-pyruvate transaminase-1	2.6.1.2	*GPT1*	17,282	6	49	40	14,108	1
Phosphoglycerate kinase-1	2.7.2.3	*PGK1* Male	2,163	0	0	0	2,163	
		Female	4,566	0	0	0	4,566	
			767,665		700	567	667,404	5

[a] Parentage exclusion.

No rare variants were encountered in HB A2, ESB, PGM3, and PGK1, but in the other protein systems rare variants were seen in either or both groups of children. There are 4 proteins in which more than 10 types of rare variant were encountered, 16 in PGM1, 14 in TF excluding the D_{CHI} variant, 11 in HP and 10 in PGD. In total, 147 types of rare electrophoretic variants were identified in 1,233 children, 700 of proximally

TABLE II.   Results of Examinations for the Occurrence of Mutations Altering Electrophoretic
Mobility: Data from Children of Distally Exposed Parents

Protein	EC no.	Locus symbol	Total loci screened	Rare variants		Variants, both parents examined	Equiv- alent locus tests	Excep- tional chil- dren
				No. of types	Total			
Haptoglobin		*HP*	20,926	9	15	12	16,741	1
Transferrin		*TF*	21,212	11	93	63	14,369	1[a]
Ceruloplasmin		*CP*	21,196	4	10	8	16,957	
Albumin		*ALB*	21,212	5	33	25	16,070	1[a]
Hemoglobin A1		*HBA1* +*HBA2*	42,408	1	1	0	0	
		HBB	21,204	0	0	0	21,204	
Hemoglobin A2		*HBD*	21,190	0	0	0	21,190	
Adenosine deaminase	3.5.4.4	*ADA*	21,204	2	9	8	18,848	1
6-Phosphogluconate dehydrogenase	1.1.1.44	*PGD*	21,208	4	9	5	11,782	1
Adenylate kinase-1	2.7.4.3	*AK1*	21,066	1	3	3	21,066	
Phosphoglucomutase-1	2.7.5.1	*PGM1*	21,144	12	60	43	15,153	
Phosphoglucomutase-2	2.7.5.1	*PGM2*	21,152	4	14	10	15,109	
Phosphoglucomutase-3	2.7.5.1	*PGM3*	6,900	0	0	0	6,900	
Acid phosphatase-1	3.1.3.2	*ACP1*	20,370	1	2	2	20,370	
Triosephosphate isomerase	5.3.1.1	*TPI*	18,452	3	4	4	18,452	
Nucleoside phosphorylase	2.4.2.1	*NP*	20,530	1	18	11	12,546	
Esterase A1	3.1.1.1	*ESA1*	20,066	3	20	17	17,056	
Esterase B	3.1.1.1	*ESB*	19,420	0	0	0	19,420	
Esterase D	3.1.1.1	*ESD*	20,362	1	1	1	20,362	
Peptidase A	3.4.11.–	*PEPA*	21,152	1	11	7	13,460	
Peptidase B	3.4.11.–	*PEPB*	21,218	2	11	4	7,716	
Glucosephosphate isomerase	5.3.1.9	*GPI*	21,218	5	75	63	17,823	1[a]
Isocitrate dehydrogenase-1	1.1.1.42	*IDH1*	21,176	3	18	15	17,647	
Lactate dehydrogenase	1.1.1.27	*LDHA*	21,196	0	0	0	21,196	
		LDHB	21,196	2	2	2	21,196	
Malate dehydrogenase-1	1.1.1.37	*MDH1*	21,212	2	3	1	7,071	
Carbonic anhydrase-1	4.2.1.1	*CA1*	21,118	2	3	3	21,118	
Carbonic anhydrase-2	4.2.1.1	*CA2*	21,172	1	2	0	0	
Glucose-6-phosphate dehydrogenase	1.1.1.49	*G6PD* Male	1,786	1	1	0	0	
		Female	4,152	5	8	7	3,633	
Glutamate-oxaloacetate transaminase-1	2.6.1.1	*GOT1*	16,346	4	56	43	12,551	
Glutamate-pyruvate transaminase-1	2.6.1.2	*GPT1*	16,334	8	51	40	12,811	
Phosphoglycerate kinase-1	2.7.2.3	*PGK1* Male	2,224	0	0	0	2,224	
		Female	4,840	0	0	0	4,840	
			637,562		533	397	466,881	6

[a] Parentage exclusion.

exposed and 533 of distally exposed parents. Because of death or lack of cooperation, it was not always possible to test both parents of a child with a rare variant. Both parents could be examined for 567 children (81%) of the former group and 397 children (74%) of the latter group. In most of these cases, a variant identical with that of the child was detected in one (two in a few cases) of the parents.

The term "exceptional child" in Tables I and II is applied to a child who has a variant not observed in either parent, the presence of the variant in the child being confirmed by duplicate, independent tests. There are 5 and 6 exceptional children among the children of proximally exposed and the distally exposed, respectively. However, the test battery described earlier indicated a discrepancy between legal and biological parentage for 2 and 3 of these children, respectively. We are thus left with 3 putative mutants in each group. Description of the 6 presumptive mutants is as follows:

1) A slowly migrating variant of GPT1 was detected in a female child of proximally exposed Hiroshima parents. This enzyme is a dimer. The abnormal phenotype consisted of three bands which are interpreted as corresponding to the normal homodimer, a heterodimer of one normal and one mutant polypeptide and the homodimer of the mutant polypeptide. The phenotype is similar to that of a rare hereditary variant of this enzyme encountered in Nagasaki, which we have termed 1-6NG1. The mobility of the mutant homodimer is identical with that of the homodimer of 6NG1, but staining intensity of the former is weaker than that of the latter. The mutant will be described in greater detail elsewhere (*37*). Neither of the parents nor a younger sister of the proposita showed the abnormal phenotype. There was no parentage exclusion with the complete battery of tests. (Mother's gonad exposure: 1.3 rad of gamma, 0.1 rad of neutrons. Father was not exposed.)

2) A slowly migrating variant of PGM2 was encountered in a male child of parents both of whom were proximally exposed in Nagasaki. The abnormal phenotype consisted of the three bands associated with the PGM2 1 phenotype and a variant band which migrated identically or slightly cathodally to the *d*-band of PGM1. This mutant has been designated PGM2 9NG2 (*33*) (Fig. 1). On starch gel electrophoresis, the mutant

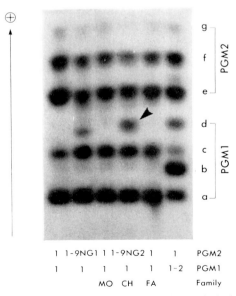

FIG. 1. Starch gel electrophoresis patterns obtained during family study for a mutant of PGM2 encountered in a child of proximally exposed parents

PGM2 1, normal (composed of e-, f-, g-bands); PGM2 1-9NG1, 1 and 9NG1 (a hereditary variant); PGM2 1-9NG2, 1 and 9NG2 (a mutant); MO, mother; CH, child; FA, father.

band migrates slightly anodal to the band of a hereditary variant, PGM2 9NG1, but to the same position as that of the other variant, PGM2 9HR1. However, on thin layer polyacrylamide gel isoelectric focusing, PGM2 9NG1, PGM2 9NG2, and PGM2 9HR1 are clearly distinguishable. Neither of the parents nor two siblings exhibited the abnormal phenotype. No parentage discrepancy was revealed by the complete battery of tests. (Mother's gonad exposure: 91 rad of gamma, 0.2 rad of neutrons. Father's gonad exposure: 6.5 rad of gamma.)

3) A rapidly migrating variant of NP was detected in a male child of proximally exposed Nagasaki parents. The abnormal phenotype consisted of a set of bands associated with the NP 1 phenotype and a set of rapidly migrating bands which exhibited a mobility identical to that of the bands associated with the NP 2 phenotype, a hereditary variant. The mutant will be described in detail elsewhere (40). Neither of the parents exhibited the abnormal bands. There was no parentage exclusion with the full battery of tests. (Mother's gonad exposure: 0.4 rad for gamma; Father's dose: 0.)

4) A rapidly migrating variant of HP was encountered in a female child of parents who were distally exposed in Nagasaki. The abnormal phenotype consisted of a set of bands associated with the HP 2 phenotype and a set of bands with a slightly faster mobility than the HP 2 bands. This mutant will be further characterized and described elsewhere (2). Neither of the parents nor four siblings exhibited the unusual bands on repeated determinations, and the bands do not correspond to any variant encountered in the course of the study. No parentage discrepancy was revealed by the complete battery of tests.

5) A slowly migrating variant of PGD was detected in a male child of distally exposed Hiroshima parents, neither of whom exhibited the trait. This enzyme is a dimer. The abnormal phenotype consisted of three bands, interpreted as corresponding to the normal homodimer, a heterodimer of one normal and one mutant polypeptide, and the homodimer of the mutant polypeptide. The mutant isozyme designated PGD HR4 migrates more slowly than the type C isozyme that occurs in 19% of the population,

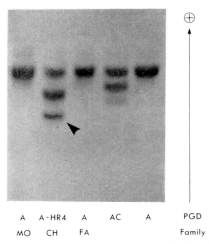

FIG. 2. Polyacrylamide gel electrophoresis patterns obtained during family study for a mutant of PGD detected in a child of distally exposed parents

A, normal; AC, A and C (a polymorphic variant); A-HR4, A and HR4 (a mutant); MO, mother; CH, child; FA, father.

and it migrates more slowly than any other variant isozyme of PGD encountered in the study (Fig. 2). The mutant will be described in detail elsewhere (40). There was no parentage exclusion with the complete battery of tests.

6)   A rapidly migrating variant of ADA was detected in a male offspring of parents neither of whom were in Nagasaki at the time of the bomb. The normal phenotype of this enzyme (ADA 1) under our electrophoretic conditions consists of three bands. The mutant phenotype consists of five bands. The two more anodal bands are variant, and the two more cathodal bands correspond to ADA 1. The central band is interpreted as an overlap of the third band of type 1 with the first band of the mutant. The phenotype appears identical to that of the rare type 1–6 variant (27). There was no exclusion of paternity with the full battery of test systems.

As described above, the 6 putative mutations occurred in 6 different proteins among which genetic polymorphism is observed in GPT1, HP, PGD, and ADA.

Findings in the Enzyme Activity Measurements

Among the children examined by electrophoresis, 4,989 of the proximally exposed parents and 5,026 of the distally exposed were examined with respect to the activity of 9 erythrocyte enzymes. The results are shown in Table III. The numbers for "total loci screened" were calculated as those in Tables I and II except for LDH. Though LDH is a tetramer consisting of two A-subunits and two B-subunits, 80% of LDH activity is contributed by the B-subunit, and any variant detected would involve that unit. Thus, the entry for LDH is twice the number of determinations for activity. In the previous report (35), the number of locus tests of G6PD and pyruvate kinase were included in the calculation of equivalent locus tests, but they are excluded here since they are thought to be inappropriate to a search for mutation resulting in the loss of enzyme activity for the following reasons:

1)   Because of nonrandom inactivation of the X chromosome bearing the variant allele in a female, it is sometimes difficult to confirm the genetic nature of a variant of a sex-linked trait by examining blood samples from both parents. An example encountered in our electrophoretic study has already been described in which a son and his maternal grandmother exhibited an electrophoretic variant of G6PD while his mother's G6PD was normal (15). Similarly, in family studies for a few G6PD variants with activity ≤66% of normal, G6PD activity of both parents was at the normal level, and we could not determine whether the variants were the results of mutation or nonrandom inactivation of variant alleles. However, in a family study for a PGK1 variant encountered in 3 male siblings, the PGK1 activity of their mother was 49% and the inheritance of the variant was confirmed though PGK1 is also a sex-linked trait.

2)   We detected many children having PK variants though the coefficient of variation for PK activity in our population was larger than 16%. In most of these cases, the PK activity in one of the parents was less than 66% of normal and the genetic nature of the variant was confirmed. However, in several variants, a recessive-type inheritance (*i.e.*, low × low → very low) was suggested by family studies.

Variants were encountered in 26 children of the proximally exposed parents and 21 children of the distally exposed. From all of the children, second samples were obtained and the existence of the variants was confirmed. Blood samples from both parents were available for 24 children in the former group and 18 in the latter. In all of them,

TABLE III.   Results from Examinations of Erythrocyte Enzymes

Enzyme	EC no.	Locus symbol		Children Total loci screened
6-Phosphogluconate dehydrogenase	1.1.1.44	PGD		9,598
Adenylate kinase-1	2.7.4.3	AK1		9,520
Triosephosphate isomerase	5.3.1.1	TPI		6,774
Glucosephosphate isomerase	5.3.1.9	GPI		9,978
Lactate dehydrogenase	1.1.1.27	LDHB		9,624
Glutamate-oxaloacetate transaminase-1	2.6.1.1	GOT1		4,876
Phosphoglycerate kinase-1	2.7.2.3	PGK1	Male	2,371
			Female	4,810
Glyceralde-3-phosphate dehydrogenase	1.2.1.12	GAPD		560
Hexokinase	2.7.1.1	HK		4,232
				62,343

heredity was confirmed except for one presumptive mutant of TPI. Description of the putative TPI mutant encountered in a female child of proximally exposed Nagasaki parents is as follows: the TPI activity of the propositus was 65% of normal, 3.9 standard deviations below the mean. The mother, father, and a younger brother exhibited 92%, 100%, and 104% of normal activity, respectively. The electrophoretic pattern of all of them was normal. There was no parentage discrepancy with the complete battery of tests. (Mother was not exposed. Father's gonad exposure: 11 rad of gamma.)

Calculation of Mutation Rate

The total number of locus tests is shown by system in the column headed "total loci screened" of Tables I, II, and III. Considerations paid in calculating the numbers were described earlier. However, only when both parents of a child with a variant were examined do we have data suitable for a rigorous treatment of the mutation rate. The number of rare variants and the frequency of such family studies are shown in Tables I, II, and III. We estimate for each system the number of alleles that have been effectively screened for mutation ("equivalent locus tests") as follows:

$$\text{total loci screened} \times \frac{\text{number of variants, both parents examined}}{\text{total number of variants}}$$

All of the number of loci screened of a polypeptide for which no variants have been encountered are credited as contributing to locus tests.

With these conventions, we can calculate that a series of electrophoretic examinations on the children of proximally exposed parents provides 667,404 "equivalent locus tests," while the number obtained from the distally exposed group is 466,881. In the children of proximally exposed parents, 3 mutations among 667,404 equivalent locus tests yield a mutation rate for electromorphs of 0.45×10^{-5} per locus per generation. The error in this estimate is substantial at the 95% confidence limits, the lower and upper bounds being 0.1×10^{-5} and 1.3×10^{-5}, respectively, on the assumption that the number of mutations corresponds to a Poisson variable. The mutation rate based on 3

for the Occurrence of Mutations Resulting in the Loss of Activity

of proximally exposed parents			Children of distally exposed parents			
Variants confirmed		Equivalent locus tests	Total loci screened	Variants confirmed		Equivalent locus tests
Total	Both parents examined			Total	Both parents examined	
0	0	9,598	9,890	4	4	9,890
3	3	9,520	9,626	1	1	9,626
6	6	6,774	6,370	3	3	6,370
11	9	8,164	10,052	3	3	10,052
2	2	9,624	9,820	0	0	9,820
2	2	4,876	5,544	7	4	3,168
0	0	2,371	2,363	3	3	2,363
0	0	4,810	4,996	0	0	4,996
1	1	560	722	0	0	722
1	1	4,232	4,734	0	0	4,734
26	24	60,529	64,117	21	18	61,741

TABLE IV.   The Mutation Rates Observed in This Study

	Children of proximally exposed parents	Children of distally exposed parents	Total
Electromorphs			
No. of children examined	13,052	10,609	23,661
Equivalent locus tests	667,404	466,881	1,134,285
Mutations	3	3	6
Mutation rate per locus per generation	0.45×10^{-5}	0.64×10^{-5}	0.53×10^{-5}
95% confidence limits			
Lower limit	0.09×10^{-5}	0.13×10^{-5}	0.19×10^{-5}
Upper limit	1.31×10^{-5}	1.88×10^{-5}	1.15×10^{-5}
Deficiency variants			
No. of children examined	4,989	5,026	10,015
Equivalent locus tests	60,529	61,741	122,270
Mutation	1	0	1
Mutation rate per locus per generation	1.65×10^{-5}	0	0.82×10^{-5}
95% confidence limits			
Lower limit	0.04×10^{-5}	0	0.02×10^{-5}
Upper limit	9.20×10^{-5}	4.85×10^{-5}	4.56×10^{-5}

mutations among 466,881 equivalent locus tests in the children of distally exposed is 0.64×10^{-5} per locus per generation, with 95% confidence interval of 0.1×10^{-5} and 1.9×10^{-5} (Table IV).

With respect to mutation resulting in the loss of enzyme activity, the same conventions were employed. In the children of proximally exposed, on the basis of one putative mutation among 60,529 equivalent locus tests, we estimate the mutation rate to be 1.65×10^{-5} per locus per generation with 95% confidence interval of 0.04×10^{-5} and 9.20×10^{-5}. No mutation was encountered in the children of the distally exposed parents among 61,741 equivalent locus tests (Table IV).

If the results of these two approaches are combined, only numerators should be added. Then, the mutation rate in the proximally exposed group is 0.60×10^{-5} per locus

TABLE V.   Results of Examinations for the Occurrence of Mutations Altering
Electrophoretic Mobility in Other Populations

Locality	Population	Locus tests	Mutation	Reference
United Kingdom	Caucasian	133,478	0	14
West Germany	Caucasian	225,000	1	1
United States	Caucasian	218,376	0	a
	American Black	18,900	0	a
Central and South America	Amerindian	118,475	0	b
Marshall Islands	Micronesian	1,897	0	24
		716,126	1	

[a] H. W. Mohrenweiser and J. V. Neel, unpublished data.
[b] Unpublished data.

per generation with 95% confidence interval of 0.2×10^{-5} and 1.5×10^{-5} on the basis of 4 mutations among 667,404 equivalent locus tests. The mutation rate in the distally exposed group does not change. It should be emphasized that these "rates" are not normative values in any respect. A normative value for nucleotide-substitution plus deficiency-states would require equal numbers of the two types of observations and correction for the fact that only approximately 1/3 of all nucleotide substitutions result in variants detectable by electrophoresis.

There is a possibility that the mutation rates obtained above are inflated by undetected discrepancies between legal and biological parentage. We estimated the frequency with which undetected nonpaternity contributes to the apparent mutation rate according to the equation of $IW(1-D)$, where I=frequency of nonpaternity in the population under consideration, W=average frequency at the loci under consideration of alleles responsible for rare variants, and D=probability of detecting nonpaternity with the battery of exclusion tests employed (29). We have estimated $I=0.0045$ and $D=0.992$ (26). $W=0.0009$ was calculated from the data obtained in the present study (see Tables I and II). Then, the *a priori* probability that an undetected parentage discrepancy (essentially, discrepancy between legal and biological paternity) is the cause of the apparent mutation becomes $0.0045 \times 0.0009 \times 0.008$, or 0.3×10^{-7}. Thus undetected parentage discrepancies should not inflate the mutation rate to the extent that an adjustment is necessary.

DISCUSSION

In addition to the "exceptional" children listed in Tables I and II, there were encountered a small number of apparent exceptional children who on further study were found to be "false positives." These resulted from such factors as: (a) a mislabelling of a sample, (b) the existence of an electromorph with low and variable activity, (c) the existence of a variant with mobility which is very similar to that of the normal protein, or (d) non-random inactivation of the X chromosome bearing the variant allele in a female. The detection of such events was guaranteed by a variety of procedures. (a)A mis-labelling of a sample was easily detected since it had been our rule to confirm the existence of a variant by repeat examinations using a sample preserved in liquid nitrogen and a second fresh sample. When mislabelling was confirmed, we examined all the samples which were taken or processed on the same day as the mislabelled sample was taken or processed and in this way could usually detect the true carrier of the variant. If no error was detected at this point, family studies would detect the "false positives". With respect to (b) low and variable activity, repeat studies using fresh samples and overloading the gels were useful. For (c) a similar mobility to that of normal, polyacrylamide gel electrophoresis and polyacrylamide gel isoelectric focusing which could separate the variant from the normal protein better were employed to detect the variant in the parents (34). For (d) non-random inactivation of X chromosome bearing the variant, an expanded family study was carried out. We could confirm the heredity of several cases of electrophoretic variants of G6PD detected in male children whose mothers were apparently normal by examining their maternal grandparents or uncles (15).

Excluding our study and a small scale study on Marshall Islanders (24), there are no studies in which electrophoresis was employed to examine the occurrence of induced mutations in a human population. However, there are several studies in which proteins were examined for spontaneous mutations by electrophoresis. Table V summarizes the results of those. Among a total of 716,126 locus tests, they yield only one putative mutant of α-globin in a series from West Germany in which α-, β-, and γ-globin of newborn children were examined by isoelectric focusing using 8M-urea containing polyacrylamide gel (1). The technique used in other studies was starch gel electrophoresis. Number of locus tests in each study was small compared with those obtained in the present study.

It is apparent that a major effort has yielded only a handful of mutations, equally distributed among the two sets of children. The possibility of such an outcome was well understood when the study was undertaken. However, the question of the genetic effects of the atomic bombs, especially of hidden (recessive) effects, is of such importance that the effort was felt to be justified. One would, of course, not wish to rest an opinion concerning the genetic effects of the bombs on this study alone, but when the new estimates of gonad doses become available, our results can be combined with those of other studies conducted during the past 40 years for a rounded view of this subject.

It should be noted that if this type of study were to be initiated today, the techniques employed for detecting both electrophoretic and activity variants would undoubtedly be somewhat different. For instance, polyacrylamide gel electrophoresis and polyacrylamide gel isoelectric focusing would probably replace starch gel electrophoresis wherever these were feasible (1), and a new generation of highly automated enzyme analysis equipment would certainly replace the type of centrifugal fast analyzer employed in this study. However, once a study of this nature is initiated, it is important that the technique be held as constant as possible over the years, so that the data may be said to be truly homogeneous.

We note, finally, that there are techniques now under development which should yield a larger return per unit effort. One of these is two-dimensional polyacrylamide gel electrophoresis of the protein contents of blood plasma, erythrocytes, platelets, and lymphocytes, coupled with computerized image analysis (25, 39). The other possibility is the direct examination of the DNA for genetic damage, an approach which, in principle, could greatly increase the genetic information obtained from each individual subject but which still is only in the very early stages (8). Recently, we have initiated a program to establish permanent cell lines of lymphocytes from approximately 1,000 families composed of proximally exposed and distally exposed atomic bomb survivors, their spouses and children and preserve them in liquid nitrogen for future use since the population is rapidly becoming unavailable.

REFERENCES

1. Altland, K., Kaempfer, M., Forssbohm, M., and Werner, W. Monitoring for changing mutation rates using blood samples submitted for PKU screening. *In* "Human Genetics, Part A: The Unfolding Genome," ed. B. Bonné-Tamir, pp. 277–287 (1982). Alan R. Liss, Inc., New York.

2. Asakawa, J., unpublished.

3. Auxier, J. A. Physical dose estimates for a-bomb survivors—studies at Oak Ridge, U.S.A. *J. Radiat. Res.*, **16** (Suppl.), 1–11 (1975).

4. Awa, A. A., Honda, T., Neriishi, S., Sofuni, T., Shimba, H., Ohtaki, K., Nakano, M., Kodama, Y., Itoh, M., and Hamilton, H. B. Cytogenetic study of the offspring of atomic bomb survivors, Hiroshima and Nagasaki, unpublished.

5. Betke, K., Beutler, E., Brewer, G. J., Kirkman, H. N., Luzzatto, L., Motulsky, A. G., Ramot, B., and Siniscalco, M. Standardization of procedures for the study of glucose-6-phosphate dehydrogenase, report of a WHO scientific group. *WHO Tech. Rep. Ser.*, **366** (1967).

6. Beutler, E. "Red Cell Metabolism, A Manual of Biochemical Methods," 2nd ed. (1975). Grune and Stratton, New York.

7. Beutler, E., Blume, K. G., Kaplan, J. C., Löhr, G. W., Ramot, B., and Valentine, W. N. International Committee for Standardization in Haematology: recommended methods for red cell enzyme analysis. *Br. J. Haematol.*, **35** (Suppl.), 331–340 (1977).

8. Delehanty, J., White, R. L., and Mendelsohn, M. L. Approaches to determining mutation rates in human DNA. *Mutat. Res.*, **167**, 215–232 (1986).

9. Ferrell, R. E., Ueda, N., Satoh, C., Tanis, R. J., Neel, J. V., Hamilton, H. B., Inamizu, T., and Baba, K. The frequency in Japanese of genetic variants of 22 proteins. I. Albumin, ceruloplasmin, haptoglobin, and transferrin. *Ann. Hum. Genet.*, **40**, 407–418 (1977).

10. Garriott, M. L. and Grahn, D. Neutron and γ ray effects measured by the micronucleus test. *Mutat. Res. Let.*, **105**, 157–162 (1982).

11. Goriki, K., unpublished.

12. Grahn, D., Lee, C. H., and Farrington, B. F. Interpretation of cytogenetic damage induced in the germ line of male mice exposed for over 1 year to ^{239}Pu alpha particles, fission neutron, and ^{60}Co gamma rays. *Radiat. Res.*, **95**, 566–583 (1983).

13. Grahn, D., Carnes, B. A., Farrington, B. H., and Lee, C. H. Genetic injury in hybrid male mice exposed to low doses of ^{60}Co γ-rays and fission neutrons. I. Response to single doses. *Mutat. Res.*, **129**, 215–229 (1984).

14. Harris, H., Hopkinson, D. A., and Robson, E. B. The incidence of rare alleles determining electrophoretic variants: data on 43 enzyme loci in man. *Ann. Hum. Genet.*, **37**, 237–253 (1974).

15. Kageoka, T., Satoh, C., Goriki, K., Fujita, M., Neriishi, S., Yamamura, K., Kaneko, J., and Masunari, N. Electrophoretic variants of blood proteins in Japanese. IV. Prevalence and enzymologic characteristics of glucose-6-phosphate dehydrogenase variants in Hiroshima and Nagasaki. *Hum. Genet.*, **70**, 101–108 (1985).

16. Kerr, G. D. Organ dose estimates for the Japanese atomic bomb survivors. *Health Phys.*, **37**, 487–508 (1979).

17. Kerr, G. D., Hashizume, T., and Edington, C. W. Historical Review. *In* "US-Japan Joint Reassessment of Atomic Bomb Radiation Dosimetry in Hiroshima and Nagasaki. Final Report," pp. 1–13 (1987). The Radiation Effects Research Foundation, Hiroshima.

18. Lewis, S. E. and Johnson, F. M. The nature of spontaneous and induced electrophoretically detected mutations in the mouse. *In* "Genetic Toxicology of Environmental Chemicals: Part B," ed. K. Ramel, B. Lambert, and J. Magnussen, pp. 359–365 (1986). Alan R. Liss, New York.

19. Milton, R. C. and Shohoji, T. Tentative 1965 radiation dose estimation for atomic bomb survivors. *ABCC Tech. Rep.*, 1–68 (1968).

20. Mohrenweiser, H. W. Frequency of enzyme deficiency variants in erythrocytes of newborn infants. *Proc. Natl. Acad. Sci. U.S.A.*, **78**, 5046–5050 (1981).

21. Neel, J. V. and Schull, W. J. "The Effect of Exposure to the Atomic Bombs on Pregnancy Termination in Hiroshima and Nagasaki," National Academy of Science-National Research Council, Publication No. 461 (1956). Washington, D. C.

22. Neel, J. V., Kato, H., and Schull, W. J. Mortality in the children of atomic bomb survivors and controls. *Genetics*, **76**, 311–326 (1974).

23. Neel, J. V., Satoh, C., Hamilton, H. B., Otake, M., Goriki, K., Kageoka, T., Fujita, M., Neriishi, S., and Asakawa, J. Search for mutations affecting protein structure in children of atomic bomb survivors: Preliminary report. *Proc. Natl. Acad. Sci. U.S.A.*, **77**, 4221–4225 (1980).

24. Neel, J. V., Mohrenweiser, H., Hanash, S., Rosenblum, B., Sternberg, S., Wurzinger, K. H., Rothman, E., Satoh, C., Goriki, K., Krasteff, T., Long, M., Skolnick, M., and Krzesicki, R. Biochemical approaches to monitoring human populations for germinal mutation rates: I. Electrophoresis. *In* "Utilization of Mammalian Specific Locus Studies in Hazard Evaluation and Estimates of Genetic Risk," ed. F. de Serres and W. Sheridan, pp. 71–93 (1983). Plenum Publ. Co., New York.

25. Neel, J. V., Rosenblum, B. B., Sing, C. F., Skolnick, M. M., Hanash, S. M., and Sternberg, S. Adapting two-dimensional gel electrophoresis to the study of human germ-line mutation rates. *In* "Two-dimensional Gel Electrophoresis of Proteins," ed. J. E. Celis and R. Bravo, pp. 259–306 (1984). Academic Press, New York.

26. Neel, J. V., Satoh, C., Goriki, K., Fujita, M., Takahashi, N., Asakawa, J., and Hazama, R. The rate with which spontaneous mutation alters the electrophoretic mobility of proteins. *Proc. Natl. Acad. Sci. U.S.A.*, **83**, 389–393 (1986).

27. Radam, G., Strauch, H., and Prokop, O. Ein seltener Phänotyp im Adenosindesaminase-Polymorphismus: Hinweis auf die Existenz eines neuen Allels. *Humangenetik*, **25**, 247–250 (1974).

28. Radiation Effects Research Foundation. "US-Japan Joint Reassessment of Atomic Bomb Radiation Dosimetry in Hiroshima and Nagasaki. Final Report," (1987). The Radiation Effects Research Foundation, Hiroshima.

29. Rothman, E. D., Neel, J. V., and Hoppe, F. M. Assigning a probability for paternity in apparent cases of mutation. *Am. J. Hum. Genet.*, **33**, 617–628 (1981).

30. Russell, W. L. X-ray-induced mutations in mice. *Cold Spring Harbor Symp. Quant. Biol.*, **16**, 327–336 (1951).

31. Satoh, C., Ferrell, R. E., Tanis, R. J., Ueda, N., Kishimoto, S., Neel, J. V., Hamilton, H. B., and Baba, K. The frequency in Japanese of genetic variants of 22 proteins. III. Phosphoglucomutase-1, phosphoglucomutase-2, 6-phosphogluconate dehydrogenase, adenylate kinase, and adenosine deaminase. *Ann. Hum. Genet.*, **41**, 169–183 (1977).

32. Satoh, C., Neel, J. V., Yamashita, A., Goriki, K., Fujita, M., and Hamilton, H. B. The frequency among Japanese of heterozygotes for deficiency variants of 11 enzymes. *Am. J. Hum. Genet.*, **35**, 656–674 (1983).

33. Satoh, C., Takahashi, N., Asakawa, J., Masunari, N., Fujita, M., Goriki, K., Hazama, R., and Iwamoto, K. Electrophoretic variants of blood proteins in Japanese. I. Phosphoglucomutase-2 (PGM2). *Jpn. J. Hum. Genet.*, **29**, 89–104 (1984).

34. Satoh, C., Takahashi, N., Kaneko, J., Kimura, Y., Fujita, M., Asakawa, J., Kageoka, T.,

Goriki, K., and Hazama, R. Electrophoretic variants of blood proteins in Japanese. II. Phosphoglucomutase-1 (PGM1). *Jpn. J. Hum. Genet.*, **29**, 287–310 (1984).

35. Satoh, C., Goriki, K., Asakawa, J., Fujita, M., Takahashi, N., Hamilton, H. B., Hazama, R., and Neel, J. V. Evaluation of genetic effects of radiation of atomic bombs at the protein level. *Jpn. J. Hum. Genet.*, **31**, 184 (Abst.) (1986).

36. Satoh, C., Goriki, K., Asakawa, J., Fujita, M., Takahashi, N., Hazama, R., Hamilton, H. B., and Neel, J. V. Effects of atomic bomb radiation on the induction of gene mutation. Abstract for 7th International Congress of Human Genetics, 1986, West Berlin.

37. Satoh, C., unpublished.

38. Schull, W. J., Neel, J. V., Otake, M., Awa, A., Satoh, C., and Hamilton, H. B. Hiroshima and Nagasaki: Three and a half decades of genetic screening. *In* "Environmental Mutagens and Carcinogens," ed. T. Sugimura and S. Kondo, pp. 687–700 (1982). Alan R. Liss, Inc., New York.

39. Skolnick, M. M. and Neel, J. V. An algorithm for comparing two-dimensional electrophoretic gels, with particular reference to the study of mutation. *In* "Advances in Human Genetics," ed. H. Harris and K. Hirschhorn, Vol. 15, pp. 55–160 (1986). Plenum Publishing Co., New York.

40. Takahashi, N., unpublished.

41. Tanis, R. J., Ueda, N., Satoh, C., Ferrell, R. E., Kishimoto, S., Neel, J. V., Hamilton, H. B., and Ohno, N. The frequency in Japanese of genetic variants of 22 proteins. IV. Acid phosphatase, NADP-isocitrate dehydrogenase, peptidase A, peptidase B and phosphohexose isomerase. *Ann. Hum. Genet.*, **41**, 419–428 (1978).

42. Ueda, N., Satoh, C., Tanis, R. J., Ferrell, R. E., Kishimoto, S., Neel, J. V., Hamilton, H. B., and Baba, K. The frequency in Japanese of genetic variants of 22 proteins. II. Carbonic anhydrase I and II, lactate dehydrogenase, malate dehydrogenase, nucleoside phosphorylase, triosephosphate isomerase, hemoglobin A and hemoglobin A2. *Ann. Hum. Genet.*, **41**, 43–52 (1977).

CHROMOSOME LOCALIZATION OF NEWLY ISOLATED PROTOONCOGENES IN *src* FAMILY

Michihiro C. Yoshida

*Chromosome Research Unit, Faculty of Science, Hokkaido University**

Chromosomal localization of seven newly isolated human protooncogenes of the tyrosine kinase family has been accomplished by the combined use of human-mouse cell hybrids, Southern blotting, and *in situ* hybridization. At least four c-*yes* genes (*yes*-1, *yes*-2, *fgr*, and *syn*) have been isolated from a human gene library with a v-*yes* DNA segment as a screening probe. The c-*yes*-1, a proto-*yes* gene, was assigned to 18q21.3. The c-*yes*-2, a processed pseudogene, was mapped to 22q12 by *in situ* hybridization. The c-*fgr*, the same gene as *src*-2, was located on 1p34-p36. The c-*syn* gene was mapped to chromosome 6 and its precise localization was assigned to the region q21. A novel v-*erb*B-related gene, c-*erb*B-2, was localized on 17q21. Two *ros*-related genes, c-*ros*-1 and c-*ros*-2, were localized to 6q22 and 13q12, respectively. Furthermore, the current mapping information of human protooncogenes and related oncogenes is presented.

During the last several years, more than two dozen human protooncogenes (cellular oncogenes) have been identified by the homology of their nucleotide sequences to retroviral oncogenes, those regions of certain retroviral genomes believed to be responsible for induction of cancers and neoplastic transformation of cultured cells (*2, 32*). Chromosome localization studies have shown that the positions of these protooncogenes on human chromosomes often correspond to specific breakpoints involved in chromosome rearrangements seen in cancer and leukemia (*3, 11, 23, 29, 36*). It is not known whether all or most of these chromosome rearrangements are associated with gene rearrangements that provide genomic derangements in malignancies. Burkitt's lymphoma is the most prominent example and analyzed by cytogenetic and molecular genetic methods. In the specific translocations in Burkitt's lymphomas c-*myc* oncogene rearranges with immunoglobulin genes and undergoes activation in the translocation-carrying cells (*28*). Recently, several new protooncogenes of the tyrosine kinase family have been isolated in Japan. Several tyrosine kinase oncogenes play a crucial role for regulation of normal cell growth or differentiation and for neoplastic transformation. The newly isolated protooncogenes, therefore, are potentially of importance in development and tumorigenesis in mammals. In this section, chromosomal localization of these newly isolated human protooncogenes is described.

Strategies for Chromosome Localization of Protooncogenes

Several strategies have been developed to map single gene sequences to distinct chromosomes. Some of the most widely used and most effective techniques are (i) in-

* Kita 10 Nishi 8, Kita-ku, Sapporo 060, Japan (吉田廸弘).

terspecific somatic cell hybridization, (ii) chromosome fractionation, and (iii) *in situ* hybridization. Detailed procedures of each technique should be obtained from the cited references.

In the first method, human cells are fused with rodents carrying appropriate genetic markers that permit selection of hybrid cells. With cell growth and division, there is loss of human chromosomes from the hybrid cells. Since the loss of human chromosomes is approximately random, clones of such hybrid cells are isolated with different human chromosome constitution. Correlation of the presence of protooncogene sequences examined by Southern blot technique and retention of specific human chromosomes of each clone permits their mapping to specific human chromosomes. Through the use of human cells with chromosome rearrangements, such as translocations and deletions, genes can be regionally mapped to specific chromosomal segments.

The second method, chromosome fractionation, has been accomplished by use of a fluorescent activated cell sorter (FACS), although chromosome separation has severe limitations. The degree of chromosome separation is critically dependent on the resolving power of the machine used, the compactness and aggregation of the chromosomes, and which fluorescent DNA binding dye is used. Currently 14–18 of the 23 human chromosomes can be separated. The application of restriction enzyme digestion and Southern blot analysis to the DNA obtained from sorted chromosomes has permitted the mapping of certain genes (*14*).

The third method is the *in situ* hybridization to chromosomes. Recent advances in *in situ* hybridization techniques have made it possible to identify single-copy DNA sequences to specific chromosome sites at the light microscopic level (*8*). The radio-labeled probes after nick-translation are directly hybridized to homologous sequences on metaphase chromosomes on a microscope slide. Hybridization conditions have also been improved with use of dextrane sulfate to increase the hybridization rate and 70% formamide at 70°C to denature the chromosomal DNA without destroying chromosome morphology. After exposure to autoradiographic emulsion, silver grains identify the chromosome site. While this is the most direct method of ascertaining genes, there may be certain technical limitations when mapping single copy genes, which are related to the problem of signal strength from the probe and its cross hybridization to other DNA segments. More effective mapping is done, therefore, in combination with somatic cell hybridization or chromosome fractionation through which the gene can be mapped to a chromosome and then regionally mapped through the use of *in situ* hybridization technique.

The localization of genes to chromosomes or parts of chromosomes follows the banding pattern of the chromosomes. The nomenclature for human chromosomes identifies each of the chromosomes by a number with the shorter arm identified as p and the long arm as q. Within each one, the long and short regions are identified and are given numbers.

Chromosomal Localization of Protooncogenes

1)   Chromosomal localization of c-yes-1 and c-yes-2

The human c-*yes*-1 protooncogene has been identified as a proto-*yes* gene of an avian sarcoma virus Y73 which induces fibrosarcomas in chicken, and c-*yes*-2 as a processed pseudogene of c-*yes*-1 (*25*). The localization of c-*yes*-1 gene was first accomplished

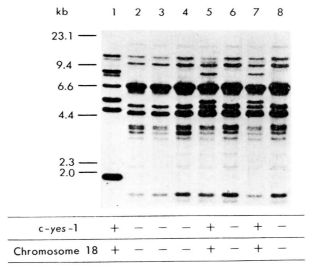

FIG. 1. Hybridization of v-*yes* probe to *Eco*RI-digested DNA from human-mouse hybrids (*25*)

Lane 1, normal human fibroblastic cells; lanes 2, 3, 4, 6, and 8, negative hybrids lacking human chromosome 18; lanes 5 and 7, positive hybrids carrying human chromosome 18.

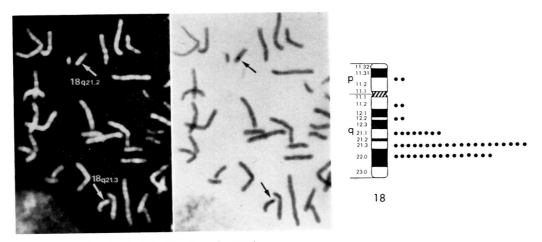

FIG. 2. *In situ* hybridization of c-*yes*-1

Partial Q-banded (left), and conventional Giemsa-stained (middle) metaphase. The arrows indicate silver grains on chromosome 18. Idiogram (right) showing the grain distribution on chromosome 18 and the significant number of grains at the q21.3.

by examining man-mouse somatic cell hybrids (*25*). The DNA from 24 hybrid clones was digested with *Eco*RI and subjected to Southern blot analysis with a ^{32}P-labeled probe, 1.5 kb long, that contained about 85% of the v-*yes* gene. Ten *Eco*RI fragments specific to humans were observed, two of which, 8.7- and 5.7-kb fragments, were classified as c-*yes*-1 and assigned to chromosome 18 (Fig. 1). Further localization of this gene was accomplished by *in situ* hybridization using a cloned c-*yes*-1 probe containing a 0.5 kb fragment (*34*). Of 215 silver grains in 100 metaphases examined, 43 were located on 18q21-q22 with a peak at band 18q21.3 (Fig. 2).

In examining the c-*yes*-1 gene location in relationship to chromosome aberrations associated with tumors, a remarkable coincidence between the c-*yes*-1 locus and the breakpoint 18q21.3 was reported in certain types of follicular lymphomas which are known frequently to be associated with a translocation t(14; 18) (q32; q21) (*5, 19, 36*). However, no transcription of the c-*yes*-1 gene was detected in FL18 cells established from a follicular lymphoma containing a t(14; 18) (*27*), although the c-*yes* gene was actively transcribed in adenocarcinoma cells of the human pancreas UVCA and epidermoid carcinoma A431 cells (*25, 27*).

The chromosomal location of a c-*yes*-2 gene was also accomplished by Southern blot analysis of the same hybrid clone panel as above described. With a v-*yes* probe, the 1.9-kb *Eco*RI fragment was assignable to chromosome 6 (*25*). However, *in situ* hybridization studies using a cloned *yes*-2 probe demonstrated that c-*yes*-2 was located on chromosome 22 at band q11 (Yoshida *et al.*, unpublished data). At present, the inconsistency in these two sets of experiments is hard to rationalize. One possible explanation is that probes used in the experiments were different.

2)   Location of c-fgr on human chromosome 1

The *fgr* gene in the *src* family has been identified as an oncogene of Gardner-Rasheed feline sarcoma virus. The amino acid sequence of the v-*fgr* product was deduced from nucleotide sequence data. The carboxyl-terminal half of the oncogene product showed highest homology with that of the v-*yes* product (*2, 32*).

The human c-*fgr* gene was isolated from a human gene library by using v-*yes* probe (*20*), and found to be a cellular homology of the oncogene of Gardner-Rasheed feline sarcoma virus (*21*). The exon-intron structure of the c-*fgr* gene was identical with that of the c-*src* gene, and the actin gene-like sequence of the viral *fgr* gene is not present in the c-*fgr* gene, indicating that the *fgr* and *src* genes originated by duplication of a prototype gene (*20*).

The chromosomal localization of the c-*fgr* gene was determined using human-mouse hybrids (*21*). Twelve hybrid clones were examined for the presence of human 11-kb *Hin*dIII-digested DNA fragment that cross-hybridized to a human c-*fgr*-specific

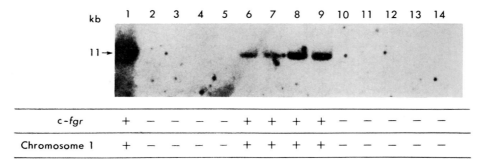

Fig. 3.   Southern blot analysis of human c-*fgr* gene in *Hin*dIII-digested DNA of human-mouse hybrids (*21*)

Lane 1, human placenta; lanes 2–5, and 10–13, negative hybrids lacking human chromosome 1; lanes 6–9, positive hybrids carrying human chromosome 1; lane 14, mouse cell line.

probe by Southern blotting. There were four hybrid clones that contained the human c-*fgr* gene and all contained human chromosome 1 (Fig. 3). For confirmation of this result, the same Southern blot filter was rehybridized with a human N-*ras*-specific probe after washing out the c-*fgr*-specific probe, since the human N-*ras* gene has been located on chromosome 1. The DNA of the hybrid clones that retained the human c-*fgr* sequence were also found to contain the N-*ras*-specific sequence. Furthermore, the relative intensities of the bands detected with each probe of the c-*fgr* and N-*ras* genes appeared to be correlated well. Therefore, the human c-*fgr* gene is located on chromosome 1.

Le Beau *et al.* (*15*) used *in situ* hybridization with a c-*src* probe and localized the *src* gene to two distinct regions, 1p34-p36 and 20q12-q13. The locus identified on chromosome 1 represents the c-*src*-2 locus, and this gene was isolated by Parker *et al.* (*22*) who showed that the nucleotide sequence of the two predicted exons of the c-*src*-2 gene corresponds to exons 11 and 12 of the c-*src* gene. Recently, Nishizawa *et al.* (*21*) demonstrated that the restriction maps of the c-*src*-2 and c-*fgr* seemed to resemble each other, and that the exon-intron structures of the two are identical with that of the c-*src* gene, at least in their sequenced regions. In addition, the sequence of the c-*src*-2 gene shows extensive homology with that of v-*fgr* (94% nucleotide sequence and 95% amino acid sequence homology), and the presence of the sequence of exon 12 reported by Parker *et al.* (*22*). From all of these results, the c-*src*-2 gene is referred as to the c-*fgr* gene (*21*). Therefore, c-*fgr* is located on 1p36.1-p36.2.

The expression of the c-*fgr* gene was examined in human placenta and A431 epidermoid carcinoma, K562 chronic myelogenous leukemia, and IM-9 leukemic cells by RNA blot hybridization. Among these tumor cells the mRNA was detected in only IM-9 with relatively higher expression (*21*). However, no amplification and rearrangement of the c-*fgr* gene was detected in IM-9 cells.

3) Location of c-syn on chromosome 6

A novel v-*yes*-related oncogene, *syn*, was isolated from a human gene library using v-*yes* DNA segment as a screening probe (*27*). The *syn* gene encoded a protein-tyrosine kinase which resembled the v-*yes* and c-*src* proteins in primary structure, indicating that the *syn* is a new member of the tyrosine kinase oncogene family. The name *syn* is derived from the *src/yes*-related novel oncogene (*26*). The restriction map and nucleotide sequence analysis of the *syn* gene were distinct from those of genomic clones of the c-*yes*-1, c-*yes*-2, c-*fgr*, and c-*src* genes (*27*).

The chromosomal localization of c-*syn* was determined first by Southern blot analysis of 14 human-mouse hybrids with ^{32}P-labeled *Kpn*I-*Dra*I fragment generated from the c-*syn* genomic clone. This probe hybridized with an 8-kb *Hind*III fragment of the human c-*syn* gene. The c-*syn* was detected in all seven hybrids that contained human chromosome 6 and was absent in the seven clones that lost chromosome 6 (*27*).

To obtain a more precise localization of the *syn* gene, *in situ* hybridization was performed using a *Stu*I 2.1 kb fragment (*35*). Specific hybridization of 99 metaphase spreads revealed that 23% of the 169 independent sites showing grains occurred over chromosome 6. Examination of the grain distribution along chromosome 6 showed that most of the grains (62%) were located on 6q21 (Fig. 4).

It has been noted that the location of this gene is near a very frequent breakpoint found in acute lymphocytic leukemia, del(6) (q21q25), and ovarian carcinoma, t(6; 14)

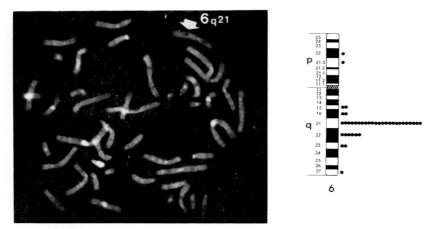

FIG. 4. *In situ* hybridization of c-*syn* gene
Left: the arrow points to a silver grain at 6q21. Right: silver grain distribution
along chromosome 6 showing significant clustering at the q21.

(q21; q24). This may suggest a possible effect of the chromosomal rearrangement at 6q21 on activation of the *syn* gene in these human cancers.

The *syn* gene showed a 2.8-kb mRNA transcript at various levels in human tumor cell lines of A431, K562, IM-9, and FL18 follicular lymphoma, although it was not detected in pancreas adenocarcinoma UCVA cells (*27*). The size of the *syn* transcript differed from those of the c-*yes* and c-*fgr* mRNAs, and their expression was also different in each tumor cell line analyzed from the same filter (*27*). Comparison of the hybridization blots of these mRNAs suggests that the expression of these related genes is distinctly regulated in each of the cells examined.

Localization of c-erbB-2

An avian erythroblastosis virus H strain contains an oncogene, v-*erb*B, that was a truncated version of the epidermal growth factor (EGF) receptor (*33*). Recently, a v-*erb*B-related gene, c-*erb*B-2, was isolated from a human gene library (*26*). The c-*erb*B-2 gene is apparently distinct from the EGF receptor gene, since transcripts of the two genes differ from each other in length and because the amino acid sequence predicted from the nucleotide sequence of cloned c-*erb*B-2 gene is very similar to the corresponding region of the EGF receptor (*26, 31*). A recently isolated *neu* oncogene from rat neuroblastoma (*1*) was found to be very similar to the c-*erb*B-2 gene through nucleotide and amino sequence analyses indicating that these two are the same gene (*33*).

The localization of the human c-*erb*B-2 gene was accomplished using two methods. First, metaphase chromosomes were sorted, immobilized on nitrocellulose filters, and hybridized with a human c-*erb*B-2 cloned DNA probe (*6*). The result suggested that the probe hybridized to a fraction contained chromosomes 16, 17, and 18. By analyzing chromosomes from a cell line that contained a t(17; 22) translocation, it was shown that the gene was now on two chromosomes of different sizes, the normal chromosome 17 and the derivative t(17; 22) chromosome, indicating that the c-*erb*B-2 is located on chromosome 17. To localize the c-*erb*B-2 gene more precisely, *in situ* hybridization was used. Analysis of 85 metaphase cells revealed that 23.5% (20 of 85) of the silver grains were located on chromosome 17. Of these 20 grains, 15 (75%) were located on band q21-q22 with the largest accumulation of grains at band 17q21.3 (*6*). A human version of the *nue* oncogene was also recently mapped on human chromosome 17 at q21 (*24*).

Several rearrangements have been associated with 17q21-q22, especially involving acute promyelocytic leukemia (APL) (*19*). DNA from seven cases of APL was subjected to Southern blot analysis for the possible involvement of the c-*erb*B-2 gene in this leukemia. However, no evidence is available to support any alterations of c-*erb*B-2 structure or transcription in neoplastic cells containing alterations in the 17q21-q22 region (*6*); nor was any structural alteration at the locus of c-*erb*B-2 confirmed by *in situ* hybridization to t(15; 17) chromosomes of APL (10). Further analysis of 30 human cancerous cell lines for the altered structures of this gene demonstrated that amplification and elevated expression of the c-*erb*B-2 gene was found in an MKN-7 gastric cancer cell line, suggesting a possible role of the c-*erb*B-2 gene in transforming epithelial cells or in the malignancy of transformed epithelial cells.

Chromosomal Localization of ros-related Genes

Recently two human sequences related to the v-*ros* oncogene of UR2 sarcoma virus have been isolated (*16, 17*); one, designated c-*ros*-1, corresponds to the c-*ros* and the other, designated c-*ros*-2, contains a portion of a tyrosine kinase domain not identical to any other known kinase genes. Matsushime *et al.* (*17*) localized the c-*ros*-1 gene. Using *Eco*RI-*Bam*HI-digested DNA from 15 human-mouse hybrids, they were able to detect a 0.8-kb fragment in three clones which retained human chromosome 6. One discordant hybrid clone in this hybrid panel contained c-*ros*-1, but it lacked karyotypic evidence of chromosome 6. However, this clone appeared to contain human major histocompatibility complex (HLA)-DRB gene and thus must contain some of chromosome 6 translocated to another chromosome. Therefore, c-*ros*-1 gene has been assigned to chromosome 6. *In situ* hybridization confirmed this assignment and more rigidly substantiated sublocalization of this gene on 6q22 (Satoh *et al.*, paper submitted). Since the 6q22 is a broad band, prometaphase-chromosomes at 500–550 band level were analyzed. A significant amount of grains was found on the negative subband at q22.2, suggesting that the c-*ros*-1 is most probably located on 6q22.2.

The c-*ros*-2 gene was found to be located on chromosome 13 by use of the same hybrids as those by which the c-*ros*-1 was mapped (Satoh *et al.*, paper submitted). To regionally localize this gene, *in situ* hybridization was performed. Specific hybridization was observed over 13q12.

The assignment of c-*ros*-1 to 6q22 suggests that this oncogene might be implicated in the pathogenesis of various ovarian carcinomas in which various rearrangements on the long arm of chromosome 6 were found (*19*). The mapping of the c-*ros*-2 to 13q12 also suggests that this oncogene might be implicated in acute nonlymphocytic leukemia, dysmyelopoietic syndrome, or myelofibrosis/myelosclerosis in which a specific breakpoint at 13q12 was seen (*19*).

Cellular DNAs prepared from human placenta, mouse thymus, chicken liver, fish testis, and adult *Drosophila melanogaster* were hybridized to the c-*ros*-2 probe (*17*).

TABLE I. Human Oncogene Mapping[a]

Chromosome	Oncogene	Chromosomal region	Source or homologous v-*onc*
1	*FGR*	1p36.1-p36.2	v-*fgr*
	LCK	1p32-p35	lymphocyte-specific protein tyrosine kinase
	BLYM	1p34	Avian lymphoma virus-derived transforming sequence
	LMYC	1p32	v-*myc* homolog, lung cancer derived
	NRAS	1p22, 1p13	v-*ras*
	SKI	1q21.1-q24	v-*ski*
2	*NMYC*	2p24	v-*myc* neuroblastoma derived
	REL	2p13-cen	v-*rel*
	LCA	2q14	Liver cancer derived
3	*RAF1*	3p25	*raf*-1
	FIM3	3q27	Friend-murine leukemia virus integration site 3 homolog
4	*KIT*	4q11-q22	v-*kit*
	RAF1P1	4p16.1	v-*raf* 1 pseudogene
5	*FMS=CSF1R*	5q34-q33	v-*fms*, colony stimulating factor 1 receptor
6	*PIM*	6p21	*pim*-1
	KRAS1P	6p12-p11	v-Ki-*ras*-1
	SYN=FYN	6q21	v-*yes*-related
	ROS	6q22.2	v-*ros*-related
	MYB	6q22-q23	v-*myb*
7	*ERBB=EGFR*	7p12-p13	v-*erb*B, epidermal growth factor receptor
	MET	7q31	*met* chemically transformed cell line derived
	RAL	7p22-p15	simian leukemia viral (v-ral) oncogene homolog (*ras* related)
8	*MOS*	8q11, 8q22	v-*mos*
	MYC	8q24	v-*myc*
9	*ABL*	9q34	v-*abl*
11	*HRAS1*	11p15.5	v-Ha-*ras*1
	WAGR[b]	11p13	Wilms' tumor/aniridia/gonadoblastoma/retardation
	BCL1[c]	11q13.3	B-cell leukemia-1
	ETS1	11q23.3	v-*ets*
	SEA	11q13	*sea*
12	*KRAS2*	12p12.1	v-Ki-*ras*2
	INT1	12q12-q14	v-*int1*
13	*FLT*	13q12	v-*ros*-related
	RB1[b]	13q14.1	Retinoblastoma 1
14	*FOS*	14q24.3-q31	v-*fos*
	AKT1	14q32	v-*akt*-1
	TCL1[c]	14q32	*tcl*-1
15	*FES*	15q25-q26	v-*fes*
17	*ERBA1*	17q11-q22	v-*erb*-A
	ERBB2	17q21-q22	v-*erb*-B
	NGL	17q11-q12	Rat neuro- or glioblastoma derived
18	*YES1*	18q21.3	v-*yes*
	BCL2[c]	18q21.3	B-cell lymphoma-2
19	*MEL*	19p13.2-q13.2	*mel*
20	*SRC*	20q12-q13	v-*src*
21	*ETS2*	21q22.3	v-*ets*
22	*BCR*[c]	22q11	Breakpoint cluster region (chronic myeloid leukemia)
	YES2	22q11	c-*yes*-1 pseudogene
	SIS=PDGFR	22q12.3-q13.1	v-*sis*
	EWS[b]	22q11	breakpoint of Ewing sarcoma
X	*HRAS2*	Xpter-q28	v-Ha-*ras*2
	ARAF1	Xp21-q11	v-*raf*

[a] From HGM8 (*9*), McKusick (*18*), and personal communication.
[b] Chromosome breakpoint.
[c] Sequences isolated from breakpoint.

The result indicated phylogenetical conservation of the c-*ros*-2 sequence in a variety of animals.

Concluding Comments

With their identification and isolation, mapping of protooncogenes has rapidly

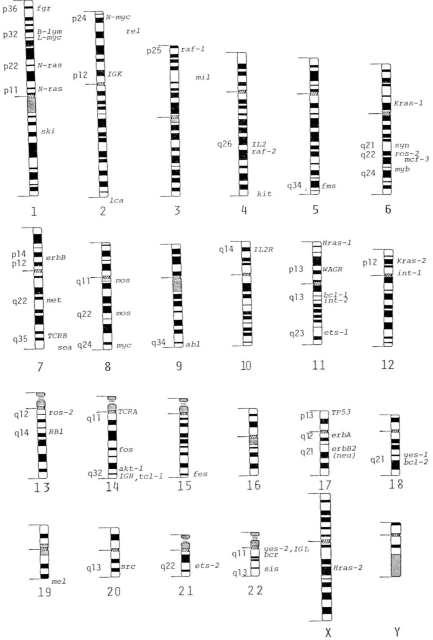

FIG. 5.   The chromosomal localization of human protooncogenes and cancer related genes, summarized from Human Gene Mapping 9 (*cf. Cytogenet. Cell Genet.*, **46**, 1987).

progressed. Current mapping information of human protooncogenes is summarized in Table I and Fig. 5. The table also lists the cancer-related genes such as transforming genes isolated from tumor cells by DNA transfection assay (for example: *BLYM* (*4*)), by isolating DNA sequences that occur amplified many-fold in tumor cells (example: *NMYC* (*12*)), and by identifying the sequences translocated into immunoglobulin genes (example: *BCL1* (*30*)) or breakpoint cluster region (example: *BCR* (*7*)). Although the chromosomal sites of specific cancer-breakpoints are not listed in Fig. 5, most of the sites correspond to those of protooncogenes (*19*, *23*, *36*). Such gene mapping information will reveal whether there is a positive effect on the activation of oncogenes, since chromosomal rearrangements such as translocations involve two precise breakpoints—one of them the likely site of a protooncogene that becomes deregulated or activated as a result of chromosomal rearrangements. In fact, the activation of oncogenes as a result of chromosome translocations has been demonstrated in Burkitt's lymphomas and chronic myelogenous leukemias (*7*, *13*, *28*). While other mechanisms including single point mutations, promoter insertion, and gene amplification have been applied to oncogene activation, gene mapping information will provide insight into the origin and evolutionary relationships of oncogenes or cancer-related genes.

Acknowledgments

This review was initiated from studies made with Professor Kumao Toyoshima, Dr. Tadashi Yamamoto, Dr. Masabumi Shibuya and their colleagues of the Institute of Medical Science, The University of Tokyo, to whom I am grateful. My sincere thanks are also due to Professor Motomichi Sasaki for invaluable contributions. This work was supported by Grants-in-Aid for Cancer Research from the Ministry of Education, Science and Culture, Japan.

Note Added in Proof

The gene symbols, *syn* and *ros*-2, used in this paper have been changed to *fyn* and *flt*, respectively. After submission of this paper, two articles on c-*yes*-2 (*Jpn. J. Cancer Res.* (*Gann*), **79**, 710–717, 1988) and on c-*ros*-1 and *flt* (*Jpn. J. Cancer Res.* (*Gann*), **78**, 772–775, 1987) were published.

REFERENCES

1. Bargmann, C. I., Hung, M. C., and Weinberg, R. A. The *neu* oncogene encodes an epidermal growth factor receptor-related protein. *Nature*, **319**, 226–230 (1986).
2. Bishop, J. M. Cellular oncogenes and retroviruses. *Annu. Rev. Biochem.*, **52**, 301–354 (1983).
3. Chaganti, R.S.K. Cytogenetic basis of human cancer. *J. Genet.*, **64**, 59–67 (1985).
4. Diamond, A., Cooper, G. M., Ritz, J., and Lane, M. A. Identification and molecular cloning of the human Blym transforming gene activated in Burkitt's lymphomas. *Nature*, **305**, 112–116 (1983).
5. Fukuhara, S., Rowley, J. D., Variakojis, D., and Swee, D. L. Chromosome abnormalities in poorly differentiated lymphocytic lymphoma. *Cancer Res.*, **39**, 3119–3128 (1979).
6. Fukushige, S., Matsubara, K., Yoshida, M. C., Sasaki, M., Suzuki, T., Semba, K., Toyoshima, K., and Yamamoto, T. Localization of a novel v-*erb*B-related gene, c-*erb*B-2, on human chromosome 17 and its amplification in a gastric cancer cell line. *Mol. Cell. Biol.*, **6**, 955–958 (1986).

7. Groffen, J., Stephenson, J. R., Heisterkamp, N., de Klein, A., Bartram, C. R., and Grosveld, G. Philadelphia chromosomal breakpoints are clustered within a limited region, *bcr*, on chromosome 22. *Cell*, **36**, 93–99 (1984).

8. Harper, M. E. and Saunders, G. F. Localization of single copy DNA sequences on G-banded human chromosomes by *in situ* hybridization. *Chromosoma*, **83**, 431–439 (1981).

9. HGM8: Human Gene Mapping 8 (1985). *Cytogenet. Cell Genet.*, **40**, Nos. 1–4 (1985).

10. Kaneko, Y., Homma, C., Maseki, N., Sakurai, M., Toyoshima, K., and Yamamoto, T. Human c-*erb*B-2 remains on chromosome 17 in band q21 in the 15; 17 translocation associated with acute promyelocytic leukemia. *Jpn. J. Cancer Res. (Gann)*, **78**, 16–19 (1987).

11. Klein, G. Specific chromosomal translocations and the genesis of B cell derived tumors in mice and men. *Cell*, **32**, 311–315 (1983).

12. Kohl, N. E., Kanda, N., Schreck, R. R., Bruns, G., Latt, S. A., Gilbert, F., and Alt, F. W. Transposition and amplification of oncogene-related sequences in human neuroblastomas. *Cell*, **35**, 359–367 (1983).

13. Konopka, J. B., Watanabe, S. M., and Witte, O. N. An alteration of the human c-*abl* protein in K562 leukemia cells unmasks associated tyrosine kinase activity. *Cell*, **37**, 1035–1042 (1984).

14. Lebo, R. V., Carrano, A. V., Burkhart-Schults, K., Dozy, A. M., Yu, L-C., and Kan, Y. W. Assignment of human β-, γ-, and δ-globin genes to the short arm of chromosome 11 by chromosome sorting and DNA restriction enzyme analysis. *Proc. Natl. Acad. Sci. U.S.A.*, **76**, 5804–5808 (1979).

15. Le Beau, M. M., Westbrook, C. A., Diaz, M. O., and Rowley, J. D. Evidence for two distinct c-*src* loci on human chromosomes 1 and 20. *Nature*, **312**, 70–71 (1984).

16. Matsushime, H., Wang, L., and Shibuya, M. Human c-*ros*-1 gene homologous to the v-*ros* sequences of UR2 sarcoma virus encodes for a transmembrane receptor-like molecule. *Mol. Cell. Biol.*, **6**, 3000–3004 (1984).

17. Matsushime, H., Yoshida, M. C., Sasaki, M., and Shibuya, M. A possible new member of tyrosine kinase family, human *frt* sequence, is highly conserved in vertebrates and located on human chromosome 13. *Jpn. J. Cancer Res. (Gann)*, **78**, 655–661 (1987).

18. McKusick, V. A. "Mendelian Inheritance in Man" (1986). Johns Hopkins Univ. Press, Baltimore and London.

19. Mitelman, F. Clustering of breakpoints to specific chromosomal regions in human neoplasia. A survey of 5,345 cases. *Hereditas*, **104**, 113–119 (1986).

20. Nishizawa, M., Semba, K., Yamamoto, T., and Toyoshima, K. Human c-*fgr* gene does not contain coding sequence for actin-like protein. *Jpn. J. Cancer Res.*, **76**, 155–159 (1985).

21. Nishizawa, M., Semba, K., Yoshida, M. C., Yamamoto, T., Sasaki, M., and Toyoshima, K. Structure, expression, and chromosomal location of the human c-*fgr* gene. *Mol. Cell. Biol.*, **6**, 511–517 (1986).

22. Parker, R. C., Mardon, G., Lebo, R. V., Varmus, H. E., and Bishop, J. M. Isolation of duplicated human c-*src* genes located on chromosome 1 and 20. *Mol. Cell. Biol.*, **5**, 831–838 (1985).

23. Rowley, J. D. Human oncogene locations and chromosome aberrations. *Nature*, **301**, 290–291 (1983).

24. Schechter, A. L., Hung, M.-C., Vaidyanathan, L., Weinberg, R. A., Yang-Feng, T. L., Francke, U., Ullrich, A., and Coussens, L. The *neu* gene: an *erb*B-homologous gene distinct from and unlinked to the gene encoding the EGF receptor. *Science*, **229**, 976–978 (1985).

25. Semba, K., Yamanashi, Y., Nishizawa, M., Sukegawa, J., Yoshida, M. C., Sasaki, M. C., Yamamoto, T., and Toyoshima, K. Location of the c-*yes* gene on the human chromosome and its expression in various tissues. *Science*, **227**, 1038–1040 (1985).

26. Semba, K., Kamata, N., Toyoshima, K., and Yamamoto, T. A v-*erb*B-related protoon-

cogene, c-*erb*B-2, is distinct from the c-*erb*-1/EGF receptor gene and is amplified in a human salivary gland adenocarcinoma. *Proc. Natl. Acad. Sci. U.S.A.*, **82**, 6497–6501 (1985).

27. Semba, K., Nishizawa, M., Miyaji, N., Yoshida, M. C., Sukegawa, J., Yamanashi, Y., Sasaki, M., Yamamoto, T., and Toyoshima, K. *yes*-related protooncogene, *syn*, belongs to the protein-tyrosine kinase family. *Proc. Natl. Acad. Sci. U.S.A.*, **83**, 5459–5463 (1986).
28. Showe, L. C. and Croce, C. Translocation mechanisms in B- and T-cell neoplasias. *Cancer Rev.*, **2**, 18–33 (1986).
29. Tereba, A. Chromosomal localization of protooncogenes. *Int. Rev. Cytol.*, **95**, 1–43 (1985).
30. Tsujimoto, Y., Yunis, J. J., Onorato-Showe, L., Erikson, J., Nowell, P. C., and Croce, C. M. Molecular cloning of the chromosomal breakpoint of B-cell lymphomas and leukemias with the t(11; 14) chromosomal translocation. *Science*, **224**, 1403–1406 (1984).
31. Ullrich, A., Coussens, L., Hayflick, J. S., Dull, T. J., Gray, A., Tam, A. W., Lee, J., Yarden, Y., Libermann, T. A., Schlessinger, J., Downward, J., Mayes, L. V., Whittle, N., Waterfield, M. D., and Seeburg, P. H. Human epidermal growth factor receptor cDNA sequence and aberrant expression of the amplified gene in A431 epidermoid carcinoma cells. *Nature*, **309**, 418–425 (1984).
32. Varmus, H. E. The molecular genetics of cellular oncogenes. *Annu. Rev. Genet.*, **18**, 553–612 (1984).
33. Yamamoto, T., Ikawa, S., Akiyama, T., Semba, K., Nomura, N., Miyajima, N., Saito, T., and Toyoshima, K. Similarity of protein encoded by the human c-*erb*-B-2 gene to epidermal growth factor receptor. *Nature*, **319**, 230–234 (1986).
34. Yoshida, M. C., Sasaki, M., Mise, K., Semba, K., Nishizawa, M., Yamamoto, T., and Toyoshima, K. Regional mapping of the human protooncogene c-*yes*-1 to chromosome 18 at band q21.3. *Jpn. J. Cancer Res. (Gann)*, **76**, 59–562 (1985).
35. Yoshida, M. C., Satoh, H., Sasaki, M., Semba, K., Yamamoto, T., and Toyoshima, K. Regional location of a novel *yes*-related proto-oncogene, *syn*, on human chromosome 6 at band q21. *Jpn. J. Cancer Res. (Gann)*, **7**, 1059–1061 (1986).
36. Yunis, J. J. Chromosomal rearrangements, genes, and fragile sites in cancer: Clinical and biologic implications. *In* "Important Advances in Oncology 1986," ed. V. T. DeVita, S. Helman, and S. A. Rosenberg, pp. 93–128 (1986). J. B. Lippincott Company, Philadelphia.

AUTHOR INDEX

SUBJECT INDEX